MANUAL OF

PEDIATRIC CRITICAL CARE

Narendra C. Singh, BSc, MB, BS, FRCPC, FAAP, FCCM
Associate Professor of Pediatrics
University of Western Ontario, London, Ontario
Director, Pediatric Critical Care Unit
Children's Hospital of Western Ontario
London, Ontario, Canada

D1374199

W.B. Saunders Company
A Division of Harcourt Brace & Company
Philadelphia London Toronto Montreal Sydney Tokyo

W.B. SAUNDERS COMPANY
A Division of Harcourt Brace & Company

The Curtis Center
Independence Square West
Philadelphia, Pennsylvania 19106

Library of Congress Cataloging-in-Publication Data

Manual of pediatric critical care / [edited by] Narendra C. Singh.

p.   cm.

ISBN 0–7216–5949–7

1. Pediatric intensive care—Handbooks, manuals, etc.
2. Pediatric emergencies—Handbooks, manuals, etc.   I. Singh, Narendra
    C.   [DNLM: 1. Critical Care—in infancy & childhood—handbooks.
    2. Critical Care—methods—handbooks.   3. Emergencies—in infancy &
    childhood—handbooks.   4. Emergency Medicine—methods—handbooks.
    WS 39 M2946 1997]

RJ370. M364 1997   618.92′ 0028—dc20

DNLM/DLC   96–7417

MANUAL OF PEDIATRIC CRITICAL CARE   ISBN 0–7216–5949–7

Printed in the United States of America.

Last digit is the print number: 9   8   7   6   5   4   3   2

My every day is filled with the love of my children, Rohana and Amar, who give me the strength and motivation to confront every new day and every new challenge. To my parents, Chetram and Hema Singh, whose unlimited, selfless dedication to their children has always guided me.

CONTRIBUTORS

P. DAVID ADELSON, MD

Assistant Professor, Department of Neurosurgery, University of Pittsburgh School of Medicine, Pittsburgh; Attending Neurosurgeon, Children's Hospital of Pittsburgh, Pittsburgh, Pennsylvania
Severe Traumatic Brain Injury in Children

PAUL R. ATKISON, MD, PhD, FRCP(C)

Associate Professor of Pediatrics, University of Western Ontario, London, Ontario; Director, Pediatric Transplant Program, Children's Hospital Western Ontario, London, Ontario, Canada
Diabetic Ketoacidosis

CATHERINE BURKE-TREMBLAY, RRT

Consultant, Clinical Trainer in Respiratory Therapy
Use of Nitric Oxide in Pulmonary Hypertension

STANLEY CALDERWOOD, MD, FRCPC

Assistant Professor of Hematology and Oncology, University of Toronto, Toronto; The Hospital for Sick Children, Toronto, Ontario, Canada
Bone Marrow Transplantation

JOSEPH A. CARCILLO, MD

Assistant Professor of Anesthesiology, Critical Care Medicine, and Pediatrics, University of Pittsburgh School of Medicine, Pittsburgh; Associate Director, Pediatric Intensive Care Unit, Children's Hospital of Pittsburgh, Pittsburgh, Pennsylvania
Septic Shock

ROBERT S. B. CLARK, MD

Assistant Professor, Department of Anesthesia/Critical Care Medicine, University of Pittsburgh School of Medicine, Pittsburgh; Associate Director, Pediatric Intensive Care Unit, Children's Hospital of Pittsburgh, Pittsburgh, Pennsylvania
Severe Traumatic Brain Injury in Children

HEIDI J. DALTON, MD

Director, Pediatric ECMO, Georgetown University, Washington, DC
Extracorporeal Membrane Oxygenation

ANNIK DE JAEGER, DGHV, CK

Assistant Professor, Department of Pediatrics, Rÿksuniversiteit Gent,
Belgium; Assistant Professor, Department of Pediatrics, Universitair
Ziekenhuis Gent, Belgium
Hepatic Failure

CATHERINE A. FARRELL, MD, FRCPC

Assistant Clinical Professor of Pediatric Critical Care, Université de
Montréal, Montreal; Medical Coordinator, Pediatric Intensive Care Unit,
Hôpital Sainte-Justine, Montreal, Quebec, Canada
Meningitis and Encephalitis

TIMOTHY C. FREWEN, MD, FRCP(C)

Professor of Pediatrics, University of Western Ontario, London, Ontario;
Vice President, Academic Medical and Dental Affairs, London Health
Sciences Centre, London, Ontario, Canada
Brain Death

BRADLEY P. FUHRMAN, MD

Professor of Pediatrics and Anesthesiology, State University of New York at
Buffalo; Chief, Pediatric Critical Care, Children's Hospital of Buffalo,
Buffalo, New York
Cardiogenic Shock and Congestive Heart Failure in Infants and Children;
Postoperative Cardiac Care for Congenital Heart Disease

JOHN B. GORDON, MD, CM

Associate Professor of Pediatrics, Medical College of Wisconsin,
Milwaukee; Associate Medical Director, Pediatric Intensive Care Unit,
Children's Hospital of Wisconsin, Milwaukee, Wisconsin
Use of Nitric Oxide in Pulmonary Hypertension

JERRIL GREEN, MD

Clinical Fellow, Pediatric Critical Care, Childrens Hospital of Pittsburgh,
Pittsburgh, Pennsylvania
Postoperative Management of the Liver Transplant Recipient

ALLAH B. HAAFIZ, MD

Senior Resident, Department of Pediatrics, University of Florida Health
Science Center and Wolfson Children's Hospital, Jacksonville, Florida
The Critically Ill Child; Acute Pain Management

LYNN J. HERNAN, MD

Assistant Professor of Pediatrics and Anesthesiology, State University of New York at Buffalo; Associate Director, Pediatric Intensive Care Unit, Children's Hospital of Buffalo, Buffalo, New York
Cardiogenic Shock and Congestive Heart Failure in Infants and Children; Postoperative Cardiac Care for Congenital Heart Disease

R. MORRISON HURLEY, MD, MSc, FRCPC

Professor and Chairman, Department of Pediatrics, University of Western Ontario, London, Ontario; Chief of Pediatrics and Pediatric Nephrology, Children's Hospital of Western Ontario, London, Ontario, Canada
Renal Failure

JAMES S. HUTCHISON, MD, FRCPC, FAAP

Assistant Professor of Pediatrics, University of Ottawa, Ontario; Attending Physician, Pediatric Critical Care, Childrens Hospital of Eastern Ontario, Ontario, Canada
Near-Drowning

PHILIP JOCHELSON, MD

Division Director, Clinical Research, Alliance Pharmaceutical Inc, San Diego, California
Lower Airway Disease

GARY I. JOUBERT, BSc, MD, FRCPC, FAAP

Assistant Professor, Department of Pediatrics, University of Western Ontario, London, Ontario; Director of Pediatric Emergency and Ambulatory Care, Children's Hospital of Western Ontario, London, Ontario, Canada
Hemodynamic Management

NIRANJAN KISSOON, MD, FCCM, FRCPC, FAAP

Professor, Department of Pediatrics, University of Florida, Jacksonville; Director, Pediatric Intensive Care Unit, Wolfson Children's Hospital, Jacksonville, Florida
The Critically Ill Child; Acute Pain Management

PATRICK M. KOCHANEK, MD

Associate Professor, University of Pittsburgh School of Medicine, Department of Anesthesiology/Critical Care Medicine, Pittsburgh; Associate Director, Pediatric Intensive Care Unit and Director, Pediatric Critical Care Research, Children's Hospital of Pittsburgh, Pittsburgh; Director, Safar Center for Resuscitation Research, Pittsburgh, Pennsylvania
Severe Traumatic Brain Injury in Children

JONATHAN B. KRONICK, MD, PhD, FRCPC, FAAP

Associate Professor of Pediatrics, University of Western Ontario, London, Ontario; Attending Physician, Pediatric Critical Care Unit and Genetic Metabolic Service, Children's Hospital of Western Ontario, London, Ontario, Canada
Acute Upper Airway Obstruction; Inherited Metabolic Disease

JACQUES LACROIX, FRCPC, FAAP

Professor, Department of Pediatrics, Université de Montréal, Montréal; Chief, Division of Pediatric Intensive Care, Hôpital Sainte-Justine, Montréal, Québec, Canada
Hepatic Failure

RICHARD J. LEE, LRCP, MRCS, FRCPC

Associate Professor, Departments of Anesthesia and Pediatrics, University of Western Ontario, London, Ontario; Associate Professor, Departments of Anesthesia and Pediatrics, Children's Hospital of Western Ontario, London, Ontario, Canada
Airway Management

MARC D. LeGRAS, BSc, MD, CM, FRCPC, FACC

Pediatric Cardiologist, Children's Cardiac Center, Legacy Emanuel Children's Hospital Portland, Oregon; formerly Assistant Professor of Pediatrics, University of Western Ontario, London, Ontario; Director of Pediatric, Electrophysiology and Pacing, Children's Hospital of Western Ontario, London, Ontario, Canada
Arrhythmias in the Pediatric Intensive Care Unit; Temporary Cardiac Pacing

BRYAN D. MAGWOOD, BSc, MD, FRCPC

Resident, Pediatric Critical Care Medicine, University of Western Ontario, London, Ontario; Children's Hospital of Western Ontario, London, Ontario, Canada
Central Venous Access; Pulmonary Artery Lines

DONALD W. MARION, MD

Associate Professor of Neurological Surgery, University of Pittsburgh School of Medicine, Pittsburgh; Neurosurgeon, Presbyterian University Hospital, Pittsburgh, Pennsylvania
Severe Traumatic Brain Injury in Children

DOUGLAS G. MATSELL, MD, CM, FRCPC

Assistant Professor of Pediatrics, University of Western Ontario, London, Ontario; Pediatric Nephrologist, Children's Hospital of Western Ontario, London, Ontario, Canada
Pediatric Renal Transplantation

KARIN A. McCLOSKEY, MD

Associate Professor of Pediatrics, University of Texas Southwestern Medical Center at Dallas Southwestern Medical School, Dallas; Attending Physician, Pediatric Emergency Medicine, Childrens Medical Center, Dallas, Texas
Interhospital Transport of the Critically Ill Child

F. NEIL McKENZIE, MB, ChB, FRCS(C)

Professor of Surgery, Division of Cardiothoracic Surgery, University of Western Ontario, London, Ontario; London Health Sciences Center University Campus, London, Ontario, Canada
Pediatric Heart Transplantation

MICHELLE McNEILL, MD

Resident, Pediatric Critical Care Medicine, University of Western Ontario, London, Ontario, Chief of Pediatric Cardiovascular Surgery, Children's Hospital of Western Ontario, London, Ontario, Canada
Intraosseous Infusions; Endotracheal Intubation

ALAN H. MENKIS, MD, FRCS(C)

Associate Professor, Department of Surgery and Pediatrics, University of Western Ontario, London, Ontario; Chief of Pediatric Cardiovascular Surgery, Children's Hospital of Western Ontario, London, Ontario, Canada
Pediatric Heart Transplantation

RICHARD J. NOVICK, MD, MSc, FRCS(C), FACS

Associate Professor, Departments of Surgery, Division of Cardiothoracic Surgery, University of Western Ontario, London, Ontario; London Health Sciences Centre, University Campus, London, Ontario, Canada
Pediatric Heart Transplantation

YVES OUELLETTE, MD, PhD, FRCPC

Assistant Professor of Pediatrics, University of Western Ontario, London, Ontario; Attending, Children's Hospital of Western Ontario, London, Ontario, Canada
Lower Airway Disease

MICHELE C. PAPO, MD, MPH

Assistant Professor of Pediatrics and Anesthesiology, State University of New York at Buffalo; Associate Director, Pediatric Intensive Care Unit, Children's Hospital of Buffalo, Buffalo, New York
Cardiogenic Shock and Congestive Heart Failure in Infants and Children; Postoperative Cardiac Care for Congenital Heart Disease

B. LOUISE PARKER, MD, FRCPC

Resident, Pediatric Critical Care Medicine, University of Western Ontario, London, Ontario; Children's Hospital of Western Ontario, London, Ontario, Canada
Brain Death; Needle Cricothyroidotomy; Tracheostomy; Needle Thoracentesis and Chest Tube Insertion

ANTHONY L. PEARSON-SHAVER, MD

Associate Professor of Pediatrics, Medical College of Georgia, Augusta; Medical Director, Pediatric Transport Team and Co-Director, Pediatric Intensive Care Unit, Medical College of Georgia Hospital and Clinics and Children's Medical Center, Augusta, Georgia
Poisoning

HERSCHEL C. ROSENBERG, MD, FRCP(C)

Associate Professor of Pediatrics, University of Western Ontario, London, Ontario; Pediatric Cardiologist, Children's Hospital of Western Ontario, London, Ontario, Canada
Cardiovascular Pharmacology

B. CATHERINE ROSS, MD, FRCPC

Resident, Pediatric Critical Care Medicine, University of Western Ontario, London, Ontario; Children's Hospital of Western Ontario, London, Ontario, Canada
Pericardiocentesis; Lumbar Puncture; Arterial Line Insertion

CHRISTOPHER G. SCILLEY, MD, FRCSC

Assistant Professor, Department of Plastic Surgery, University of Western Ontario, London, Ontario; Medical Director, Thompson Burn Unit, London Health Sciences Centre, London, Ontario, Canada
Burn Injury

SAMI D. SHEMIE, MD, CM, FRCPC

Assistant Professor of Pediatrics, University of Toronto, Toronto; Director of Residency Training, Critical Care Medicine, Hospital for Sick Children, Toronto, Ontario, Canada
Cardiovascular Monitoring

NARENDRA C. SINGH, BSc, MB, BS, FRCPC, FAAP, FCCM

Associate Professor of Pediatrics, University of Western Ontario, London, Ontario; Director, Pediatric Critical Care Unit, Children's Hospital of Western Ontario, London, Ontario, Canada
Airway Management; Lower Airway Disease; Use of Nitric Oxide in Pulmonary Hypertension; Status Epilepticus; Jugular Bulb Catheterization

RAM N. SINGH, MD, FRCPC

Assistant Professor of Pediatrics, Intensive Care, and Anesthesia, Ottawa University, Ottawa, Ontario, Canada
Trauma Management

CURT M. STEINHART, MD, FCCM

Professor of Pediatrics, Surgery, and Anesthesiology and Chief, Section of Pediatric Critical Care Medicine, Medical College of Georgia, Augusta; Medical Director, Pediatric Intensive Care Unit, Medical College of Georgia Hospital and Clinics and Children's Medical Center, Augusta, Georgia
Poisoning

DAVID M. STEINHORN, MD

Assistant Professor of Pediatrics, State University of New York at Buffalo; Associate Director, Pediatric Intensive Care Unit, Childrens Hospital of Buffalo, Buffalo, New York
Guidelines for Nutritional Support of Critically Ill Children

ANN THOMPSON

Professor, Anesthesiology/CCM and Pediatrics, Department of Critical Care Medicine, University of Pittsburgh, Pittsburgh; Director, Pediatric Critical Care Unit, Childrens Hospital of Pittsburgh, Pittsburgh, Pennsylvania
Postoperative Management of the Liver Transplant Recipient

SHEKHAR T. VENKATARAMAN, MB, BS

Assistant Profesor, Departments of Anesthesiology/Critical Care Medicine and Pediatrics, University of Pittsburgh School of Medicine, Pittsburgh; Associate Director, Pediatric Intensive Care Unit and Medical Director, Respiratory Care, Children's Hospital of Pittsburgh, Pittsburgh, Pennsylvania
Assessment of Oxygenation and Ventilation; Principles of Mechanical Ventilation

HEATHER J. VOSPER, BSc(Hon), BSc(Pharm), PharmD

Clinical Pharmacist, Pediatric Critical Care Unit, Children's Hospital of Western Ontario, London, Ontario, Canada
Pediatric Formulary

MARK K. WEDEL, MD, JD, FACP

Division Director, Medical Research, Alliance Pharmaceutical Corporation; Attending Physician, Critical Care Medicine, Scripps Clinic and Research Foundation, La Jolla, California
Lower Airway Disease

IDO YATSIV, MD

Assistant Director, Pediatric Intensive Care Unit, Hadassah Hebrew University Medical Center, Jerusalem, Israel
Central Nervous System Monitoring

PREFACE

Pediatric Critical Care as a subspecialty has undergone tremendous growth in the past 30 years. Although pediatric critical care units treat the majority of critically ill children, a number of children are managed in emergency rooms and adult critical care units. With a better understanding of the uniqueness of the critically ill child and the advent of newer modalities of therapy, there is an increasing need for the dissemination of this information. There are a number of excellent texts that detail the uniqueness of the pediatric physiology and its implications in terms of pathophysiology, clinical presentation, monitoring, and treatment modalities. These texts, however, are primarily written for physicians who have a primary role in pediatric critical care. In view of the comprehensive nature of such texts, the immediate practical needs of trainees, noncritical care physicians, nurses, respiratory therapists, and other health care providers are often not met.

The objectives of this text are to provide background information along with a practical and user friendly reference guide for health care providers who treat critically ill children. A comprehensive overview of pediatric critical care topics, for example, pediatric head injuries, resuscitation, trauma, seizures, and asthma, will assist the health care provider and the emergency room staff in the treatment of critically ill children. Other topics more relevant to the critical care staff include cardiovascular and respiratory monitoring, postoperative cardiac care, organ transplantation, and mechanical ventilation. In addition, newer modalities of therapy including nitric oxide, high frequency oscillation, and liquid ventilation have also been included.

It should be recognized that the management of the critically ill child is very much a multidisciplinary task. Therefore, in keeping with this format, this text attempts to meet the immediate needs of all health care providers that are involved in the care of the sick child.

NARENDRA C. SINGH

ACKNOWLEDGMENTS

I would like to thank Carole Gaily and Vanessa Freer for their assistance in the preparation of this book. I would like to thank Dr. Tim Frewen for his mentorship, guidance, and friendship over the years. I would also like to recognize my other colleagues, Dr. Jonathan Kronick, Dr. Richard Lee, and Dr. Yves Ouellette, for their support and contributions to this book. I also want to thank the multidisciplinary team in our pediatric ICU for guidance in the management of critically ill children and their families.

NARENDRA C. SINGH

CONTENTS

7

8

9

12

13

1

The Critically Ill Child

ALLAH B. HAAFIZ, MD
NIRANJAN KISSOON, MD, FCCM, FRCP(C), FAAP

Critical illness is defined as derangement in physiology with the potential to result in significant morbidity and mortality without prompt and appropriate intervention. A common denominator of critical illness in children is cardiopulmonary compromise. This typically occurs as a result of progressive deterioration of respiratory and circulatory function during the course of various diseases, as outlined in Figure 1–1 and Table 1–1. Early recognition, anticipatory supportive intervention, and institution of definitive therapy may interrupt the pathophysiologic process leading to cardiopulmonary arrest. For optimal outcome, delivery of cardiopulmonary support should be expeditious, with limited history and laboratory data and often without a definitive diagnosis.

A critically ill child can present in a variety of settings, including prehospital, a primary care physician's office, and an emergency department. Similarly, a child on a general ward or in a critical care unit may undergo rapid cardiopulmonary deterioration, necessitating prompt attention.

Although the approach to correction of cardiopulmonary derangements should follow accepted guidelines, the extent of intervention that can be offered will vary with the setting and is limited by the availability of resources (e.g., equipment and personnel). For example, treatment of a patient with ineffective respirations in the office environment will entail an activation of emergency medical services. In the critical care environment, this patient may receive more sophisticated investigations and monitoring. Patients in the prehospital setting are especially vulnerable to further deterioration due to the less-than-optimal environment for monitoring and therapy.

Prompt attention by a skilled pediatric transport team and accurate triage of the patient can avoid crucial delay in the start of definitive treatment. Another factor that ensures appropriate and prompt therapy and referral is the use of protocols. This is true for the majority of tertiary care emergency departments affiliated with training programs with limited hours of on-site pediatric attending coverage. In this chapter, we discuss the common diseases leading to rapid deterioration and approach to the management of the final common manifestation, that is, cardiopulmonary failure.

1

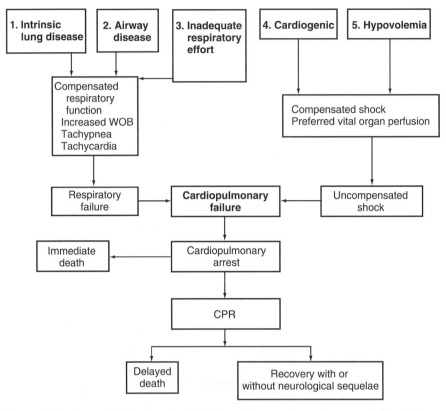

Figure 1–1. Pathway of deterioration in critical illness. Common diseases in groups 1 through 5 are outlined in Table 1–1. WOB, work of breathing.

Pathophysiology

Respiratory failure or shock may be the pathophysiologic expression of primary disease states (see Fig. 1–1 and Table 1–1). If untreated, the two entities may be indistinguishable and merge into cardiopulmonary failure. The spectrum of clinical features results from *inadequate oxygen delivery* and *impaired clearance of tissue metabolites*. For example, in shock, lactic acid accumulates as a consequence of anaerobic glycolysis; whereas in respiratory failure, acute respiratory acidosis develops as pulmonary gas exchange is impaired. The entire process of cardiorespiratory failure can be viewed as a continuum from compensated to decompensated, amplifying vital organ compromise leading to multiple target organ dysfunction (Fig. 1–2).

SHOCK

Shock is a clinical syndrome that results from *failure of the cardiovascular system to adequately meet the metabolic demands of vital organs and tissues.*

Table 1–1. COMMON CONDITIONS PRESENTING AS CARDIOPULMONARY FAILURE

1. Intrinsic lung diseases
   Pneumonia
   Adult respiratory distress
     syndrome
   Loss of lung volume
    Pleural effusion
    Pneumothorax
2. Airway diseases
   Bronchiolitis
   Acute severe bronchial asthma
   Laryngotracheobronchitis
   Epiglottitis
   Foreign body aspiration
3. Inadequate respiratory effort
   Sepsis
   Severe trauma
	Poisoning
	   Guillain-Barré syndrome
	   Poliomyelitis
	4. Cardiogenic shock
	   Myocarditis
	   Congenital heart diseases
	   Hypoxic myocardial dysfunction
	   Cardiac tamponade
	5. Hypovolemia
	   Gastrointestinal losses
	   Burns
	   Diabetic ketoacidosis
	   Hemorrhage
	   Distributive (relative
	    hypovolemia)

See Figure 1–1 (numbers relate to those in Fig. 1–1).

Children have an enormous potential to compensate for decreased stroke volume by increasing heart rate. Accordingly, *tachycardia* is the compensatory manifestation of early normotensive shock. *Hypotension is a late sign* and indicates failure of compensatory mechanisms. At this late stage, the augmented vasomotor tone is impaired as H^+ ions continue to accumulate in the tissues. This will lead to *arteriolar dilatation* and, consequently, peripheral pooling, especially in septic shock. Further *hypoxic-ischemic damage* to endothelial cells triggers the cascade of disseminated intravascular coagulation and microvascular occlusion. At the cellular level, ATPase-dependent and ATPase-nondependent membrane dysfunction leads to irreversible shock. The central nervous system is particularly vulnerable to global ischemic damage because of its high basal metabolic rate. (Detailed accounts of cardiogenic and septic shock are given in Chapters 7 and 9, respectively.)

RESPIRATORY FAILURE

Respiratory insufficiency may occur as a result of *primary pulmonary pathology* or *extrapulmonary disease* (see Fig. 1–1 and Table 1–1). The resultant hypoxemia alone or in conjunction with hypercarbia impairs metabolic and physiologic functioning of the myocardium and central nervous system. If not treated, severe hypoxemia and acidemia disrupt physiologic adjustments of multiple organs, including the cardiovascular system. Acute respiratory failure is the cause of as much as *50% of infant mortality* and is the most common reason for admissions to the pediatric intensive care unit.

Two stages of respiratory insufficiency can be recognized. During the early stage, the child is anxious and shows paradoxical irritability. Signs of increased work of breathing, such as flaring of the alae nasi and intercostal and subcostal

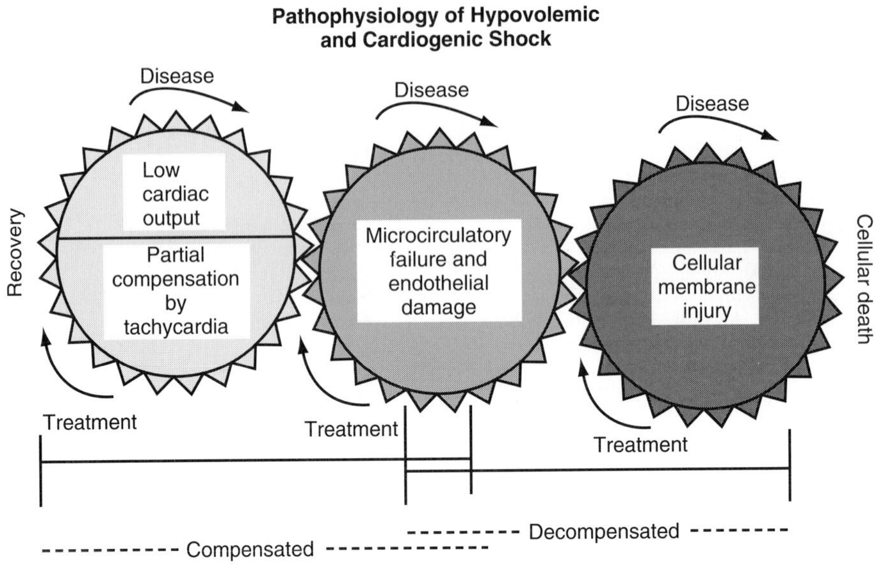

**Pathophysiology of Hypovolemic
and Cardiogenic Shock**

Figure 1–2. Outline of the complex interactions and relationship of clinical symptomatology and cellular processes that may result in cellular death. If the patient is promptly treated, recovery may result as a favorable response to therapy.

retractions, are obvious during this phase. Decreased work of breathing and blunting of sensorium are the signs of the progressive stage of respiratory failure. If untreated, this will lead to cardiopulmonary failure. There are several unique features that put infants at high risk for respiratory failure. Infants have a smaller trachea; a soft thoracic cage; poorly developed intercostal muscles; a short, flat diaphragm; and fewer pores of Kohn for collateral ventilation. In addition, infants are prone to experience a disproportionate decrease in airway diameter with an increase in thickness of respiratory mucosa. Furthermore, they have uncoordinated movements of diaphragm and ribs during rapid eye movement sleep. Respiratory distress is also more likely to precipitate exhaustion because their inherently high metabolic rate increases their energy demands. The etiology, pathophysiology, and management treatment of two types of respiratory failure are summarized in Table 1–2.

Management

The optimal approach to the management of critical illness necessitates treatment of the underlying condition; for example, asthma or pneumonia must be treated to prevent deterioration beyond the compensated state (see Fig. 1–1). Failure to adequately treat the underlying condition and to prevent deterioration will trigger a cascade leading to cardiopulmonary failure and arrest (see Fig. 1–1).

Table 1–2. MAJOR FORMS OF ACUTE RESPIRATORY FAILURE

Feature	Type I	Type II
Etiology	Pneumonia, atelectasis, pulmonary embolism, pulmonary edema, adult respiratory distress syndrome	Head injury, chest wall dysfunction, sedation, burns, severe asthma, Guillain-Barré syndrome, myasthenia gravis, poliomyelitis
Pathophysiology	Impaired gaseous diffusion, ventilation-perfusion defect	Alveolar hypoventilation
Characteristic	↓ Pao_2 Normal or low $Paco_2$	↓ Pao_2 ↓ $Paco_2$
Treatment	Supplemental oxygen, artificial airway and ventilation Address underlying disease	Artificial airway and ventilation Address underlying disease

When this occurs, *cardiorespiratory support takes priority over definitive therapy or occurs simultaneously.*

Available equipment and investigative facilities are limited in the setting of private offices. Therefore, prompt referral and transport should be arranged. During the interim, attention must be paid to airway and breathing. A plan of action for emergency department and critical care is given in Figure 1–3. In essence, effective intervention is accomplished through dynamic therapeutic decision making based on evolving clinical and laboratory data. This requires ongoing individualized clinical and laboratory monitoring as well as anticipation of complications of disease and interventions. Although critical care medicine is typically non-organ based, it may require a variety of organ-based input.

CARDIOPULMONARY RESUSCITATION

A patient with severe cardiopulmonary compromise requires immediate resuscitation to prevent global hypoxic-ischemic damage. Cardiopulmonary resuscitation requires an organized approach, ideally under the supervision of health care personnel who are experienced in both resuscitation techniques and the drugs required (Table 1–3). In the office setting, the maneuvers of basic life support, such as airway and artificial breathing, should be instituted with prompt activation of emergency medical services. In the prehospital setting (e.g., trauma, drowning), basic and advanced life support (including intubation and ventilation) may be offered depending on the personnel expertise, available resources, and existing protocols of the emergency medical service for children (EMS-C) system. In the hospital, advanced life support is provided according to the protocols. Regardless of the setting, the practice and protocols should be in keeping with the guidelines of the American Heart Association and the American Academy of Pediatrics. These guidelines for resuscitation are outlined in Figure 1–4.

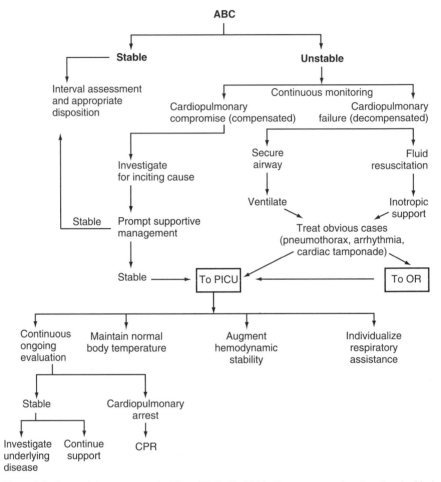

Figure 1–3. Approach to management of the critically ill child in the emergency department and critical care unit.

POSTRESUSCITATION CARE

After initial cardiopulmonary stabilization, the patient requires close monitoring and ongoing vital organ support. This may necessitate the transfer of the patient to a tertiary pediatric critical care unit. Ideally, this transport should be done by a team with the equipment and skills to administer care as an extension of the critical care unit. Frequent assessments, inotropic support, ventilation, prevention of hypothermia, and treatment of inciting causes are very important elements of postresuscitation care. Commonly used drugs in the immediate postresuscitation and stabilization periods are summarized in Table 1–4.

Table 1–3. DRUGS USED IN PEDIATRIC CARDIOPULMONARY RESUSCITATION

Drug	Dose	How Supplied	Remarks
Epinephrine hydrochloride		1:10,000 (0.1 mg/mL)	Most useful drug in cardiac arrest; 1:1000 must be diluted
Bradycardia	0.001 mg/kg (0.1 mL/kg)		
Asystolic or pulseless arrest	*First dose* IV/IO: 0.01 mg/kg (1:10,000) ET: 0.1 mg/kg (1:1000) Doses as high as 0.2 mg/kg may be effective *Subsequent doses* IV/IO/ET: 0.1 mg/kg (1:1000) Doses as high as 0.2 mg/kg may be effective		Be aware of effective dose of preservative administered (if preservatives are present in epinephrine preparation) when high doses are used
Atropine sulfate	0.02 mg/kg IV (0.2 mL/kg)	0.1 mg/mL	*Minimum dose:* 0.1 mg (1 mL); use for bradycardia after assessing ventilation *Maximum dose:* infants and children up to 0.5 mg; adolescents up to 1.0 mg
Lidocaine hydrochloride	1 mg/kg IV	10 mg/mL (1% solution) 20 mg/mL (2% solution)	Use for ventricular arrhythmias *only*
Bretylium tosylate	5 mg/kg IV	50 mg/mL	Use if lidocaine is not effective; repeat dose with 10 mg/kg if first dose is not effective
Sodium bicarbonate	1 mEq/kg IV (1 mL/kg)	1 mEq/mL (8.4% solution)	Infuse slowly and only when ventilation is adequate
Calcium chloride	20 mg/kg IV (0.2 mL/kg)	100 mg/mL (10% solution)	Use only for hypocalcemia, calcium channel blocker overdose, hyperkalemia, or hypermagnesemia; give slowly

8

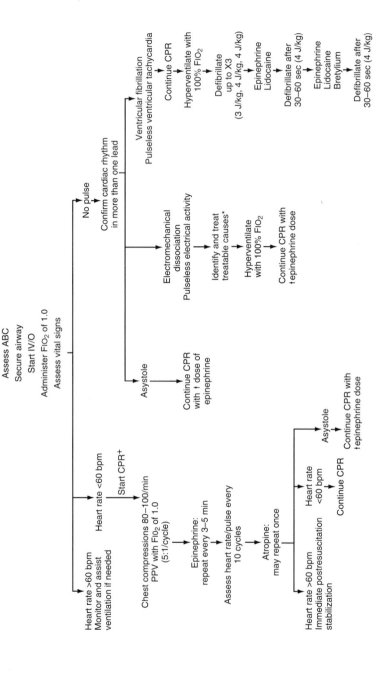

Figure 1–4. Decision tree for advanced pediatric life support. * Treatable causes of electromechanical dissociation and pulseless electrical ability include severe hypoxemia, acidosis, and hypovolemia; cardiac tamponade; and profound hypothermia. †Doses of all medications used in CPR are outlined in Table 1–4.

Table 1–4. DRUGS USED IN IMMEDIATE POSTRESUSCITATION
AND STABILIZATION PERIODS

Drug	Dosage	How Supplied	Remarks
Epinephrine	0.1–1.0 µg/kg/min	1 mg/mL (1:1000)	*
Dopamine hydrochloride	2–20 µg/kg/min	40 mg/mL	*
Dobutamine	5–20 µg/kg/min	250 mg/vial	*
Isoproterenol	0.1–1.0 µg/kg/min	1 mg/5 mL	*
Lidocaine	20–50 µg/kg/min	40 mg/mL (4% solution)	Use lower infusion dose with shock, liver disease

All drugs are given by continuous infusion and are titrated to desired hemodynamic effect.
*In some instances, higher doses or combination therapy is used.

Differential Diagnosis

The differential diagnosis of critical illness in children is broad (see Fig. 1–1 and Table 1–1). However, the likely diagnoses will vary with the practice setting. For example, in a pediatric office setting, children with respiratory emergencies, such as asthma and bronchiolitis, are generally seen. Trauma and near-drowning victims, on the other hand, are more likely to be seen in the prehospital setting or emergency department (Table 1–5). In many cases, the diagnosis is obvious or not important for initial life-saving measures. A more important consideration in the initial assessment is the degree of cardiopulmonary or central nervous system compromise and the need for immediate aggressive therapy. Institution of therapy may precede the definitive diagnosis or occur concurrently and may be independent of the inciting etiology. After the initial stabilization, it is important to search for a diagnosis to determine whether definitive therapy is warranted. The approach to diagnosis in the critically ill child is unique because therapies (e.g., antibiotics for presumed sepsis) should be instituted before obtaining a diagnosis.

Laboratory Investigations

The scope of investigations in the critically ill child is broad and consists of investigations of altered homeostasis as well as those for establishment of a definitive diagnosis.

HEMODYNAMIC AND FUNCTIONAL STABILIZATION

These investigations may include a complete blood count, serum electrolytes, glucose albumin, chest radiography, urinalysis, and arterial blood gas analysis. Occasionally, a computed topography of the head is indicated to rule out increased intracranial pressure, intracranial masses, or hemorrhage. This list is not exhaustive,

Table 1–5. DIAGNOSIS AND PRIORITIES IN MANAGEMENT IN VARIOUS SETTINGS

Health Care	Conditions Encountered	Priorities	Comments
Prehospital care provider	Trauma, seizure, burns, near-drowning, respiratory diseases	All interventions of ALS when required Transport to appropriate emergency facility	Unlimited scope Communication with command center is crucial
Emergency department	EMS transfers as above Emergencies related to virtually every organ system (respiratory and CNS), infections, dehydration and shock, sepsis, sickle cell crises, toxicological emergencies, allergic reactions, and child abuse	All interventions of ALS when required Thorough clinical and laboratory evaluation Involve and coordinate multidisciplinary services	Unlimited scope Liaison among PICU, referrals, and transport Written protocols and algorithm for triage, treatment, and ongoing monitoring
Physician's office	Predominantly infectious (sepsis, meningitis) and upper and lower respiratory diseases	BLS Activate EMS First dose of antibiotics if suspect sepsis and meningitis	Limited scope Communicate with transporting and receiving facilities
Critical care unit	Referral from all of the above	ALS Sophisticated monitoring Multidisciplinary approval	Unlimited scope

ALS, advanced life support; EMS, emergency medical services; CNS, central nervous system; BLS, basic life support; PICU, pediatric intensive care unit.

and further investigations may be warranted depending on the specific clinical situation.

ESTABLISHMENT OF PRIMARY DISEASE

A detailed history of present and past illnesses, physical examination, and observation during initial stabilization will assist in determining the need for and type of investigations to establish a definitive diagnosis. For example, lumbar puncture for examination of the cerebrospinal fluid may be necessary but should be deferred until cardiopulmonary stability is ensured.

ONGOING MONITORING

Rapid alterations may occur in clinical and laboratory parameters during critical illness. Ongoing monitoring is mandatory to provide prompt and dynamic interventions to facilitate a favorable outcome; these investigations include both physiologic and therapeutic drug monitoring.

Physiologic Monitoring

Monitoring of the central venous and arterial pressures and cardiac output may be necessary in patients who are candidates for or show evidence of compromised cardiovascular function or in patients who are on inotropic support. Patients who are mechanically ventilated require further monitoring of airway pressure and indices of oxygenation and ventilation as well as parameters pertaining to pulmonary status (e.g., compliance, resistance, airway pressures). Similarly, patients with central nervous system dysfunction may require intracranial pressure monitoring or continuous electroencephalographic monitoring to avoid undetected rebounds in respective physiologic functions. The frequency of ongoing laboratory investigations should be determined by the clinical course of the patient.

Therapeutic Drug Monitoring

The critically ill child may require multiple drugs for a variety of conditions. For example, it is not unusual for a patient to be receiving concurrently ionotropes, antibiotics, anticonvulsants, diuretics, neuromuscular blocking agents, and oxygen. Drug administration in a critically ill child may be conducted with the use of target effect or target concentration strategies. In target effect strategy, the dose of the drug is tailored to a desired clinical effect. For example, the dose of neuromuscular blocking agent is increased until a therapeutic effect (e.g., paralysis) is achieved. The drug should be discontinued if toxicity supervenes or the desired effect is not achieved with the recommended doses. When target concentration strategy is used, the dose of the drug is adjusted to achieve a desired therapeutic level. For example, antibiotics (e.g., gentamicin, vancomycin) may be titrated to an optimal serum concentration rather than merely an easily recognizable clinical effect.

Prognosis

The prognosis of a critically ill child depends on multiple variables, including the degree and duration of vital organ system involvement, status and duration of cardiovascular decompensation, promptness of intervention, and primary disease process. In most cases in which cardiopulmonary resuscitation is successful in restoring the spontaneous circulation, the ultimate outcome will depend on the degree and duration of the insult to the central nervous system.

BIBLIOGRAPHY

Chameides L (ed): Textbook of Pediatric Advanced Life Support. Hartford, CT, American Heart Association/American Academy of Pediatrics, 1990.
Goetting MG: Mastering pediatric cardiopulmonary resuscitation. Pediatr Clin North Am 41:1147, 1994.
Kissoon N: Triage and transport of the critically ill child. Crit Care Clin 8:37, 1992.
Kissoon N, Vidyasagar D: Cardiopulmonary resuscitation: Shock and dehydration: Transportation issues. Ind J Pediatr 58:91, 1991.
Kissoon N, Walia MS: The critically ill child in the pediatric emergency department. Ann Emerg Med 18:30, 1989.
McCrory JH, Downs CE: Resuscitation of the child. In Holbrook PR (ed): Textbook of Pediatric Critical Care. Philadelphia, WB Saunders, 1993, pp 71–84.

2

Airway Management

NARENDRA C. SINGH, BSc, MB, BS, FRCPC, FAAP
RICHARD J. LEE, LRCP, MRCS, FRCPC

Respiratory failure accounts for a significant number of life-threatening situations in children, and proper airway management can often limit the progression of or reverse the disease process. It is therefore imperative that physicians be familiar with the unique nature of the pediatric airway and with the necessary equipment and drugs and have a systematic approach to managing a compromised pediatric airway.

Pathophysiology

The likelihood of successful airway support in a pediatric patient will increase with knowledge of the pediatric airway. The differences between the child and the adult place the child at an increased risk for the development of respiratory failure (Fig. 2–1). Because of certain structural differences, there is greater likelihood of an increase in airway obstruction and a decrease in lung volume. The child is more susceptible to respiratory muscle fatigue and, because of higher resting oxygen consumption, is more likely to develop tissue hypoxia. Physicians should have knowledge of certain anatomic differences that may influence the likelihood of a smooth intubation (Table 2–1).

Equipment

Before a physician attempts to secure the airway, the necessary equipment should be available. Table 2–2 provides guidelines for the type of equipment and the appropriate size for the various age groups.

Drugs to Facilitate Intubation

Intubation in a cardiac arrest situation does not require the use of drugs; however, in an awake patient, the proper use of drugs will facilitate the procedure.

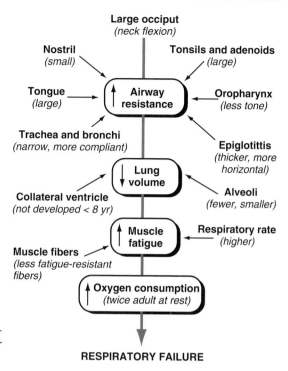

Figure 2–1. Anatomic and physiologic differences in respiratory function between adults and children.

Drugs will decrease the patient's anxiety, pain, and discomfort and can prevent worsening of the primary disease (e.g., increased intracranial pressure [ICP]). The use of drugs that are unfamiliar to the clinician should be avoided because respiratory depression in the presence of an unsuccessful intubation may have dire consequences.

Atropine administration is recommended before all pediatric intubations to decrease secretions and to blunt the bradycardia associated with stimulation, hypoxia, and following succinylcholine administration. Atropine is used at a dose

Table 2–1. ANATOMIC DIFFERENCES AND IMPLICATIONS FOR INTUBATION

Large occiput	With a large occiput, the head flexes at the neck and obstructs the airway; therefore, the "sniffing position" is optimal to align the airway
Anterior larynx	Difficult to perform blind intubation; more difficulty in visualizing cords; straight blade may facilitate intubation; cricoid pressure may improve visualization
Cricoid ring	Narrowest part of the airway; therefore, cuffed tubes are usually not necessary in children less than 8 years old
Short trachea	Intubation of the right bronchus is common

Table 2–2. EQUIPMENT AND SIZES

Equipment	Size
Oral airway	The length of the oropharyngeal airway equals the distance from the angle of the mandible to the angle of the mouth.
Suction catheter	Soft (8F–16F)
	Adult Yankauer (one size)
	Pediatric Yankauer (one size)
Endotracheal tube	
Cuffed	$4 + \dfrac{\text{Age (yr)}}{4}$
Uncuffed	
	Diameter of little finger
	Diameter of nares
Laryngoscope blade	
Curved	Preterm: Miller 0
Straight	Newborn: Miller 1
	1–2 yr: Miller 1.5
	3–8 yr: Miller 2.0
Magill forceps	Neonatal
	Pediatric
	Adult

of 0.01 to 0.02 mg/kg, with a minimum dose of 0.1 mg because less than this may cause paradoxical bradycardia.

SEDATING AGENTS

In awake patients, consideration should be given to the use of a sedating agent before intubation. Some agents have the potential to benefit the primary condition; whereas others can worsen the clinical situation (Table 2–3).

Benzodiazepines. Of the benzodiazepines, *diazepam* is most frequently used; however, it is slower acting and has a longer duration of action than *midazolam*. *Lorazepam* is slower acting and has a longer duration of action than diazepam. *Flumazenil* (0.01 mg/kg) may reverse the sedation from benzodiazepines but may not clinically reverse the respiratory depression.

Opiates. *Fentanyl* has a more rapid onset and shorter duration of action than *morphine*. Because of decreased histamine release, fentanyl is less likely to cause hypotension and, therefore, is useful in patients with borderline hemodynamic function. The chest wall rigidity that occurs after fentanyl use can be prevented by slow administration of the drug and reversed with the use of naloxone or a muscle relaxant. The respiratory depression that occurs with both fentanyl and morphine can be reversed with the use of naloxone.

Barbiturates. *Thiopental* has a rapid onset and short duration of action. It is advantageous in patients with increased ICP because it decreases the cerebral metabolic rate of oxygen ($CMRO_2$) and cerebral blood flow (CBF), which results in decreased ICP. It should be avoided in patients with borderline hemodynamic function because it causes hypotension as a result of both vasodilation and myocardial depression.

Table 2–3. SEDATING AGENTS

Agent	Clinical Use	Comments
Diazepam (0.1–0.2 mg/kg) O: 1–3 min D: 10–20 min	Elective intubation, seizures	Good amnesia, respiratory depression
Midazolam (0.05–0.15 mg/kg) O: 1–3 min D: 10 min	Elective intubation, seizures	Good amnesia, respiratory depression, short duration
Fentanyl (1–2 μgm/kg) O: 30–60 sec D: 30 min–4 hr	Elective intubation, airway obstruction	Less hypotension, reversible respiratory depression
Morphine (0.1–0.2 mg/kg) O: 2–5 min D: 4–6 hr	Elective intubation, airway obstruction	Hypotension, reversible respiratory depression
Thiopental (2–5 mg/kg) O: 10–20 sec D: 10–30 min	Increased intracranial pressure	Rapid onset, hypotension, bronchospasm
Ketamine (1–2 mg/kg) O: 15–20 sec D: 10–20 min	Hypotension, asthma	Increases intracranial pressure, less respiratory depression, hallucinations and dreams

O, onset; D, duration.

Ketamine. *Ketamine* produces rapid sedation, amnesia, and analgesia. It is advantageous in patients with bronchospasm and hypotension due to its sympathomimetic properties, which result in bronchodilatation and increased heart rate, blood pressure, and cardiac index. Owing to increased secretions, patients should be given *atropine* as a prophylaxis. Because ketamine may cause increased ICP and numerous hallucinations, it should be avoided in patients with elevated ICP; prophylactic *lorazepam* may prevent the psychic sensations. It also causes an increase in secretion that may be prevented with the use of atropine.

MUSCLE RELAXANTS

Muscle relaxants should be avoided if the patient has a difficult airway (e.g., upper airway obstruction) or cannot be effectively bag-and-mask ventilated after receiving the sedating agent (Table 2–4).

Short-Acting Depolarizing Agents. *Succinylcholine* has a rapid onset and short duration, making it the most commonly used muscle relaxant. Pretreatment with atropine is recommended to prevent bradycardia. The use of succinylcholine should be avoided in patients with a history of malignant hyperthermia, and it can result in hyperkalemia in patients with upper motor neuron lesions, neuromuscular disease, burns, crush injuries, or severe intra-abdominal sepsis. In patients with acute burns or trauma, succinylcholine may be used because the potassium-releasing action begins at 2 to 5 days and persists for 2 to 3 years after the injury.

Long-Acting Nondepolarizing Agents. Long-acting *pancuronium* has a slower onset but longer duration of action. The drug may increase heart rate and blood pressure.

Table 2–4. MUSCLE RELAXANTS

Agent	Clinical Use	Comments
Succinylcholine (1–2 mg/kg) O: 30–60 sec D: 3–12 min	Elective intubation, rapid-sequence intubation	Bradycardia, increased intracranial pressure (older patients), hyperkalemia
Atracurium (0.5 mg/kg) O: 2.5–4 min D: 20–45 min	Hemodynamic instability	Little hemodynamic effect
Vecuronium (0.1 mg/kg) O: 1–4 min D: 30–60 min	Hemodynamic instability	Least hemodynamic effect
Pancuronium (0.1–0.15 mg/kg) O: 1–5 min D: 50–90 min	Extended paralysis	Tachycardia
Rocuronium (0.6–1.2 mg/kg) O: 1–2 min D: 20–50 min	Hemodynamic instability	Rapid onset of action

O, onset; D, duration.

Intermediate-Acting Nondepolarizing Agents. *Vecuronium, atracurium,* and *rocuronium* have a distinct advantage in that they produce the fewest hemodynamic side effects.

Systemic Approach to the Pediatric Airway

BASIC AIRWAY MANEUVERS

Although airway management often includes endotracheal intubation, simple maneuvers may help create a patent airway, alleviating the need for endotracheal intubation.

Positioning of Patient

The tongue may commonly cause airway obstruction; therefore jaw thrust or other maneuvers should be attempted to elevate the tongue from the posterior pharynx (Fig. 2–2). If the infant is vomiting, then positioning on his or her side decreases the likelihood of aspiration.

Suctioning of Airway

Suctioning of the nares and oropharynx should be done if the above maneuvers fail or the patient is vomiting. Because neonates and infants are primarily nasal breathers, suctioning of the nares and nasopharynx is essential.

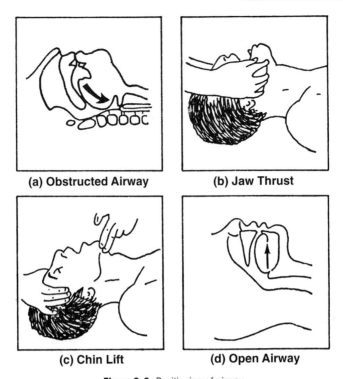

(a) Obstructed Airway   (b) Jaw Thrust

(c) Chin Lift   (d) Open Airway

Figure 2–2. Positioning of airway.

100% Oxygen

If the patient is breathing, a mask with 100% oxygen should be placed on the face. In the apneic patient, bag-and-mask ventilation with 100% oxygen should be initiated.

Oropharyngeal Airway

An oropharyngeal airway may be used in the unconscious patient to elevate the tongue forward. It is inserted by placing the tube in the mouth with the concavity superior and rotating it 180° to avoid pushing the tongue posteriorly. A *soft nasopharyngeal airway* may also be used in the semiconscious patient.

Have Maneuvers Been Successful?

If it has been established that the airway is patent, then breathing must be assessed, with institution of bag-and-mask ventilation if necessary. If the above maneuvers have been unsuccessful, they may be repeated while preparations are being made for intubation.

INTUBATION

In addition to the inability to establish patency of the airway, there are numerous indications for intubation (Table 2–5).

Sequence of Orotracheal Intubation

1. Use a *cardiorespiratory monitor* and *pulse oximeter* if available.
2. Have all *drugs and equipment available.*
3. Place the patient in a *sniffing position.* By slightly extending the patient's head onto the neck and slightly flexing the neck in relation to the trunk, optimal positioning of the mouth, pharynx, and larynx will be created to facilitate intubation.
4. In *preoxygenation,* administer 100% oxygen via a mask to the breathing patient. In an apneic patient, begin bag-and-mask ventilation with 100% oxygen.
5. After receiving *atropine* (0.01 mg/kg; min 0.1 mg), the child should become transiently tachycardic.
6. After *sedation* (see Table 2–3) and before paralysis, a proper seal should be obtained with the mask, and it should be possible to bag-and-mask ventilate.
7. Avoid administering *muscle relaxants* (see Table 2–4) if the airway is difficult (e.g., airway obstruction) or you are not absolutely confident that endotracheal intubation will be successful (e.g., unable to bag-and-mask ventilate).
8. *Open mouth* and *insert laryngoscope* with the right thumb on the bottom teeth and the index finger on the top teeth; the mouth is opened with use of the scissors maneuver. The laryngoscope is held with the left hand, and the blade is introduced into the right side of the mouth and moved to the center while the tongue is swept to the left side.
9. *Visualize the vocal cords,* using one of the following methods.

Straight Blade
   a. The blade may be gradually introduced with upward traction along the shaft of the laryngoscope until the epiglottis is in view and then elevated to allow visualization of the cords.

Table 2–5. INDICATION FOR ENDOTRACHEAL INTUBATION

Poor respiratory effort
Central: drugs, infection, trauma
Spinal injury
Chest wall deformity (kyphosis)
Upper airway disease: croup, epiglottitis
Lower airway disease: pneumonia, bronchiolitis, asthma
Control of other symptoms
Increased intracranial pressure
Shock: removal of respiratory effort

b. Alternatively, the blade may be introduced all of the way into the esophagus and gradually withdrawn until the cords are visualized.

Curved Blade

Both of the above techniques may be used; however, the tip of the curved blade is inserted into the vallecula, and traction along the body of the laryngoscope will elevate the epiglottis and bring the cords into view. In contrast, the straight blade directly elevates the epiglottis.

10. *Insert the endotracheal tube* (ETT) to the right of the curvature of the blade (not through the curvature) to maintain adequate visualization of the cords. Cricoid pressure may help to visualize the cords.
11. *When should the attempt be aborted?* If the child desaturates or becomes bradycardic, then bag-and-mask ventilation should be reinstituted. As a guideline, the duration of the attempt should not exceed the length of time the physician is able to hold his or her breath.
12. To *determine whether the ETT is in the correct position,* directly visualize the tube between the cords. This is the most reliable method. Other methods involve auscultation of the chest and epigastrium, symmetrical chest movements, stable vital signs, end-tidal carbon dioxide monitoring, Trach-mate magnetic detector, and chest radiograph.

Nasotracheal Intubation

Intubation using a nasotracheal tube (NTT) is not recommended in the emergency situation or in patients with suspected basal skull fracture. It is used in patients who require prolonged intubation because it is easier to immobilize and prevents the patient from biting on the ETT. The sequence of intubation is the same as for orotracheal intubation and can be done by either of two methods.

1. After lubrication, the ETT is passed through the nares into the oropharynx. The tube is then visualized with the use of laryngoscopy and picked up 1 cm from the tip with Magill forceps. The tip is inserted through the cords, with an assistant helping to push the tube distal to the cords.
2. Oral intubation may be done before nasotracheal intubation and is advantageous because the patient is more stable and the procedure does not have to be hurried. The above method is followed *except* that the tip of the nasotracheal tube is lined up with the oral tube as it enters the cords and the nasotracheal tube is inserted as the oral ETT is withdrawn.

Intubation under Specific Clinical Situations

Specific clinical situations require special consideration because the technique and drug that are used have the potential to benefit the situations (Table 2–6).

All children presenting to the emergency department should be assumed to have a *full stomach,* and therefore, a rapid-sequence induction should be performed to prevent aspiration (Table 2–7). In patients with *increased ICP,* a similar technique will blunt the rise in ICP with intubation. Both *lidocaine* and *thiopental,* alone or in combination, are recommended because both may further blunt the rise in ICP with stimulation. In isolated hypotension without increased ICP, *ketamine*

Table 2–6. INTUBATION IN SPECIAL CLINICAL SITUATIONS

Clinical Situation	Technique/Drugs	Comments
Full stomach	Rapid-sequence induction (see Table 2–7)	Lidocaine is not necessary
Hypovolemia	Atropine, *ketamine*, succinylcholine	Ketamine: increased blood pressure and cardiac index
Status asthmaticus	Atropine, *ketamine*, succinylcholine	Ketamine: bronchodilator
Increased intracranial pressure	Rapid-sequence induction (see Table 2–7)	Lidocaine, thiopental: decreased intracranial pressure
Airway obstruction (e.g., croup) Awake Obtunded Anxious and hypoxic	**Do not paralyze** Inhalation anesthetic Bag-and-mask ventilate (intubate if unsuccessful) If inhalation is not quickly available, then use narcotic to sedate and then intubate	Narcotic is reversible if intubation is unsuccessful

is the drug of choice because it may increase heart rate, blood pressure, and cardiac output. Due to its bronchodilator property, it is also useful in facilitating intubation of asthmatics.

Airway obstruction in children is one of the most anxiety-provoking situations for a clinician. Patients with airway obstruction should not be paralyzed for intubation because an unsuccessful intubation may have dire consequences. If the

Table 2–7. RAPID-SEQUENCE INDUCTION

1. Have monitor equipment and drugs available
2. Preoxygenation
   If breathing, 100% O_2 by mask
   If apneic, bag-and-mask ventilate with 100% O_2
3. Premedicate
   Atropine (0.01–0.02 mg/kg; min 0.1 mg)
   Lidocaine (1–1.5 mg/kg)
   Pancuronium (defasciculating dose, 0.01 mg/kg)
4. Achieve mask seal
   Bag-and-mask ventilate only if apneic
5. Cricoid pressure by assistant
6. Sedating agent
   Thiopental (2–4 mg/kg), avoid in hypotension
7. Muscle relaxant
   Succinylcholine (1–2 mg/kg)
8. Intubate
   Begin bag ventilation
9. Decompress stomach
   Nasogastric tube

*Not needed for patient less than 8 to 10 years old.

child is awake and there is sufficient time, inhalation anesthesia administered in the operating room is the technique of choice. If the child is obtunded, bag-and-mask ventilation is often successful, followed by intubation. If the child is awake and is in impending failure (e.g., anxious and hypoxic), then a sedating agent (e.g., *morphine, fentanyl*), which can be reversed, may facilitate the intubation. If the intubation is unsuccessful, then the narcotic can be reversed with *naloxone*.

BIBLIOGRAPHY

Kissoon N, Singh NC: Airway management and ventilatory support. *In* Reisdorff EJ, Roberts MR, Wiegenstein JG (eds): Pediatric Emergency Medicine. Philadelphia, WB Saunders, 1992, pp 51–67.

Singh NC, Kissoon N. Croup and epiglottis. *In* Surpure JS (ed): Synopsis of Pediatric Emergency Medicine. Reading, MA, Andover Medical Publishers, 1993, pp 23–32.

Thompson AE. Pediatric airway management. *In* Fuhrman BP, Zimmerman JJ (eds): Pediatric Critical Care. St. Louis, Mosby–Year Book, 1992, pp 111–128.

3

Hemodynamic Management

GARY I. JOUBERT, BSc, MD, FRCPC, FAAP

Shock and hypoxia are the two major causes of mortality and morbidity in infants and children. *Shock* is defined as inadequate tissue perfusion to supply oxygen and nutrients to meet the metabolic demands of the tissue and remove cellular waste. The physician should note that this definition is not based on a minimum blood pressure required for tissue perfusion. The early recognition and treatment of shock will prevent unnecessary morbidity and mortality. In this chapter, I review primarily hypovolemic shock, the pathophysiology of its clinical presentation, investigations, and management. Cardiogenic (Chapter 7.3) and septic shock (Chapter 9.1) are discussed elsewhere.

Pathophysiology

Perfusion to tissue is maintained by cardiac output. *Cardiac output* is determined by two parameters: stroke volume and heart rate.

Stroke volume is the result of preload (ventricular end-diastolic volume), the amount of afterload (resistance) against which the myocardial pump must pump, and myocardial contractility (as determined with the use of Starling's law).

Heart rate, the other determinate of cardiac output, is under the control of the vagus nerve (increased vagal tone results in decreased heart rate) and circulating catecholamines, which cause increased heart rate and myocardial contractility. In neonates and infants, the ability to increase stroke volume is limited; as a result, *cardiac output is predominantly dependent on heart rate.*

Afterload is systemic (peripheral) vascular resistance. Peripheral vascular resistance is under the control of the sympathetic nervous system and circulating catecholamines.

Blood pressure is a function of cardiac output and peripheral vascular resistance.

Shock is the result of a failure of the above normal physiologic mechanisms to maintain adequate cardiac output. Regardless of the underlying etiology of shock, the end result is either an absolute or a functional state of hypovolemia. This state of hypovolemia activates a variety of physiologic responses that attempt, in the acute phase, to compensate for the diminished cardiac output. These responses exert their effects through biochemical and inflammatory mediators on the microvasculature.

Microvasculature

Microcirculatory changes occur as a result of shock. The changes are mediated through a change in sympathetic tone and vasoactive substances that act on precapillary sphincters and arteriolar smooth muscle. Their combined action results in muscle contraction, which leads to increases in precapillary shunting and local tissue hypoxia. This eventually gives rise to local tissue capillary breakdown and a capillary leak phenomenon.

Biochemical mediators are released from numerous cell and tissue types. Their release starts a physiologic cascade, resulting in the eventual obliteration and degradation of capillary integrity.

Types of Shock

The three major types of shock are hypovolemic, distributive, and cardiogenic. Although the underlying pathophysiology in all three types of shock is similar (absolute or functional hypovolemia), the pathways that lead to this ultimate end point are different. These differences form the bases for the different therapeutic interventions.

Hypovolemic Shock

Hypovolemic shock, the most frequent clinical form of shock, is defined as an absolute loss of volume from the vascular tree. This loss of volume can be classified into three groups:

1. Loss of blood volume (hemorrhagic)
2. Loss of body water (dehydrational)
3. Loss of plasma

Distributive Shock

Distributive shock results in a functional hypovolemic state in which the total circulating volume has been redistributed. This redistribution can occur within the vascular tree (i.e., loss of autoregulation of the capillary bed) or outside the vascular tree (capillary leak syndrome) or represent a combination. Distributive shock can be thought of as resulting from either of two major pathologic states:

1. Septic shock (see Chapter 9.1)
2. Neurogenic shock

Cardiogenic Shock

Cardiogenic shock occurs when the heart is unable to maintain cardiac output secondary to pump failure. Pump failure may be intrinsic to myocardial muscle failure or extrinsic, resulting in inability of the ventricle to fill or empty.

Compensated Shock

Compensated shock is the state of tissue hypoperfusion in which the adaptive physiologic responses attempt to maintain central organ perfusion at the expense of peripheral perfusion. Blood pressure may be maintained or only slightly decreased, with perfusion to the extremities markedly decreased.

Decompensated Shock

Decompensated shock is the state in which the adaptive physiologic responses can no longer compensate for tissue hypoperfusion and central organ perfusion is no longer maintained, leading to organ failure. This state is often irreversible.

Clinical Evaluation

The clinical evaluation of shock is based on both historical and clinical assessment. Tables 3–1 and 3–2 provide reviews of the signs and symptoms associated with the various types of shock. Note that in the early phases of hypovolemic and distributive shock, the clinical signs are often subtle. The infant and child can compensate with increased sympathetic tone and tachycardia to offset acute volume loss. Once volume loss exceeds 40% of circulating blood volume, the circulatory system can no longer compensate, at which point decompensated shock develops.

Table 3–1. CLINICAL SIGNS OF SHOCK

Type of Shock	Heart Rate	Blood Pressure	Periphery	Urine
Hypovolemic	Early sign: increased	Initially increased, then decreased	Cool extremities, poor capillary refill	Decreased, to oliguric
Distributive	Early sign: increased	Decreased	Cool/warm extremities, poor capillary refill	Decreased, to oliguric
Cardiogenic	Tachycardia,* bradycardia*	Decreased	Cool extremities, poor capillary refill	Decreased, to oliguric

*Depends on underlying mechanism.

Table 3–2. CLASSIFICATION OF HEMORRHAGIC SHOCK

Sign or Symptom	Class 1	Class 2	Class 3	Class 4
Blood volume loss	10–15%	20–25%	30–35%	>40%
Pulse	>100	>150	>150	>150
Respiratory rate	Normal	Increased	Tachypneic	Tachypneic or apneic
Capillary refill (sec)	<5	5–10	10–15	>20
Blood pressure	Normal	Increased pulse pressure	Decreased	Severely decreased
Mentation	Normal	Anxious	Confused	Coma
Orthostatic hypotension	+	+ +	+ + +	+ + +
Urine output (mL/kg/hr)	1–3	0.5–1	<0.5	None

Investigations

Investigations are summarized in Table 3–3.

Management

Shock is managed aggressively, with the goal of therapy directed at the return of normal cardiac output (organ perfusion) regardless of the underlying mechanism causing the shock (Table 3–4).

As is the case in all acute resuscitative efforts, of paramount importance are the establishment of a *patent airway,* ensuring ventilation (either spontaneous or controlled), and *access to the vascular system.*

Intravascular access is established using the largest bore intravenous catheter

Table 3–3. LABORATORY INVESTIGATIONS IN SHOCK

Blood	Imaging	Open (in Trauma Patient or Patient with Other Diagnosis)
CBC with differential	Chest radiograph	CAT scan head/abdomen
Blood urea nitrogen	Pelvis in trauma patient	
Creatinine	Abdomen in trauma patient	
Blood glucose	Long bones in trauma patient	Two-dimensional echocardiogram, if needed
Blood cultures		
Blood gases		
Electrolytes		
Lactate		
Liver transaminases		
PT (INR)/PTT		
Amylase (trauma)		

Table 3–4. PRIORITIES IN THE MANAGEMENT OF SHOCK

Airway patent:
    Ensure airway is patent
    May require intubation
    Always intubate early
Breathing:
    Ensure adequate ventilation (spontaneous or controlled)
    Ensure that chest movement is adequate
Circulation (Tables 3–1 and 3–2) and vascular access (see Chapter 11.8)
    Intravenous
    Intraosseous: age less than 6 years
Fluid resuscitation
    See flow diagram (Fig. 3–1)
    Fluid choice: normal saline or Ringer's lactate
Inotropic therapy (see Chapter 7.5, Cardiovascular Pharmacology)
Monitor
    Blood pressure: noninvasive/invasive
    Urine output
    Heart rate
    Respiratory rate
    Oxygen saturation
    Placement of a Foley catheter
    Central venous pressure

that the particular vein will accept. In infants and young children (less than 6 years old), access to the vascular system can be achieved with the intraosseous technique (see Chapter 11.1).

Postresuscitative Fluid Management

After acute fluid resuscitation and stabilization of the patient, there is a need for ongoing fluid management (Fig. 3–1). Fluid requirements after resuscitation include maintenance fluids and replacement of fluid losses.

MAINTENANCE FLUIDS

Maintenance fluids is defined as the amount of fluid required to maintain normal fluid dynamics (hydration) (Table 3–5).

Table 3–5. MAINTENANCE FLUID

Weight	Fluid (mL/kg body weight/24 hr)	Infusion Rate (mL/kg/hr)
0–10 kg	100	4
10–20 kg	150	2
>20 kg	170	1

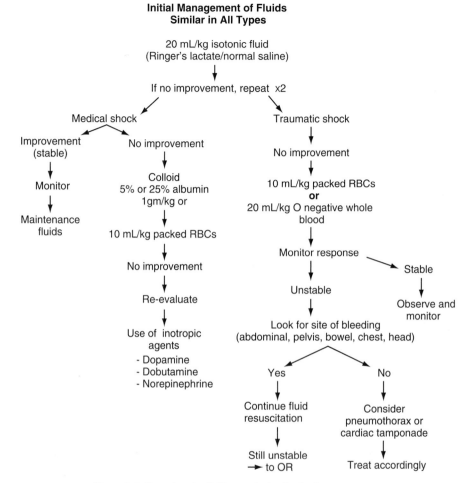

**Initial Management of Fluids
Similar in All Types**

20 mL/kg isotonic fluid
(Ringer's lactate/normal saline)

If no improvement, repeat x2

Medical shock

Traumatic shock

Improvement
(stable)

No improvement

No improvement

Monitor

Colloid
5% or 25% albumin
1gm/kg or

10 mL/kg packed RBCs
or
20 mL/kg O negative whole
blood

Maintenance
fluids

10 mL/kg packed RBCs

Monitor response

No improvement

Stable

Re-evaluate

Unstable

Observe and
monitor

Use of inotropic
agents
- Dopamine
- Dobutamine
- Norepinephrine

Look for site of bleeding
(abdominal, pelvis, bowel, chest, head)

Yes

No

Continue fluid
resuscitation

Consider
pneumothorax or
cardiac tamponade

Still unstable
→ to OR

Treat accordingly

Figure 3–1. Flow chart for fluid resuscitation in shock management.

- Maintenance fluids are linked to caloric requirements for the individual (for every 100 calories, there is a requirement for 100 mL of fluid).
- The required amount of fluid takes into account insensible losses but not additional fluid losses such as gastrointestinal losses, excessive urinary losses, excessive respiratory losses, and losses caused by increased metabolic rate (e.g., fever).

ELECTROLYTE MAINTENANCE

In addition to maintenance fluids, there is a need for the replacement and maintenance of blood electrolytes. Electrolyte maintenance is closely linked to fluid needs.

Sodium requirements are 2.5 to 3 mEq/100 mL fluid/24 hr (or 2.5 to 5 mEq/kg/day, depending in part on urinary sodium losses).

Potassium requirements are 2 to 2.5 mEq/100 mL fluid/24 hr (or 2 to 4 mEq/kg/day, depending on urinary potassium losses).

SPECIAL CONSIDERATIONS

In addition to ongoing maintenance fluid administration, there is a need to replace excessive ongoing fluid losses. This need may be due to losses in the gastrointestinal tract, in the respiratory tract in the patient receiving oxygen or ventilation, or in the urinary tract, or from increased metabolic demands, as occurs with fever. With the ongoing fluid losses, there may be an imbalance in the electrolytes that must be replaced. Electrolyte imbalance can be classified as one of three categories depending on the sodium concentration in the serum.

Types of Sodium Imbalance

Isonatremic. In the isonatremic patient, the range of serum sodium concentration is 130 to 150 mEq/L. Replacement of the fluid and sodium deficit should occur over a 24-hour period. The first half of the deficit should be replaced within the first 8 hours; the remaining half of the deficit should be replaced within the next 16 hours. Remember that both maintenance and deficit fluids are administered at a rate of total per-hour fluid volume.

Hypernatremic. In the hypernatremic patient, the serum sodium concentration is greater than 150 mEq/L. The replacement of water and sodium in a patient with hypernatremic dehydration should be a very gradual process. Fluid replacement should occur over a 48- to 72-hour period. The goal of fluid replacement is to lower the serum sodium concentration at a rate of 10 to 15 mEq/24 hr, or about 0.5 mEq/hr.

Initially, normal saline is used to replace the water deficit to prevent a rapid decrease in sodium and to replace the effective total body deficit of sodium. After urine output is reestablished and serum sodium is under control, the solution can be changed to 0.45% normal saline.

Hyponatremic. In the hyponatremic patient, the serum sodium concentration is less than 130 mEq/L. Sodium deficit can be calculated with the following formula:

Serum sodium deficit = serum sodium level sought – current serum sodium level × 0.6 (range, 0.6 to 0.8 depending on age) × body weight (kg)

The goal is to replace this sodium deficit over a 24-hour period. In the patient who is symptomatic (e.g., seizing), the serum sodium should be increased more rapidly in the acute stage. A solution of sodium chloride (3% normal saline) is used to rapidly increase the serum sodium concentration to a value of greater than 120 mEq/L).

Correction of these fluid and electrolyte imbalances requires careful and judicious use of water and salts (e.g., sodium and potassium). Life-threatening electrolyte imbalances should be corrected first, with fine tuning occurring later, using electrolyte and fluid monitoring as guidelines. Early recognition of shock in children is often challenging, as the signs and symptoms can be subtle. If clinicians depend solely on blood pressure changes to determine when to intervene, irreversible changes may occur with significant impacts on mortality and morbidity.

4

Trauma Management

RAM N. SINGH, MD, FRCPC

Trauma is the leading cause of death in children between 1 and 14 years old; and for every death, four children survive with permanent disability, resulting in significant social, emotional, and economic impact on society. Vigilant initial assessment and expert resuscitation followed by rapid triage and definitive therapy are crucial for optimum outcome.

Pathophysiology

Children are not just small adults. There are significant differences between the anatomy and physiology of adults and those of children, which have been highlighted in Chapter 2, Airway Management. The following are some of the unique aspects of pediatric trauma:

- The head is the most commonly injured system.
- Airway compromise is a serious threat.
- More than 80% of the injuries are due to blunt trauma.
- Falls and vehicular accidents account for more than 80% of the injuries.
- Multisystem injury is a rule, rather than an exception.

Trauma Center and Trauma Team

Theoretically, every seriously injured child should receive care in a pediatric trauma center staffed by a full trauma team; however, this often is not possible. The recommended composition of a pediatric trauma team includes a team leader, several other physicians, a neurosurgeon, an anesthetist, an orthopedic surgeon, emergency nurses, a respiratory therapist, and laboratory and radiology technicians. However, most hospitals do not follow these guidelines owing to limited hospital resources and because of the perception that not all members of the team may be required for the initial evaluation and resuscitation but rather should be available on demand. The Pediatric Trauma Scale (PTS) was designed for rapid assessment of injury severity and triage (see Chapter 13). A PTS score of ≤8 has been identified as an indicator of injury sufficiently severe to warrant referral to a tertiary care or pediatric trauma center.

Assessment and Management

The initial assessment and management of the trauma victim are based on principles of advanced trauma life support (ATLS) as outlined by the American College of Surgeons. The ATLS guidelines do not teach new concepts in trauma management; rather, they emphasize a systematic approach to trauma care in establishing assessment and management priorities. Although the overall strategy is to arrive at an integrated plan for treatment, the evaluation and management of a trauma victim are divided into the following four phases: primary survey, phase of resuscitation, secondary survey, and definitive care.

PRIMARY SURVEY

During the primary survey, life-threatening conditions must be identified and managed immediately. The components of the primary survey are as follows:

Airway

Assessment. The airway should be assessed for *obstruction* caused by secretion, vomitus, a foreign body, the tongue, or the soft tissues.

Management
1. *Suction* the nostrils and mouth.
2. Open the airway by the *jaw-thrust* or *jaw-lift* maneuver.
3. Avoid the *sniffing position* or *head-tilt and chin-lift* maneuver as all children with multiple injuries should be assumed to have cervical spine injury until proved otherwise.
4. Consider placing an *oral airway.*
5. Consider *intubation* and mechanical *ventilation* if the airway cannot be maintained by the above maneuvers.
6. Consider a *surgical airway* such as cricothyrotomy if intubation is not possible.

Endotracheal Intubation. Endotracheal intubation in a multiply injured pediatric patient should be performed by highly trained personnel. Indications for intubation in a multiple-trauma patient are listed in Table 4–1. Rapid sequence intubation should be attempted in these patients (this technique has been described in Chapter 2). The choice of drugs in different clinical scenarios is given in Table 4–2. A patient with multiple trauma should be intubated first orally and then, if preferred, changed to a nasal route. A nasal tube is contraindicated in the presence of basal skull fracture.

Table 4–1. INDICATIONS FOR INTUBATION IN MULTIPLE-TRAUMA PATIENTS

Airway obstruction
  Obstruction not relieved by airway maneuvering
  Surgical obstruction such as facial or neck injuries
Protection of the airway
  Prevent aspiration
  Comatose patient GCS score ≤8
To improve gas exchange
  Apnea or hypoventilation
  Significant chest trauma
To reduce work of breathing
  Hypovolemic shock
Control of increased intracranial pressure
  GCS score ≤8
  Focal neurologic deficit

GCS, Glasgow Coma Scale.

Breathing

Assessment
1. Assess respiratory rate and depth and effort of *breathing*.
2. Perform *auscultation* of chest to detect diminished air entry.
3. Detect any *asymmetry* in chest movement and expansion.
4. The possibility of *cardiac tamponade* should be ruled out at this stage.

Management
1. Deliver *supplemental oxygen* to all patients via nasal prongs or face mask at a rate of ≥12 L/min.

Table 4–2. DRUGS FOR INTUBATION IN MULTIPLE-TRAUMA PATIENTS

If patient has absent vital signs or is unstable
  No drugs

If head injury is a major concern

Patient is hypotensive	Patient is normotensive
Fentanyl 1–2 μg/kg IV	Thiopental 4–5 mg/kg
Atropine 0.01–0.02 mg/kg IV	Atropine 0.01–0.02 mg/kg IV
Lidocaine 1 mg/kg IV	Lidocaine 1 mg/kg IV
Pancuronium* 0.01 mg/kg IV (defasciculating dose)	Pancuronium* 0.01 mg/kg IV (defasciculating dose)
Succinylcholine 1–2 mg/kg†	Succinylcholine 1–2 mg/kg

If head injury is not a major concern

Patient is hypotensive	Patient is normotensive
Ketamine 1–2 mg/kg	Thiopental 4–5 mg/kg
Atropine 0.01–0.02 mg/kg	Atropine 0.01–0.02 mg/kg
Succinylcholine 1–2 mg/kg	Succinylcholine 1–2 mg/kg

*A defasciculating dose of pancuronium is not indicated in children younger than 10 years old.
†Vecuronium may be substituted for succinylcholine and pancuronium.

2. *Intubate* and mechanically *ventilate* if there is inadequate gas exchange despite a patent airway.
3. If a tension pneumothorax is identified, then a needle *thoracentesis* should be done, followed by insertion of a chest tube.

Circulation

Assessment
1. Identify exsanguinating *hemorrhage.*
2. Assess current *hemodynamic status* by examining pulse rate, pulse quality, cardiac rhythm, blood pressure, and capillary refill.
3. Establish degree of *hemorrhagic shock* based on ATLS classification (see Chapter 3).

Management
1. Control external hemorrhage by *direct pressure.*
2. Identify shock, obtain *vascular access*, and start *resuscitation* as outlined in resuscitation phase.

Disability Assessment

To identify life-threatening central nervous system injuries, a rapid neurologic assessment should be performed with the use of the pneumonic *AVPU:*

- A: *Alert*
- V: Response to *verbal* stimuli
- P: Response to *pain* only
- U: *Unresponsive*

Exposure

After the initial assessment and resuscitation, the patient's clothing should be removed to facilitate complete examination of the different systems of the body during the secondary survey. Risks of hypothermia can be avoided with the use of a radiant warmer or a warming blanket.

PHASE OF RESUSCITATION

1. Obtain *intravenous access* with the use of two large-bore catheters. No more than 90 seconds should be lost in obtaining a peripheral venous access; if unsuccessful, *intraosseous access* should be obtained. The next preferred site should be *femoral venous access*, which is often the safest and easiest to obtain.
2. An attempt should be made to *replace fluid losses* with crystalloid, colloid, or blood product. A flow sheet regarding fluid management is provided in Chapter 3, p. 27.
3. Management of life-threatening problems identified in the primary survey is continued.

4. If, despite aggressive fluid resuscitation, the patient remains unstable, immediate consideration should be given to surgical control of bleeding.
5. At this stage of assessment and resuscitation, the patient should have a minimum of *cardiorespiratory monitoring*, oxygen saturation monitoring, noninvasive blood pressure assessment every 5 minutes, and continuous temperature assessment.
6. A *urinary catheter* should be placed to measure accurate urine output.
7. An *orogastric* or *nasogastric tube* should be placed to decompress the stomach.
8. A lateral *radiograph* of the cervical spine and an anteroposterior view of chest, abdomen, and pelvis should be obtained as soon as possible.
9. *Crossmatch for blood*, initial hemoglobin, hematocrit, electrolytes, and blood gases should be obtained.

SECONDARY SURVEY

During the secondary survey, a complete head-to-toe examination is performed to identify injuries in every system of the body. Examination should be done systematically, with inspection, palpation, percussion, and auscultation. Once an injury is identified, a decision must be made in prioritizing its management in relation to other injuries. The steps in secondary survey are briefly outlined:

1. **Head and face:** The head is examined for any evidence of external injuries. The pupils are examined for any asymmetry. The ears are examined for blood behind the drums. The Glasgow Coma Scale (GCS) score is determined to assess the severity of head injury. Facial bones are examined for fractures.
2. **Neck:** The neck is examined for swelling, tenderness, or subcutaneous emphysema.
3. **Chest:** The chest should be examined for external injuries or flail segment. Palpation will identify crepitus or bony tenderness, and auscultation of the chest will help identify a pneumothorax or hemothorax.
4. **Abdomen:** Bruises or distension may indicate serious underlying organ injuries. Palpation and auscultation will help in formulation of an initial diagnosis. Rectal examination and repeated measurement of abdominal girth should be part of the routine abdominal examination.
5. **Pelvis:** Bony prominence should be examined for tenderness, fractures, and instability.
6. **Genitourinary:** The urethral meatus should be examined for blood. Urine specimens, even when clear, should be sent for microscopic examination.
7. **Extremities:** A thorough examination of the extremities should be performed to elicit bony fractures or soft tissue injuries.
8. **Thoracolumbar spine:** An examination is performed by log rolling the patient; maintaining adequate cervical-spine precautions; and looking for evidence of tenderness, swelling, or fractures.
9. **History:** The medical history should record the mechanism of injury and extent of injuries of other victims. A brief summary of the patient's past medical history, including allergies, should be obtained.

10. **Re-evaluation:** Patients should be periodically re-evaluated for any deterioration in vital signs or neurologic status.

DEFINITIVE CARE

Once the treatment for life-threatening conditions has begun or is completed, definitive care of the other injuries should be initiated. Detailed laboratory and radiologic techniques should be used to define the extent of injuries. Preparation should be made for transport to another center, an operating room, or an intensive care unit (see Chapter 5).

Assessment of Management of Individual Systems

Chest Trauma. The reported incidence of chest trauma in the pediatric population has been as high as 50%. Fortunately, most of these injuries have been minor, but at least 5 to 10% of these children have chest injuries that require immediate intervention. The most common presentations of severe chest injuries are hypoxemia, increased respiratory effort, and, sometimes, hypotension. The majority of deaths from chest trauma can be prevented if the injuries are recognized and treated immediately. Some of the common chest injuries are as follows:

Tension Pneumothorax. Tension pneumothorax is often the most devastating condition if left untreated. It can be diagnosed by observing decreased air entry and a hyperresonant and bulging chest on the affected side. In an older child, deviation of trachea and mediastinum to the opposite side can be appreciated. If pneumothorax is suspected, an immediate needle thoracocentesis should be performed, followed by chest tube placement.

Hemothorax. Hemothorax is usually detected during the secondary survey or after a routine chest radiograph. Massive hemothorax, which can be detected earlier, can also cause hypotension in extremely small children. If a massive hemothorax is diagnosed, a chest tube can be placed to improve oxygenation and ventilation.

Flail Chest. This is not a common injury in the pediatric population and is generally caused by high-velocity impact resulting in multiple rib fractures. If the diagnosis is made, treatment consists of stabilization of the fragment, possible intubation, and positive pressure ventilation.

Cardiac Tamponade. Hypotension, refractory to fluid administration, should arouse suspicion of cardiac tamponade. If suspected, immediate pericardiocentesis could be life saving.

Pulmonary Contusion/Laceration. Pulmonary contusion or laceration, unless severe, is often detected late during the investigation and stabilization of trauma. Clinical signs include hemoptysis, hypoxemia, and decreased air entry on the affected side. The chest radiograph shows diffuse opacity or atelectasis on the affected side. Treatment depends on the degree of hypoxemia; some patients require intubation and mechanical ventilation.

Abdominal Trauma. More than 90% of the abdominal injuries in children are due to blunt trauma, with the only external evidence of trauma being bruises, often due to a lap belt. Acute gastric dilation can sometimes cause massive distension of the abdomen; however, this is tympanic on percussion. Decompression of the stomach and bladder is necessary, followed by repeated examination and measurement of the abdominal girth along with repeated hemoglobin measurement. Common abdominal injuries in children are rupture of the spleen, liver, and intestine, followed by contusion or laceration of the kidneys or bladder.

If blunt abdominal trauma is suspected, an anteroposterior and cross-table lateral *radiograph* of the abdomen should be obtained to detect hollow viscous perforation. *Computed tomography* of the abdomen with contrast material will detect the majority of the injuries to the liver, spleen, and kidneys. Because most blunt abdominal injuries in children can be treated conservatively, the indications for *diagnostic peritoneal lavage* (DPL) are limited to the following:

- If the patient is undergoing another surgical procedure without a computed tomography scan of the abdomen and a serious abdominal injury is suspected.
- Before transport of an unstable patient, a positive peritoneal lavage may indicate a need for surgical intervention at the referring center.

Serial measurement of the *serum amylase* level may provide valuable information in evaluating blunt abdominal trauma, especially if pancreatic injury is suspected.

Head Trauma. Severe head injury remains the most common cause of death in the pediatric trauma patient. Chapter 8.4 addresses head trauma in the pediatric population.

Cervical Spine Trauma. Cervical spine injury with spinal cord damage, although extremely rare, is the most unfortunate complication of multiple trauma

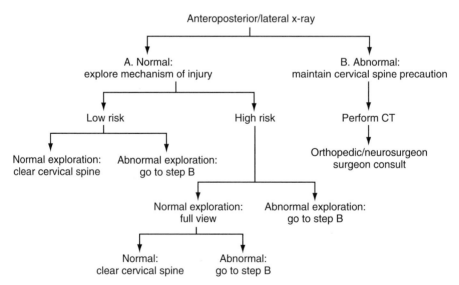

Figure 4–1. Evaluation of cervical-spine injury in a conscious patient. "High risk" includes history of high-velocity impact, serious head injury, or symptoms of spinal cord injuries. "Full view" includes anteroposterior, lateral, odontoid, flexion, and extension views of the neck.

in children. More than half of these patients never reach the hospital alive; the other half are often left with severe disabilities. Every child with multiple trauma should be assumed to have cervical spine injury until proved otherwise. Flow diagrams of evaluation of suspected cervical spine injury in conscious and unconscious patients are given in Figures 4–1 and 4–2, respectively. The clinical features of spinal injuries include local tenderness, swelling, crepitus, and hematoma. If there is underlying spinal cord damage, the patient may have pain, weakness, paresthesia, or abnormal reflexes in the extremities. In extreme cases, patients may be in spinal shock as manifested by hypotension and bradycardia. Priapism in a male child is often a helpful sign. If there is any clinical or radiological suspicion of spine or spinal cord injury, the patient should remain in cervical spine precautions, be urgently seen by an orthopedic surgeon or neurosurgeon, and be considered for therapy with high-dose methylprednisone. Because a significant number of children with spinal cord injury do not have radiologic abnormalities (spinal cord injury without obvious radiologic abnormality [SCIWORA]), a high index of suspicion is always necessary.

Genitourinary System Injuries. Renal injuries are suspected when a child has hematuria, flank pain, and tenderness. If significant injury to the kidneys is suspected, an intravenous pyelogram should be obtained as soon as the patient is stable. Renal contusion is the most common form of injury and often responds to conservative management. If there is renal laceration, early surgical intervention is required.

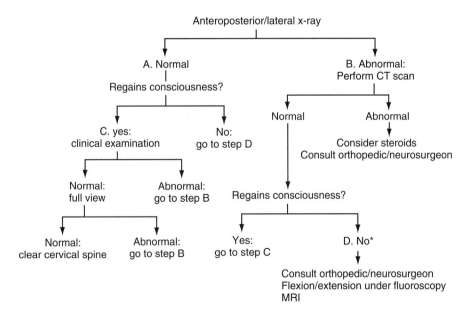

Figure 4–2. Evaluation of cervical-spine injury in an unconscious patient. "Full view" includes anteroposterior, lateral, odontoid, flexion, and extension views of the neck.
*Clearing cervical spine in an unconscious patient remains controversial; therefore, only options are provided.

Summary

In this chapter, emphasis was placed on initial evaluation and management of pediatric trauma. For detailed information on definitive assessment and current treatment of various organ systems, a list of references is provided.

BIBLIOGRAPHY

Fackler JC, Yaster M: Multiple trauma in pediatric patients. *In* Rogers MC (ed): Text Book of Pediatric Intensive Care. Baltimore, Williams & Wilkins, 1992, pp 1443–1475.

Touloukian RJ: Pediatric Trauma, 2nd ed. St. Louis, Mosby–Year Book, 1992.

Traumatic emergencies. *In* APLS: The Pediatric Emergency Course. Dallas, American College of Emergency Physicians, 1993, pp 59–84.

Pediatric trauma. *In* Advanced Trauma Life Support Course. Chicago, ATLS, 1990, pp 217–233.

5

Interhospital Transport of the Critically Ill Child

KARIN A. McCLOSKEY, MD

Interest and progress in pediatric and neonatal critical care transport have paralleled the development of sophisticated regionalized pediatric and neonatal intensive care units. Once the benefits of these units were recognized, it was necessary to have *a safe and medically sophisticated method for bringing patients to the facilities.* In the late 1960s and early 1970s, transport systems developed along two separate philosophical lines. Hospital-based helicopter transport was used for rapid movement of victims of multiple trauma from the scene of an accident to a trauma center. The concept of the "golden hour" supported the use of speedy transport for adult trauma victims. The golden hour is the defined period for successful resuscitation of the adult trauma patient. Simultaneously, specially equipped mobile intensive care unit ambulances were developed to transport premature and sick newborns to neonatal intensive care units. The lack of facilities in the field or the community for thorough stabilization and the potential need for rapid surgical intervention at a tertiary care center necessitated a *swoop-and-scoop* philosophy for helicopter teams transporting multiple-trauma victims. Delivery of a neonatal intensive care team to a referring hospital, thus beginning intensive care before transport, used a philosophy sometimes called *stay and play*, in which the transport team effectively admitted the patient to a neonatal intensive care unit and was in no hurry to depart from the referring hospital before considerable stabilization of the patient had been completed.

In the past 10 years, various combinations of both types of systems have been used for interhospital transport of pediatric and some neonatal patients. Helicopters staffed by teams transporting patients of all ages or by specialized pediatric teams have been used for interhospital transport of pediatric patients with both multiple trauma and critical medical illnesses. Some specialized pediatric teams have preferred to operate under the mobile intensive care unit system, in which stabilization times at the referring hospital average 1 hour and may range from 15 minutes to several hours. In determining an optimal team or vehicle for an individual patient, consideration must be given to *proximity to the tertiary care center,* potential *need for the physical facilities* of a tertiary care center (i.e., an operating room), *vehicles* available, *pediatric training of available teams,* and *capabilities of the referring hospital* in pediatric stabilization. No single system is likely to be optimal for every type of patient.

Preparation

Hospitals receiving transported patients and those providing an actual transport team must investigate existing regulations and guidelines for the transport of pediatric patients (see below). In developing a team, consideration must be given to the anticipated number of pediatric patients to be transported and to whether the team will be dedicated to pediatric transport or will transport patients of all ages. If the team will transport patients of all ages, then the following must be determined: the anticipated percentage of patients who will be pediatric, the specific pediatric training and experience that will be needed, the *team composition* for pediatric transport, the *vehicles* that will be used, whether the *number of anticipated transports* support the use of a dedicated transport team or whether team members have to be pulled from critical care units, and the *type of communication center* that will be required to handle incoming transport calls. The 1993 American Academy of Pediatrics guidelines for air and ground transport and the Commission on Accreditation of Air Medical Services (CAAMS) document on accreditation standards can assist in team development. The CAAMS accreditation process is currently voluntary but may represent a future standard of care.

Hospitals likely to refer pediatric patients must consider both advance and immediate preparation for transport. Advance preparation (Table 5–1) includes investigation of *local transport services* with regard to their vehicle use, *team composition, response time,* and, most important, *pediatric training* and *experience.* Advance preparation also includes *administrative protocols* for reimbursement issues, identification of tertiary centers to be used for referral, and decisions regarding what level of patient to accept for initial stabilization. The level of patient issue is relevant in only a few areas of the country. In those regions, certain hospitals are designated as basic stabilization centers for children, and other hospitals may be bypassed by the prehospital care system. In regions where such designation is not available, any hospital accepting emergency patients must be prepared to receive and stabilize all patients for up to several hours until appropriate transfer can be arranged. Advance preparation can be facilitated through communication with the most frequently used pediatric critical care unit and the transport team that it provides or recommends.

Immediate preparation (Fig. 5–1) includes obtaining transport consent; securing all lines and tubes; stabilization of the cervical spine and splinting of any fractures; preparation of blood products that may be needed during transport; and copying of all laboratory data, radiographs, and records related to the patient's stabilization. Ancillary services (e.g., social services, chaplain, translator) personnel can be called to assist the family with understanding the transport process and arranging transportation to the tertiary center.

Table 5-1. REFERRING HOSPITAL: ADVANCE PREPARATIONS—DEVELOP ADMINISTRATIVE CONTRACTS—EVALUATE AVAILABLE RESOURCES

Mode of Transport	Advantages	Limitations	Evaluate
Private automobile	Cost, preserves local resources	Loss of medical control, multiple potential time delays	Family's commitment to tertiary care, family's physical ability to get there
Local ambulance	One-way travel time, cost	Loss of local resources, decreased level of care from local emergency department	Pediatric training, pediatric equipment, pediatric experience, existence of backup local resources
Local ambulance plus nurse/physician	Improved medical control, one-way travel time	Loss of local resources, may lack portable equipment, possibility may still decrease level of care from emergency department	Pediatric training, pediatric equipment, pediatric experience, existence of backup local resources
All-age transport team (in helicopter)	Speed, expert scene response	Possibility pediatric training and experience, continuity of care, cost, difficulty with procedure in helicopter	Pediatric equipment, pediatric training, response time, how to access
Dedicated pediatric neonatal transport team	High level of pediatric training; equipment, training, and experience	Availability to all areas, sometimes limited vehicle access, cost	Available vehicles, response time, how to access

Communications

Communication is often the most crucial issue in the successful outcome of a transport. Transport communication is fraught with potential for misinterpretation or misunderstanding. In the course of treating the patient, physicians, nurses, and transport teams will be managing patient care by telephone, in unfamiliar environments, in noisy moving vehicles, and during times of great emotional stress for all concerned, especially the patient and the patient's family.

The hospital receiving pediatric patients is responsible for providing 24-hour accessibility to a physician who is able to accept a patient in transfer, provide any necessary treatment recommendations, and dispatch the transport team. Other medical personnel may assist in facilitating these efforts. Transport decisions should not be delayed because personnel have other detracting, high-priority duties.

An important part of communication on the part of the receiving hospital is a community outreach program. This gives both the team and the referring hospital

42

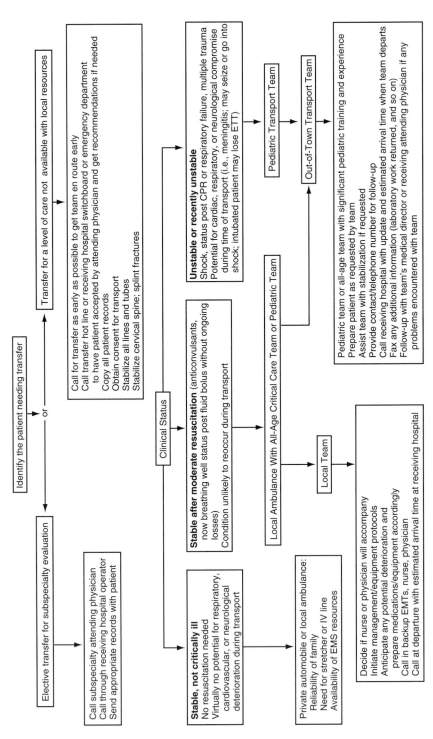

Figure 5-1. Referring hospital: immediate preparation for pediatric transport.

an opportunity to get to know each other. Expectations of both groups can be discussed during a calm time when no crisis is occurring. The actual transport process is expedited if the referring hospital has copies of the team's transport consent form, hospital admission form, and directions to the receiving hospital. Advance knowledge of what the team will expect and what resources it will need during assumption of patient care will help to prepare the staff, patient, and family. For example, some teams will want the family to stay at the referring hospital to allow direct information exchange between parents and team members, whereas others release the parents to begin the trip to the receiving hospital. Some teams will allow a family member to travel in the transport vehicle; most will not. Some teams will need continuous assistance from members of the referring hospital staff; most will try to function independently with designation of a liaison staff member for sending laboratory work, ordering radiographs, and so on. The efficiency of the entire process is enhanced if these issues are investigated before an actual transport is needed.

The referring hospital is responsible for providing a history of the patient's condition that is as complete as possible, along with current clinical status and any interventions performed. A complete set of vital signs, the patient's current mental status, and other clinical signs of neurologic, respiratory, and cardiac status must be communicated to the individual receiving the transport call. Decisions about transport and recommendations for vehicle before the team's arrival cannot be made effectively without certain basic information.

American Academy of Pediatrics Guidelines

In 1993, a Task Force of the American Academy of Pediatrics published guidelines for air and ground transportation of neonatal and pediatric patients. Topics covered in these guidelines include:

- Organization of a pediatric interfacility transport service
- Communication and the dispatch center
- Administrative issues
- Transport system personnel
- Team composition, selection, and training
- Quality improvement
- Safety
- Vehicle choice
- Equipment and medications
- Outreach education
- Transport system data collection
- Air medical physiology

Two Overriding Themes of the Guidelines Manual. The first basic theme is that there is a certain minimum capability that must be met by any team transporting a pediatric patient. This means that the guidelines apply both to dedicated pediatric teams and to teams that transport patients of all ages, including children. If a team does not have certain basic training and experience and is not capable of certain basic medical management of pediatric patients, they should defer transport to a more appropriate team. The second theme is that team composition is entirely dependent on skill levels of team members rather than on specific educational degrees obtained. Cognitive, procedural, communication, and "other" skills are defined in detail. Training modalities for achievement of each of these skills are provided.

Cognitive Skills Are the Most Difficult to Achieve and to Test. To meet this skill level, a transport team member must be experienced in diagnosis and management of pediatric life-threatening illnesses or injuries and in recognition and treatment of the most likely types of potential deterioration in a patient's condition. The skill level is generally achieved and maintained only through significant experience in caring for critically ill infants and children. Procedural skills include pediatric airway management, chest tube placement, central venous access, intraosseous line placement, peripheral vascular access, and arterial access. A very high level of expertise with procedures is necessary because they may be needed in a moving environment, which differs from the relative calm and availability of backup found in the emergency department or intensive case unit. The team should be expected to be routinely successful in performing these procedures. Appropriate communications skills include the ability to simultaneously navigate interactions between the team member and the referring hospital personnel, receiving hospital personnel, other team members, the patient, and the patient's family. Diplomacy and maintenance of a calm demeanor in a hectic atmosphere are crucial. Other skills necessary for pediatric transport include independence, flexibility, efficiency, ability to act as a team player, physical stamina, and a true understanding and enjoyment of the transport environment. Within these four skill levels, team members should function only in their own scope of practice in the base hospital and should not be expected to perform activities that they would not perform within their own hospital setting.

Vehicle and Team Options

Vehicles used for interhospital transport include private automobiles, ground ambulances (whether from the usual prehospital setting or specially outfitted for interhospital transport), helicopters, and fixed-wing jet or propeller aircraft. Each type of vehicle has its advantages and disadvantages with regard to the transport of pediatric patients. *Issues to be considered in choosing a vehicle include:*

- Available space for equipment and team members
- Travel speed
- Ability to operate in inclement weather
- Ability to allow assessment of the patient and performance of procedures in the vehicle's interior
- Ability to stop to allow patient assessment or performance of procedures
- Ability for team members to communicate with each other and with their medical control physician
- Distance to be traveled

- Geographic conditions for travel (e.g., rush hour traffic, poor roads, and mountainous terrain)
- Cost of operation

Depending on local circumstances, potential transport teams include the patient's family, a local prehospital emergency medical services crew with or without a nurse or physician from the referring hospital, a critical care transport team that transports patients of all ages, and a dedicated pediatric or neonatal critical care transport team. *Issues to consider in team choice include:*

- Severity of the patient's illness
- Likelihood of deterioration or need for major intervention during the anticipated time of transport
- Training and experience of the team in pediatric medical management
- Vehicles available to each type of team and their proximity to the referring hospital
- Any specialization or limitations defined by the team itself, that is, performance of scene flights, performance of in-transit extracorporeal membrane oxygenation, or use of a balloon pump device

Triage

Triaging patients for interhospital transport is a difficult process for both the referring and the receiving physician. A patient's condition can easily improve or deteriorate after an initial decision is made. In the interest of the patient, it is preferable to err on the side of using a higher level of transport team or vehicle than the patient's condition warrants.

The first question to be answered is, *Which patients need to be referred to another center?* This will be entirely dependent on availability of local resources to treat the patient's condition. Once a decision to transfer is made, the optimal mode of transport must be determined. Stable patients referred for elective scheduled subspecialty evaluations can clearly travel by private automobile unless they have an underlying condition or baseline status that requires stretcher transport. Patients with stable, isolated long bone fractures or relatively minor medical conditions for which inpatient staff at the referring hospital is unprepared can easily be transported by local ambulance. The difficult triage decisions arise with moderately to severely ill or injured children who have undergone an initial stabilization but who either need further stabilization or may need a sophisticated level of medical care during transport. As a general rule, with the exception of patients requiring immediate surgical intervention, *the level of pediatric care available during transport should supersede speed of the transport process.* When a dedicated pediatric team is available, it should rarely be necessary to use an all-age transport team.

No objective scoring system has been validated to determine precisely which patients need the highest level of critical care transport. In fact, the optimal scoring system will ultimately be one adaptable for local needs, as no universal system can account for the great variations in geography, distance, and referring hospital capabilities encountered by transport teams nationally. Several methods of triage are currently in use; these include the combined judgment of the referring and the receiving physician, a "common sense" approach to triage, use of an existing objective scoring system originally developed for another purpose, and use of patient status classification system.

Physician judgment is probably a quite viable method of transport triage if the determination is made by attending physicians with a working knowledge of the capabilities of the referring hospital. The system is likely to be suboptimal if decisions are made by physicians-in-training who have minimal experience in local referral or interhospital transport issues.

A *"common sense" approach to triage* results in the use of the highest available level of pediatric transport team for patients who are expected to be admitted to an intensive care unit, who have the potential for respiratory or neurologic deterioration during the anticipated time of transport, or who have recently experienced a major resuscitation effort. The philosophy for the first criterion is that if the patient needs an intensive care unit on arrival at the tertiary center, he or she will need that level of care en route. The third criterion recognizes the fact that a patient recovering from a recent resuscitation (from shock, respiratory distress, or cardiopulmonary arrest) may undergo a similar event in the succeeding hours.

Existing *objective scores* for transport triage may be useful for patients with certain specific categories of illness or injury. For example, a Glasgow Coma Scale score may be useful for triage of patients with neurologic compromise, and a Pediatric Trauma Scale score may be of benefit in patients who are victims of multiple trauma. It is inappropriate to use scores that, for example, predict outcome of patients already in a pediatric intensive care unit. To date, no existing objective scoring system has been validated for use in triage for pediatric interhospital transport.

The *patient status classification system* is the most promising method of objective triage. It can be used in conjunction with existing scoring systems. Basic clinical and interventional criteria are noted at the time of the initial telephone call. The patients are classified into one of three to six categories, with their overall classification being in the highest category of any clinical or interventional variable. For example, a system with five classification categories might put a patient with no respiratory distress into category 1; tachypnea into category 2; grunting, flaring, wheezing, or stridor into category 3; periods of apnea into category 4; and respiratory arrest into category 5. Need for intervention might place a patient with normal oxygen saturations on room air into category 1; requirement for moderate oxygen supplementation into category 2; requirement for 100% oxygen via nonrebreather mask into category 3; requirement for high-level oxygen via endotracheal tube into category 4; and poor oxygen saturations despite 100% oxygen and maximal ventilator settings into category 5. The transport system would predetermine both use of the critical care transport team and composition of that team based on the patient's highest classification category. For example, patients classified in category 1 or 2 might use a local emergency medical services system, those in category 3 might use a two-member nurse/nurse or nurse/paramedic transport team, and patients in category 4 or 5 might be predesignated to use a three-member team or a team that includes a physician.

Whatever objective form of triage system is used, there must be the option for the receiving attending physician to override the decision of the triage tool. This is especially crucial if the receiving attending physician believes that the patient needs a more sophisticated level of transport team than that indicated by the triage tool.

Summary

Successful interhospital transport of a critically ill or injured child depends on a variety of conditions that are best addressed in advance. The quality of care provided during interhospital transport is as important as that at the referring hospital and at the tertiary center in the ultimate outcome of the patient's condition. The evolution of pediatric transport as a specific medical field should help to maintain a high-level continuum of care throughout every minute of the first few hours of patient stabilization.

BIBLIOGRAPHY

American Academy of Pediatrics Committee on Pediatric Emergency Medicine: Emergency Medical Services for Children: The Role of the Primary Care Provider. Elk Grove Village, Ill, American Academy of Pediatrics, 1992.

American Academy of Pediatrics Task Force on Interhospital Transport: Guidelines for Air and Ground Transport of Neonatal and Pediatric Patients. Elk Grove Village, Ill, American Academy of Pediatrics, 1993.

Aoki BY, McCloskey K: Evaluation, Stabilization, and Transport of the Critically Ill Child. St. Louis, CV Mosby, 1992.

Accreditation Standards of the Commission on Accreditation of Air Medical Services (CAAMS) 2nd ed. Anderson, SC, 1993.

McCloskey K, Orr R: Pediatric Transport Medicine. St. Louis, CV Mosby, 1995.

6

Respiratory

6.1 Assessment of Oxygenation and Ventilation

SHEKHAR T. VENKATARAMAN, MB, BS

The primary functions of the cardiorespiratory system are to *provide adequate oxygen (O_2) to the tissues and to eliminate carbon dioxide (CO_2)* produced by the tissues. Oxygenation encompasses the entire process of O_2 transfer in the lungs through O_2 delivery to the tissues (Fig. 6–1). Similarly, removal of CO_2 involves CO_2 production by the tissues, CO_2 transport in the venous blood from the tissues, and CO_2 elimination in the lungs through ventilation (Fig. 6–1). Cardiorespiratory distress in infants and children is often associated with abnormalities in oxygenation and CO_2 removal and requires diligent monitoring.

Assessment of Oxygenation

Monitoring of oxygenation includes assessment of gas exchange in the lungs, oxygen transport to the tissues, and oxygen utilization in the tissues (Fig. 6–2).

GAS EXCHANGE IN THE LUNG: ASSESSMENT OF THE LUNG AS AN OXYGENATOR

Indexes used to assess the lung as an oxygenator are arterial O_2 tension (PaO_2), oxyhemoglobin saturation (SaO_2), intrapulmonary shunt fraction (Q_s/Q_t), alveolar-to-arterial O_2 tension difference ($PA\text{-}aO_2$), arterial-to-alveolar oxygen tension ratio (PaO_2/PAO_2), and arterial-to-fraction of inspired O_2 ratio (PaO_2/FIO_2).

The partial pressure of oxygen in the arterial blood (PaO_2) represents the net effect of O_2 exchange in the lung. At sea level, the normal PaO_2 in a newborn infant breathing room air is 40 to 70 mm Hg. With increasing age, the PaO_2 increases until it reaches an adult value of 90 to 120 mm Hg. *Hypoxemia* is a PaO_2

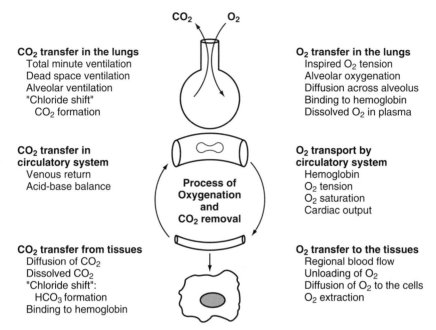

CO₂ transfer in the lungs
Total minute ventilation
Dead space ventilation
Alveolar ventilation
"Chloride shift"
CO_2 formation

**CO₂ transfer in
circulatory system**
Venous return
Acid-base balance

CO₂ transfer from tissues
Diffusion of CO_2
Dissolved CO_2
"Chloride shift":
   HCO_3 formation
Binding to hemoglobin

O₂ transfer in the lungs
Inspired O_2 tension
Alveolar oxygenation
Diffusion across alveolus
Binding to hemoglobin
Dissolved O_2 in plasma

**O₂ transport by
circulatory system**
Hemoglobin
O_2 tension
O_2 saturation
Cardiac output

O₂ transfer to the tissues
Regional blood flow
Unloading of O_2
Diffusion of O_2 to the cells
O_2 extraction

Figure 6–1. Physiology of oxygenation and ventilation. Oxygenation involves oxygen transfer in the lungs, oxygen transport and delivery to the tissues by the circulatory system, and oxygen transfer from the blood to the tissues. Ventilation involves CO_2 production by the tissues, transfer of CO_2 from the tissues to the blood, transport of CO_2 by the circulatory system to the lungs, and elimination of CO_2 by alveolar ventilation in the exhaled gas.

level lower than the acceptable range for age, whereas *hypoxia* is inadequate tissue oxygenation. For a child, a Pao_2 of <60 mm Hg may be considered hypoxemia, whereas that level may be acceptable for a newborn. Causes of hypoxemia are decreased inspired oxygen concentration, intrapulmonary shunting, right-to-left intracardiac shunts, and hypoventilation.

NONINVASIVE ESTIMATION OF Pao₂ WITH TRANSCUTANEOUS OXYGEN MONITORING

The transcutaneous oxygen tension ($TcPo_2$) is 0 to 5 mm Hg in adults without any manipulation of skin blood flow. In term infants, $TcPo_2$ is 0 to 10 mm Hg; in premature infants, $TcPo_2$ is 10 to 15 mm Hg with birth weights of 1500 to 2000 gm and approximately 15 to 25 mm Hg with birth weights of <1500 gm. $TcPo_2$ monitors have an O_2-sensing electrode and a heating element that is set to heat the surface of the skin to 42°C to 44°C. Heating the skin causes hyperemia, and when the vessels are maximally dilated, $TcPo_2$ approximates Pao_2 (Fig. 6–3). To be clinically useful, it is important to be able to detect not only normoxemia but also hypoxemia ($Po_2 <50$ mm Hg) and hyperoxemia ($Po_2 >100$ mm Hg). $TcPo_2$ has been found to correlate well with Pao_2 in the range of 30 to 200 mm Hg. Poor

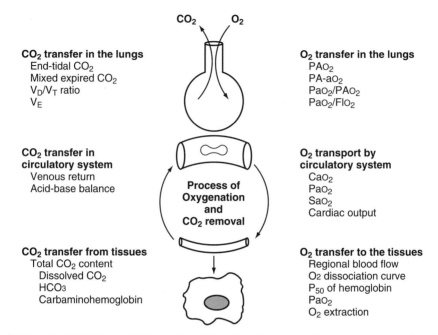

CO$_2$ transfer in the lungs
End-tidal CO$_2$
Mixed expired CO$_2$
V$_D$/V$_T$ ratio
V$_E$

O$_2$ transfer in the lungs
PAO$_2$
PA-aO$_2$
PaO$_2$/PAO$_2$
PaO$_2$/FIO$_2$

CO$_2$ transfer in circulatory system
Venous return
Acid-base balance

Process of Oxygenation and CO$_2$ removal

O$_2$ transport by circulatory system
CaO$_2$
PaO$_2$
SaO$_2$
Cardiac output

CO$_2$ transfer from tissues
Total CO$_2$ content
Dissolved CO$_2$
HCO$_3$
Carbaminohemoglobin

O$_2$ transfer to the tissues
Regional blood flow
O$_2$ dissociation curve
P$_{50}$ of hemoglobin
PaO$_2$
O$_2$ extraction

Figure 6–2. Monitoring oxygenation and ventilation. The different variables required to monitor each point in transport of O$_2$ and CO$_2$ are shown in the figure.

correlation between TcPO$_2$ and PaO$_2$ is seen with shock, acidosis, hypothermia, skin edema, cyanotic heart disease, and tolazoline infusion. Arterial index (ARI) is the ratio of TcPO$_2$ to PaO$_2$. In the newborn, the ARI is usually around 1.0, and with increasing age, the ARI decreases, with adult values of about 0.7 to 0.8. If maximal vasodilation cannot be achieved, such as with shock, then TcPO$_2$ will be lower than PaO$_2$. A low ARI is an index of the severity of circulatory dysfunction, that is, the lower the TcPO$_2$ and ARI, the greater is the circulatory dysfunction.

The arterial oxygen saturation of hemoglobin (SaO$_2$) is the percent oxyhemoglobin in the arterial blood. The oxygen dissociation curve describes the affinity with which oxygen binds to hemoglobin. Acidemia, hypercarbia, a decreased temperature, and a decreased red blood cell 2,3-diphosphoglycerate level shifts the curve to the right. Cyanosis can be detected in the nailbeds and mucosa when the deoxygenated hemoglobin concentration is $\geq$5 gm%. Detection of cyanosis is often imprecise, especially under artificial lighting. As the severity of illness increases, more precise monitoring of SaO$_2$ becomes essential.

Pulse Oximetry

According to the Beer-Lambert law, the absorbance of a light-absorbing material is directly proportional to the concentration (C) of the light-absorbing

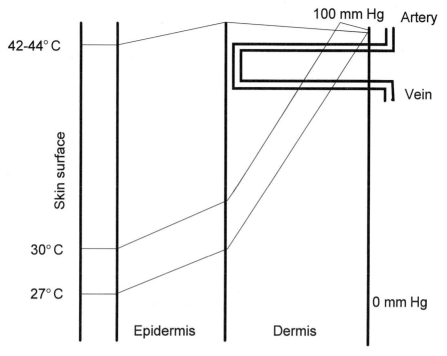

Figure 6–3. Oxygen profile through the layers of the skin.

material. Hemoglobin acts as a light-absorbing material in blood. Oxyhemoglobin absorbs light maximally at a wavelength of 660 nm, whereas deoxyhemoglobin absorbs very little at that wavelength. At 800 nm, both hemoglobins absorb equally, and at ≥ 940 nm, the reduced hemoglobin absorbs much more light than does oxyhemoglobin. When light is passed through a vascular bed, the light transmitted has nonpulatile and pulsatile components (Fig. 6–4). The nonpulsatile component is assumed to represent light transmitted across the tissues, capillaries, and veins. The pulsatile component is assumed to represent light transmitted throught the arterial bed. Therefore, the light absorbed by the pulsatile component should correspond to SaO_2. Pulse oximeters use two wavelengths of light: 660 nm (red region) and 940 nm (infrared region). A computer algorithm is generated where the ratio of light absorbance at 660 to 940 nm is empirically correlated with SaO_2 obtained through invasive blood sampling from normal adult volunteers. The resultant pulse oximetric oxygen saturation (SpO_2) has been found to correlate well with SaO_2 in critically ill patients in the range of 70% to 100%. At <70%, SpO_2 correlates with SaO_2, but there is greater variability. SpO_2 can reliably detect hypoxemia, defined as an SpO_2 value of <90%. SpO_2 is less sensitive than $tcPO_2$ in detecting hyperoxemia. *Fetal hemoglobin* does not affect SpO_2 because the absorption characteristics are similar to those of adult hemoglobin. *Carboxyhemoglobin* absorbs light maximally at 660 nm but does not absorb light at 960 nm. *As*

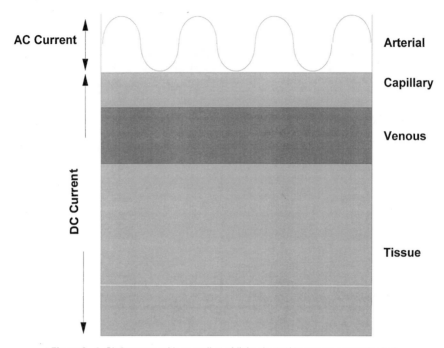

Figure 6-4. Plethysmographic recording of light absorption across a vascular bed.

carboxyhemoglobin levels increase, SpO₂ readings will overestimate SaO₂ because it assumes that the increased light absorption at 660 nm is due to oxyhemoglobin. With smoke inhalation, where increased carboxyhemoglobin is possible, co-oximetry should be performed to measure SaO₂. *Methemoglobin* aborbs light almost equally at 660 and 960 nm. This makes the ratio of the light absorbed at the 660 nm to the light absorbed at 960 nm to be 1, which corresponds to an SaO₂ value of 85%. With low methemoglobin levels (<15%), SpO₂ underestimates SaO₂. With high methemoglobin levels (>30%), the SpO₂ overestimates SaO₂. *Bilirubin* absorbs light maximally at 460 nm and therefore should have no effect on SpO₂.

Intrapulmonary shunt fraction (Q$_s$/Q$_t$) is defined as the fraction of right ventricular output that enters the left ventricle without any oxygen transfer. In the absence of intracardiac shunts, Q$_s$/Q$_t$ is calculated with the following formula:

$$Q_s/Q_t = (Cc'o_2 - Cao_2)/(Cc'o_2 - Cvo_2)$$

where Cc'o₂ is oxygen content of the pulmonary venous blood with the assumption that the lung is a perfect oxygenator, Cao₂ is arterial oxygen content, and Cvo₂ is mixed venous oxygen content. *Oxygen content is the amount of oxygen carried by a unit volume of blood and is equal to the amount bound to hemoglobin and dissolved in plasma.* Oxygen content is calculated by the following formula:

$$\begin{aligned} O_2 \text{ content} = &(\text{hemoglobin} \times 1.34 \times O_2 \text{ saturation}/100) \\ &+ (0.003 \times Po_2 \text{ of sample}) \end{aligned}$$

Intrapulmonary shunt may consist of one or more of three components: anatomic shunts, capillary shunts, and venous admixture. $Cc'o_2$ is most affected by FIO_2, Cao_2 is most affected by intrapulmonary shunting, and Cvo_2 is most affected by cardiac output and oxygen consumption. Calculation of intrapulmonary shunt requires sampling mixed venous blood, which requires a pulmonary artery catheter; calculations are cumbersome and assumes that all alveolar spaces behave equally well. When a pulmonary artery catheter is not available, then one of the indexes described below may be used as an index of shunting.

PA-ao_2, Pao_2/PAo_2, and Pao_2/FIo_2. If the lungs were a perfect oxygenator, then pulmonary venous O_2 would be identical to alveolar Po_2 (PAo_2), and if right ventricular output traverses the ideal lung, then Pao_2 would be the same as pulmonary venous O_2. PAo_2 is calculated from the following simplified alveolar gas equation:

$$PAo_2 = (PB - PH_2O) \times FIO_2 - (Paco_2/RQ)$$

where PB is the barometric pressure; PH_2O is the partial pressure of water vapor, which is 47 mm Hg when fully humidifed; and RQ is the respiratory quotient (carbon dioxide production/oxygen consumption). With intrapulmonary shunting, Pao_2 is less than PAo_2. PA-ao_2, Pao_2/PAo_2, and Pao_2/FIo_2 are indexes that determine the extent to which the Pao_2 deviates from PAo_2 as a measure of intrapulmonary shunting. The normal PA-ao_2 is usually <20 mm Hg in a child and <50 mm Hg in a newborn infant. A large PA-ao_2 represents intrapulmonary shunting or venous admixture. PA-ao_2 is affected not only by intrapulmonary shunting but also by mixed venous oxygen saturation. A major limitation of this index is that it changes unpredictably with increasing FIO_2. To compare gradients over time, FIO_2 must remain constant. To be reliable, the arterial-to-mixed venous Po_2 difference must also be constant. Unlike PA-ao_2, Pao_2/PAo_2 changes much more predicably with increasing FIO_2. Thus, it is preferred to PA-ao_2 as an index of oxygen transfer in the lung and can be used to predict changes in Pao_2 when FIO_2 is altered. Pao_2/FIO_2 is the easiest index to calculate and does not require calculation of PAo_2. The disadvantage is that it does not adjust for alveolar CO_2. At high FIO_2, this error becomes quite small. The normal Pao_2/FIO_2 in a child breathing room air at sea level is >400 mm Hg. A Pao_2/FIO_2 of <250 is an indication for supplemental oxygen, and a ratio of 100 on supplemental O_2 is usually an indication for intubation and mechanical ventilation.

ASSESSMENT OF OXYGEN TRANSPORT

Oxygen delivery ($\dot{D}o_2$) is the amount of oxygen delivered by the cardiovascular system to the tissues every minute. It is calculated by the following formula:

$$\dot{D}o_2 = Cao_2 \times CI$$

where CI is the cardiac index (in L/min/m^2). A normal $\dot{D}o_2$ in a child is approximately 650–750 mL/min/m^2. The two major determinants of $\dot{D}o_2$ are hemoglobin and cardiac index. Mild hypoxemia can be compensated by increasing hemoglobin, cardiac index, or both. If $\dot{D}o_2$ is adequate to meet the tissue O_2 demands, the absolute Pao_2 is not that critical.

ASSESSMENT OF OXYGEN UTILIZATION

Oxygen consumption ($\dot{V}o_2$) *is the amount of oxygen that is utilized by the body in a minute.* $\dot{V}o_2$ can be measured by analyzing the inspired and expired gases with a Douglas bag or with the Fick equation:

$$\dot{V}o_2 = CI\ (Cao_2 - C\bar{v}o_2)$$

Fever, thyrotoxicosis, and increased catecholamine release or administration increase the metabolic rate and increase $\dot{V}o_2$. Hypothermia and hypothyroidism tend to decrease $\dot{V}o_2$. Measurement of $\dot{V}o_2$ may be important in critically ill patients, especially those with moderately severe cardiorespiratory dysfunction. Under normal conditions, $\dot{V}o_2$ is independent of $\dot{D}o_2$. In some patients, $\dot{V}o_2$ becomes $\dot{D}o_2$ dependent. If clinically possible, $\dot{D}o_2$ should be increased until $\dot{V}o_2$ is no longer $\dot{D}o_2$ dependent.

Mixed venous oxygen saturation ($S\bar{v}o_2$) is commonly used as a measure of the balance between O_2 demand and supply. A low $S\bar{v}o_2$ usually signifies that $\dot{D}o_2$ is decreased and the body is extracting more oxygen from the blood. This is usually true in hypovolemia and cardiogenic shock. In sepsis, where there is maldistribution of peripheral blood flow, $S\bar{v}o_2$ may be normal or even high, although there may be oxygen deficits in the tissues. A high $S\bar{v}o_2$ is usually seen in hypothermia due to decreased oxygen demand. A high $S\bar{v}o_2$ can also be seen in brain death as the brain usually constitutes a major part of the total body oxygen consumption.

Assessment of Ventilation

CO_2 produced during metabolism in the tissues is transported in the venous blood in three main forms: dissolved in plasma, as bicarbonate, and bound to hemoglobin. In the lungs, CO_2 diffuses from the pulmonary capillaries into the alveolus, where minute alveolar ventilation removes the CO_2 from the alveoli. $Paco_2$ is the partial pressure of CO_2 in arterial blood and reflects the efficiency of the lung as a ventilator. Arterial $Paco_2$ measurement requires arterial blood sampling either through a puncture or through an indwelling arterial catheter.

NONINVASIVE ESTIMATION OF Paco$_2$ WITH CAPNOGRAPHY

A *capnogram* is a plot of the CO_2 concentration over time during breathing (Fig. 6–5). There are *four phases in a capnogram.* The first phase is the flat part of the capnogram, where no CO_2 is detected. This corresponds to the late phase of inspiration and the early phase of expiration. The second phase is the upstroke, or ascending, part. This corresponds to the appearance of CO_2 in the exhaled gas when the alveolar space mixes with the dead space gas. The CO_2 concentration rises rapidly during the second phase and reaches a plateau. The third phase is the plateau phase. This corresponds to alveolar gas appearing in the exhaled gas. The termination of the plateau phase is the end of expiration. The CO_2 concentration at this point is called the end-tidal CO_2 ($ETco_2$). If one assumes an ideal lung, the CO_2 tension of the blood leaving the lung should equilibrate with that in the

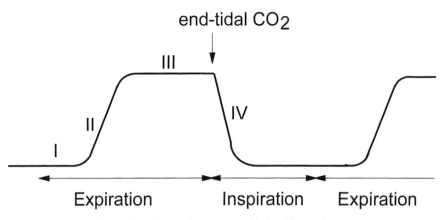

Figure 6-5. A normal capnogram with the different phases.

alveoli. Because CO_2 is 20 times as diffusible as oxygen, it is reasonable to assume that the pulmonary venous CO_2 reflects alveolar CO_2. Because the last part of the lung that empties during expiration is the alveolar space, $ETCO_2$ is a reasonable estimate of $PaCO_2$. The fourth phase is the downstroke, or descending, part. This is due to fresh gas passing across the sampling site with inspiration.

An abnormally high baseline during phase I represents rebreathing of expired CO_2 (Fig. 6–6A). A slow upstroke during phase II is due to a slow rate of sampling (only with sidestream analyzers), prolonged exhalation, or uneven emptying of the lung (Fig. 6–6B). A rising phase III with no plateau is seen with slow emptying of the alveoli and is usually seen with prolonged exhalation with lower airway obstruction (Fig. 6–6C). A high $ETCO_2$ indicates increased metabolic rate or hypoventilation (Fig. 6–6D). An abnormally low plateau indicates hyperventilation, increased alveolar dead space, decreased effective pulmonary blood flow, or contamination with fresh inflow of gas (Fig. 6–6D). An irregular plateau is the result of uneven emptying of the lungs producing fluctuating changes in expired CO_2 concentration (Fig. 6–6E). A slanted downstroke usually indicates rebreathing of exhaled CO_2 (Fig. 6–6F). Normally, arterial–to–end-tidal difference in CO_2 is <5 mm Hg. When alveolar dead space increases, arterial–to–end-tidal difference in CO_2 increases. An increased arterial–to–end-tidal CO_2 difference can also be seen with an abnormally low lung perfusion. When $ETCO_2$ is higher than $PaCO_2$, it usually indicates rebreathing of expired CO_2 or uneven emptying of the lungs.

In addition to its use as a noninvasive measure of $PaCO_2$, $ETCO_2$ is useful in assessing the efficacy of cardiopulmonary resuscitation. $ETCO_2$ is low with decreased pulmonary blood flow, and when cardiac output improves, $ETCO_2$ increases as well. Because lungs are the only source of CO_2 elimination, $ETCO_2$ can also be used to detect endotracheal or esophageal intubation. If there is reasonable pulmonary blood flow, a capnometer will detect CO_2 if the tube is endotracheal and will not detect any CO_2 if the tube is esophageal.

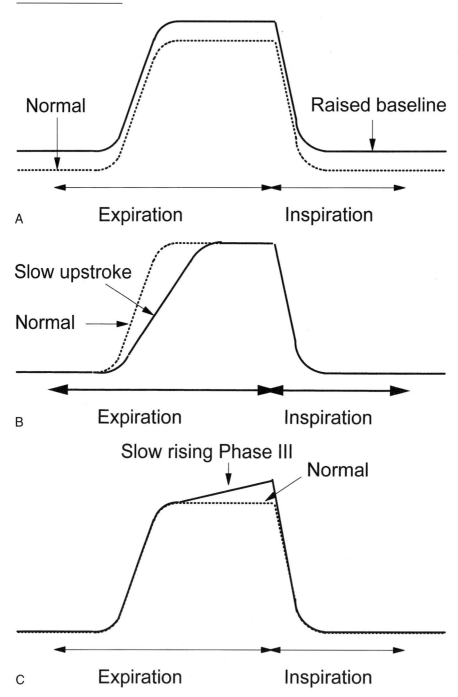

Figure 6–6. Abnormal capnograms. *A,* An abnormally high baseline during phase I. *B,* A slow upstroke during phase II. *C,* A rising phase III with no plateau.

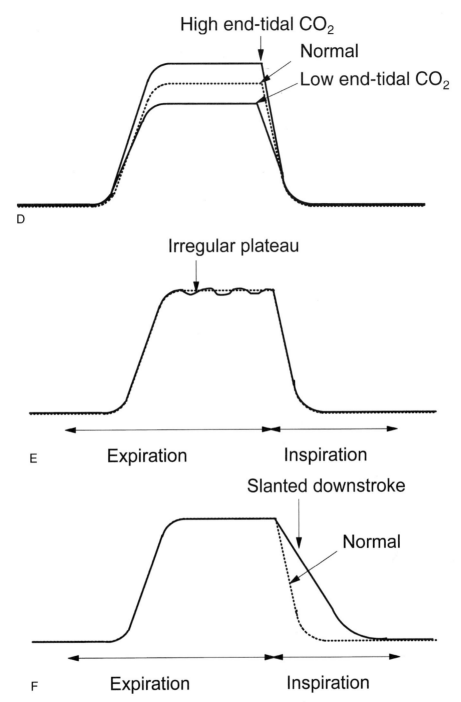

Figure 6-6. *Continued D,* A high ETco₂ and a low plateau. *E,* An irregular plateau. *G,* A slanted downstroke.

MIXED EXPIRED CO_2 FOR ESTIMATION OF PHYSIOLOGIC DEAD SPACE

With the assumption that inspired gas has no CO_2, all of the CO_2 present in the exhaled gas represents CO_2 that has diffused across the alveoli. Physiologic dead space can be calculated with the Bohr equation:

$$V_D/V_T = Paco_2 - P\bar{E}co_2/Paco_2$$

where, V_D/V_T is the dead space-to-tidal volume ratio, and $P\bar{E}co_2$ is the CO_2 tension of the mixed expired gas.

Collection and Usefulness of Blood Gases

An *arterial blood gas* is useful for determining the effectiveness of the lung as an oxygenator and a ventilator. A *venous blood gas* is useful for determining the acid-base status of the tissues. A *mixed venous blood gas* is useful in determining the circulatory status of the patient. Despite the concern of loss of oxygen through diffusion in plastic syringes, it is not a significant clinical problem if the sample is analyzed immediately. The syringe should contain heparin (≤ 0.1 mL/4 mL of blood). A high heparin concentration tends to decrease the blood sample pH. Care should be taken to not introduce air bubbles in the sample; the effect of air bubbles would be to decrease the sample Po_2 when the Po_2 is >150 mm Hg and to increase the sample Po_2 when the Po_2 is <100 mm Hg. Modern analyzers report the results corrected to a temperature of 37°C. What if the patient's temperature is 35°C or 40°C? Temperature affects gas solubility, ion dissociation, and oxygen-dissociation curve. When the temperature falls, the Po_2 and Pco_2 decrease, whereas pH increases. For example, at 37°C, at pH 7.40, Po_2 is 80 mm Hg and Pco_2 is 40 mm Hg; decreasing the temperature to 35°C increases to pH 7.43 and decreases Po_2 and Pco_2 to 70 and 37 mm Hg, respectively. The lower Pco_2 does not reflect increased alveolar ventilation but rather the effect of temperature on the solubility of CO_2 in blood. The clinical importance of temperature correction is controversial.

BIBLIOGRAPHY

Huch A, Huch R, Rooth G: Continuous transcutaneous monitoring. Advances in Experimental Medicine and Biology, Vol 220. New York, Plenum Press, 1987.
Huch R, Huch A, Lübbers DW (eds): Transcutaneous Po_2. New York, Thieme-Stratton Inc., 1981.
Kacmarek RM, Hess D, Stoller JK: Monitoring in Respiratory Care. St. Louis, Mosby-Year Book, 1993.
Payne JP, Severinghaus JW (eds): Pulse Oximetry. Heidelberg, Springer-Verlag, 1986.
Shapiro BA, Peruzzi WT, Templin R: Clinical Application of Blood Gases, 5th ed. St. Louis, Mosby-Year Book, 1994.
Spence AA (ed): Respiratory Monitoring in Intensive Care. Clinics in Critical Care Medicine, Vol 4. New York, Churchill Livingstone, 1982.
Tremper KK, Barker SJ (eds): Advances in Oxygen Monitoring. International Anesthesiology Clinics, Vol 25. Boston, Little, Brown and Company, 1987.
Tremper KK, Barker SJ: Pulse oximetry. Anesthesiology 70:98–108, 1989.

6.2 **Principles of Mechanical Ventilation**

SHEKHAR T. VENKATARAMAN, MB, BS

Mechanical ventilation is often required in cardiorespiratory distress in infants and children. I discuss briefly the physiology of inflation and deflation, the characterisitics of ventilators, different modes of ventilation, and a practical approach to the selection of ventilatory parameters. The physiology of gas exchange in the lung is described in Chapter 6.1.

Physiology

VOLUMES AND CAPACITIES

Tidal volume is the volume of gas that is moved in and out of the lungs with each breath. Normal tidal volume, during spontaneous breathing, is 6 to 8 mL/kg regardless of age. The volume of gas remaining in the lung at the end of a normal exhalation is called the *functional residual capacity* (FRC). The volume of gas that can be breathed in by a maximal inspiratory effort from a normal inspiration is called the *inspiratory reserve volume. Inspiratory capacity* is the maximum volume of gas that be inspired from FRC and is equal to the sum of the tidal volume and inspiratory reserve volume. The volume of gas that can be exhaled from FRC by a maximal expiratory effort is called the *expiratory reserve volume.* The volume of gas remaining in the lung after a maximal expiratory effort is called the *residual volume*; this volume cannot be expelled from the lung despite maximal expiration. The volume of gas that can be expired by a maximal expiratory effort after a maximal inspiratory effort is the *vital capacity* and includes the expiratory reserve volume and inspiratory capacity. The lung volume during a maximal expiration at which the airways begin to close is called the *closing volume.* When the closing volume is greater than FRC, then airways close during normal expiration and may result in atelectasis.

INFLATION AND DEFLATION

The lungs resist inflation. Impedance to lung inflation is mainly due to airway resistance and the compliances of the lung and thoracic structures. *Airway resistance* is the change in transpulmonary pressure (proximal airway pressure minus alveolar pressure) required to produce a unit flow of gas through the airways of the lung. *Lung compliance* is the change in lung volume for a unit change in transalveolar pressure (alveolar pressure minus pleural pressure). Specific lung compliance is defined as lung compliance that is normalized to lung volume or body weight, and it is similar in children and adults. *Chest compliance* is the change in thoracic cage volume produced by a unit change in transthoracic pressure (ambient pressure minus pleural pressure). A certain amount of force is required to overcome the impedance to inflation. Normal expiration is passive and is due to the elastic recoil of the lung. Elastic recoil of the lung during expiration reduces alveolar volume, and the elastic recoil of the chest and surfactant lining the alveoli tends to oppose it. The balance between these forces maintains FRC. The rate of inflation and deflation of the lung is exponential and depends on lung compliance and airway resistance. *Time constant* is the product of compliance and resistance, and it is used to define the time taken to cause a given change in lung volume. One time constant is the time taken to cause a 63% change in lung volume, and three time constants are the time taken to cause a 95% change in lung volume. The airway resistance is almost equally distributed between the upper and lower airways in the infant, whereas in the adult, the majority of the airway resistance resides in the upper airway. The airways of the infant are more collapsible than those of the older child, resulting in dynamic compression of the intrathoracic airways during forced expiration.

GAS EXCHANGE

During normal tidal breathing, gas moves from the proximal airway to the respiratory bronchioles, mostly due to bulk flow and, to a lesser extent, by diffusion. Gas exchange from the respiratory bronchioles to the alveolus occurs entirely by diffusion. Arterial oxygen tension (PaO_2) in the infant is lower than that in an adult for the same fraction of inspired oxygen (FIO_2) because of a lower diffusing capacity for oxygen. Breathing is predominantly diaphragmatic in infants and children. Abdominal distension due to moderate to severe hepatomegaly, severe ascites, or gastrointestinal obstruction impedes diaphragmatic movement during inspiration and increases the work of breathing. In infants and young children, an increase in diaphragmatic contraction force coupled with a compliant chest wall results in paradoxic breathing and ineffective ventilation. An infant's metabolic rate adjusted for weight is approximately twice that of an adult. A higher ventilatory demand, tendency toward paradoxic breathing, propensity for premature airway closure from dynamic collapse of the airways, and compliant chest wall make respiratory illnesses more life threatening in the very young.

INDICATIONS FOR MECHANICAL VENTILATION

The indications for institution of mechanical ventilation are given in Table 6–1. Hypercarbia results from minute ventilation insufficient to meet the production of CO_2. *Impending respiratory failure* is characterized by rapidly progressive respiratory distress or fatigue of respiratory muscles. It is preferable to intubate and institute mechanical ventilation before respiratory failure develops. Ventilation-perfusion mismatching and intrapulmonary shunting are the most common reasons for inadequate oxygenation in patients with respiratory disease. By decreasing the oxygen cost of breathing, mechanical ventilation can decrease cardiac work load. Mechanical ventilation may also be instituted to deliberately hyperventilate to produce hypocapnia and respiratory alkalosis, such as in patients with intracranial hypertension or pulmonary hypertension.

Table 6–1. INDICATIONS FOR MECHANICAL VENTILATION

Apnea or respiratory arrest
Ineffective ventilation (hyperbaric respiratory failure)
Definition: $PaCO_2$ >50 mm Hg with arterial pH <7.30
Decreased ventilatory drive
Ventilator pump failure
Respiratory muscle fatigue from increased work of breathing
Inadequate oxygenation (hypoxemic respiratory failure)
Definition: PaO_2 <50 mm Hg with an FIO_2 of >0.5
Alveolar space disease (pulmonary edema, pneumonia, adult respiratory distress syndrome)
Lobar disease (pneumonia, atelectasis)
Other system disease
Circulatory failure (heart failure, shock)
Poor nutrition from excessive work of breathing
Deliberate hyperventilation (intracranial hypertension, pulmonary hypertension)

MODES OF VENTILATION

There are two forms of conventional mechancial ventilation: controlled (CMV) and assisted (AMV). CMV refers to provision of ventilator breaths regardless of the patient's efforts. Ventilator breaths are initiated by a timing mechanism that divides each minute equally into a number of breaths. Intermittent mandatory ventilation (IMV) refers to a form of CMV where spontaneous breathing is permitted. Synchronized IMV refers to IMV breaths that are synchronized to the patient's breathing effort. AMV refers to the provision of a mechanical breath that is triggered by the patient's spontaneous breathing efforts. With AMV, the ventilator will not deliver a breath unless it senses a patient's breath. Assist-control ventilation refers to a combination of AMV and CMV. During inspiration, after the tidal volume is delivered, an inspiratory hold will maintain inspiratory pressure and prolong the duration of inspiration.

VOLUME-REGULATED TIME-CYCLED VENTILATION

In volume-regulated time-cycled ventilation, the tidal volume delivered per breath is controlled by the inspiratory flow rate and the inspiratory time (Table 6–2). Inspiratory flow rate required to produce a delivered tidal volume of 10 to 15 mL/kg is usually about 1 to 3 L/kg/min. *Peak inspiratory pressure* (PIP), the maximal pressure measured in the proximal airway during inspiration, is not limited. Rather, the ventilator is set to sound an alarm when the PIP in the ventilator circuit is 5 to 10 cm H_2O higher than that which generates an adequate tidal volume. PIP is increased when compliance decreases, airway resistance increases, or the artificial airway becomes occluded. This mode of ventilation provides relatively consistent tidal volumes despite changes in the patient's compliance or resistance. During IMV, with ventilators that have an inspiratory valve, the patient must open the inspiratory valve during spontaneous breathing to obtain a tidal volume. In infants and children, this may impose additional work of breathing, resulting in asynchrony and fatigue. In continuous flow ventilators, the

Table 6–2. DIFFERENCES BETWEEN VOLUME-REGULATED
AND PRESSURE-LIMITED VENTILATION

Ventilator Parameter	Volume-Regulated	Pressure-Limited
Inspiratory flow	Low (1–2 L/kg/min)	High (4–10 L/kg/min)
Peak inspiratory pressure	Variable, reached at the end of inspiration	Preset, reached early in inspiration
Tidal volume	Preset	Variable, depends on compliance and resistance
Inspiratory pause	In addition to preset inspiratory time	Part of the preset inspiratory time
Mean airway pressure	Lower	Higher

absence of an inspiratory valve allows a constant flow of gas during the expiratory phase. This decreases the work of breathing and facilitates spontaneous breathing in infants and children. It is important to note that unless continuous flow ventilation has provisions to allow higher flow rates during the expiratory phase for spontaneous breathing, the preset flow rate may not be sufficient.

PRESSURE-LIMITED TIME-CYCLED VENTILATION

In pressure-limited time-cycled ventilation, the inspiratory flow rate is high (4 to 10 L/kg/min), to allow the PIP to reach the predetermined limit early in inspiration, and the peak inflation pressure is held at that level until the onset of expiration (see Table 6–2). With ventilators that have both inspiratory and expiratory valves, the inspiratory valve closes as soon the the pressure limit is reached and prevents additional gas flow into the patient. In continuous-flow ventilators, the excess flow is vented through a pressure-limit valve in the circuit because there is no inspiratory valve. Changes in compliance or resistance will affect the tidal volume while the airway pressure remains constant.

Selection of Parameters

TIDAL VOLUME

A practical approach to determining an adequate tidal volume is to evaluate the degree of chest expansion while manually ventilating the patient and to reproduce that when the patient is connected to the ventilator. *An adequate tidal volume must produce an adequate chest rise.* The normal tidal volume regardless of age for spontaneously breathing patients is 6 to 8 mL/kg. The *effective tidal volume* (TV_{eff}) is the tidal volume that is actually delivered to the patient. During mechanical ventilation, it may be necessary to deliver a TV_{eff} of 8 to 10 mL/kg. Volume monitors such as the Bear NVM (for neonates and infants) and the Ohmeda volume monitor (for children and adults) are capable of measuring the patient's TV_{eff} directly via a pneumotachometer placed at the hub of the endotracheal tube. Ventilator circuit compliance does not affect this measurement.

During volume-controlled ventilation, when a pneumotachometer is not available, the TV_{eff} can be estimated by subtracting the compressible volume in the ventilator circuit from the delivered tidal volume. With continuous-flow ventilators, delivered tidal volume is equal to the inspiratory flow (in mL/sec) multiplied by the inspiratory time (in seconds). The compressible volume lost in the circuit can be calculated by multiplying the compliance of the ventilator circuit by the difference between PIP and positive end-expiratory pressure (PEEP). The compliance of the ventilator circuit is determined by delivering a preset tidal volume to the circuit with the patient connection occluded and then observing the pressure change in the circuit. The volume used to inflate the occluded tubing circuit divided by the pressure change produced in the circuit is the compliance of the ventilator circuit. Infants and children <10 years old are usually intubated with uncuffed endotracheal tubes. Therefore, it is not uncommon for some of the delivered tidal volume to leak around the endotracheal tube, especially at higher peak airway pressures. In the presence of a leak around the endotracheal tube, a pneumotachometer may be required to accurately measure the TV_{eff}. During pressure-limited time-cycled ventilation, tidal volume is determined by the difference between PIP and PEEP. The compliances and resistances of the lung and the ventilator circuit will ultimately determine the TV_{eff}. During pressure-limited time-cycled ventilation, TV_{eff} cannot be estimated and must be measured directly with a pneumotachometer.

VENTILATOR RATE

The rate selected depends on the age and the ventilatory requirements of the patient and subsequently should be adjusted according to the Pa_{CO_2}. The initial ventilator rate for a newborn infant usually ranges from 25 to 30/min; for a 1-year-old, 20 to 25/min; and for an adolescent, 15 to 20/min. *Inspiratory time* can be set either as a percentage of the total respiratory cycle or as a fixed time in seconds, depending on the ventilator. Inspiratory time must be selected to allow sufficient time for all lung segments to be inflated. In heterogeneous lung disease with varying regional time constants, a short inspiratory time may not be sufficient to inflate all lung segments and may contribute to underventilation and underinflation. Similarly, sufficient expiratory time must be provided for all lung segments to empty. If inspiration starts before the lung has completely emptied, this will result in air trapping and inadvertent PEEP, or "auto-PEEP." In the presence of lower airway obstruction, the expiratory time may have to be lengthened to avoid air trapping.

FRACTION OF INSPIRED OXYGEN

The required *fraction of inspired oxygen* (FIO_2) will depend on the clinical circumstance. When intrapulmonary shunting is low (<10%), Pa_{O_2} can be increased by increasing FIO_2. When intrapulmonary shunting is high (>20%), FIO_2 has very little effect on Pa_{O_2}. High FIO_2 (>70%) can cause oxygen toxicity to the lungs and exacerbate the underlying lung disease; therefore, every attempt must be made to reduce the FIO_2 to relatively "nontoxic" levels (usually <60%). Because mean airway pressure is the primary determinant of oxygenation, increased airway pressures may allow a reduction in FIO_2. During volume-regulated time-cycled ventilation, the only reliable way to increase mean airway pressure is by increasing PEEP. During pressure-limited time-cycled ventilation, mean airway pressure can be increased by increasing PIP, PEEP, or inspiratory time.

POSITIVE END-EXPIRATORY PRESSURE

The level of PEEP will depend on the clinical circumstance. The effects of PEEP include increased end-expiratory residual lung volume; increased functional residual capacity above closing volume, thereby preventing airway closure and atelectasis; maintenance of stability of alveolar segments; increased intrathoracic pressure; impedance in systemic venous return to the heart; and increased pulmonary vascular resistance through increased lung volume and intrathoracic pressure. The *optimum PEEP* is the level at which there is an acceptable balance between the desired goals and undesired adverse effects. The desired goals are improvement in oxygenation, reduction in work of breathing, improvement in lung compliance, and maximal oxygen delivery. Arbitrary limits cannot be placed on the level of PEEP or mean airway pressure that will be required to maintain adequate gas exchange. An optimal level of PEEP should allow reduction in inspired oxygen concentration to nontoxic levels while maintaing PaO_2 or SaO_2 of >60 mm Hg or >90%, respectively. When the level of PEEP is high, PIP may be limited to prevent it from reaching dangerous levels that contribute to air leaks and barotrauma. The level of PEEP selected for patients with lower airway obstruction is usually low (3 to 5 cm H_2O). High levels of PEEP are not recommended in respiratory failure due to lower airway diseases because of the concern for pulmonary barotrauma from air trapping and alveolar hyperinflation. However, in adults with severe asthma, high levels of PEEP have been shown to decrease the magnitude of air trapping and work of breathing without significant complications. In children with tracheomalacia or bronchomalacia, PEEP decreases the airway resistance by distending the airways and preventing dynamic compression during expiration.

Pathophysiologic Approach to Mechanical Ventilation

PARENCHYMAL LUNG DISEASE

Parenchymal lung disorders, such as adult respiratory distress syndrome (ARDS), idiopathic respiratory distress syndrome (IRDS), and interstitial pneumonias, are characterized by a reduced FRC, an increased closing volume above FRC, and diffuse subsegmental atelectasis. Lung volumes must be maintained above closing volume throughout the respiratory cycle to prevent atelectasis and improve ventilation-perfusion matching. The most effective method of achieving this is by increasing mean airway pressure. The optimal level of mean airway pressure required can be defined as the level that results in maximal oxygen delivery, the highest lung compliance, and the lowest intrapulmonary shunt without a significant decrease in cardiac function. As the severity of lung disease increases, the airway pressures required to maintain adequate gas exchange also increase. Mild hypercapnia may be permitted under these circumstances provided arterial pH is adequate.

RESPIRATORY PUMP FAILURE

Ventilatory rate and TV_{eff} are set to maintain normocarbia. Spontaneous breathing should be encouraged as much as possible because total control of ventilation may result in disuse atrophy of the respiratory muscles and complicate weaning from mechanical ventilation. Assisted ventilation through encouragement of spontaneous breathing may prevent disuse atrophy. The FIO_2 is usually kept to a minimum as these disorders are not associated with inadequate oxygenation. In patients who have had chronic hypoventilation, hypercarbia is often acceptable, provided arterial pH is within the normal range. Positive end-expiratory pressure/ continuous positive airway pressure (PEEP CPAP) is usually set at a relatively low level (3 to 5 cm H_2O).

AIRWAY OBSTRUCTION

Respiratory failure due to lower airway obstruction poses a special problem during mechanical ventilation. Depression of cardiac output and hypotension may occur during intubation because of the institution of positive airway pressure to already hyperinflated lungs. Volume-controlled ventilation is the preferred mode of ventilation. Pressure-control ventilation should be avoided as it results in higher mean airway pressure. Expiratory time must be sufficient to allow adequate emptying of the lung. If the expiratory time is inadequate, air trapping and hyperinflation from auto-PEEP, or inadvertent PEEP, will result. Low levels of PEEP (3 to 5 cm H_2O) are tolerated relatively well. Although some studies in adults have shown that PEEP/CPAP of ≥ 10 cm H_2O decreased air trapping and the work of breathing in patients with acute severe asthma, high levels of CPAP/ PEEP are generally not recommended in respiratory failure. PEEP/CPAP is useful in children with airway obstruction due to tracheomalacia or bronchomalacia.

HEART DISEASE

The application of PEEP/CPAP will provide relief of atelectasis. Hyperinflation should be avoided because it may increase pulmonary vascular resistance and right ventricular afterload. The oxygen cost of breathing can be reduced through a combination of controlled ventilation and sedation. Muscle relaxation may provide additional reduction in oxygen cost of breathing. A rule of thumb is that the greater the inotropic support a heart needs, the greater should be the respiratory support provided. In adults with congestive heart failure, positive intrathoracic pressure improves cardiac output due to decreased left ventricular afterload.

After open-heart surgery, many infants and children require mechanical ventilation during the postoperative period. Prolonged mechanical ventilation is more likely in infants, with complex heart lesions, prolonged bypass, prolonged circulatory arrest times, and hemodynamic instability. In the immediate postoperative period, patients should be on controlled mechanical ventilation until hemodynamic functions improve. TV_{eff} should be ≥ 10 to 12 mL/kg. PEEP should be applied to prevent and relieve atelectasis. Initially, the ventilator rate should be appropriate for the age. In patients with pulmonary hypertension or pulmonary vascular disease, hyperventilation to provide respiratory alkalosis will decrease pulmonary vascular resistance and right ventricular afterload. In patients with marginal cardiac output, high airway pressures are to be avoided. In patients who have undergone a Fontan procedure, early extubation is desirable, and if that is not possible, then spontaneous ventilation should be encouraged. Because these patients are totally dependent on venous return for their cardiac output, airway pressures must be kept at a minimum. High intrathoracic pressure may not only impede venous return but also decrease pulmonary blood flow from increased pulmonary vascular resistance.

ABDOMINAL DISTENSION

The presence of abdominal distension poses a special problem. Positive intra-abdominal pressure tends to elevate the diaphragm, decrease transpulmonary pressure in the lung bases, and decrease alveolar lung volumes in the lung bases. To maintain normal lung volumes, a greater transpulmonary pressure has to be generated; this increases the airway pressures during positive pressure ventilation and increases work of breathing during spontaneous breathing. During positive pressure ventilation, a higher transpulmonary pressure may cause hyperinflation of the apical regions while restoring normal volumes in the bases. Therapy should be directed primarily toward reducing the intra-abdominal pressure.

NEUROLOGIC DISEASES

Hyperventilation with respiratory alkalosis is a very effective method of reducing intracranial pressure. High intrathoracic pressure may impede venous return from the brain by increasing central venous pressures. Therefore, high levels of PEEP are to avoided. In patients with acute neuromuscular diseases that are self-limiting, respiratory assistance is provided to maintain adequate minute ventilation while avoiding disuse muscle atrophy by encouraging spontaneous breathing as much as possible. Neuromuscular blockade must be avoided.

Weaning and Extubation

PREREQUISITES

Weaning should be started when the *underlying disease has improved* as signaled by an improvement in gas exchange, pulmonary mechanics, or ventilation-perfusion relationships and the patient is breathing effectively. Respiratory muscle strength, endurance, work of breathing, nutritional status, and stability of the cardiovascular system are factors that determine weaning. Patients must be able to breathe effectively, protect the airway, and maintain adequate gas exchange. If the work of breathing becomes excessive, weaning should not continue.

MONITORING

As the ventilator support is decreased, the patient's effort increases. A patient's ability to tolerate this increased load is reflected in an increase in the strength and endurance of respiratory efforts. The strength of respiratory effort is monitored by the size of chest expansion that gives a qualitative assessment of tidal volume, measurement of the spontaneous tidal volume, the inspiratory pressure of the spontaneous breath, or the inspiratory pressure produced by a maximal inspiratory effort. Work of breathing is monitored by respiratory rate; use of accessory muscles; presence or absence of retractions; pressure-time index, an integrated index incorporating spontaneous inspiratory pressure, maximal inspiratory pressure, fraction of the respiratory cycle spent on inspiration, and the spontaneous tidal volume; or oxygen cost of breathing. *Oxygen cost of breathing*, the fraction of the total oxygen consumption that is consumed for respiratory efforts, can be measured with an indirect calorimeter and has been found to be a reliable predictor of work of breathing. Arterial blood gases reflect only the adequacy of gas exchange. Abnormalities in arterial blood gases usually occur late in weaning failure. The inability to tolerate the increase in respiratory load during weaning is signaled by ineffective respiratory efforts. The signs of ineffective respiratory effort are tachypnea, poor air entry, poor chest expansion, and paradoxic breathing. In adults, this is reflected as rapid, shallow breathing with a rapid respiratory rate and a very small tidal volume.

MODES OF WEANING

The ventilator rate, PEEP, and FIO_2 are decreased to minimal levels. When the ventilator rate, PEEP, and FIO_2 are reduced to low levels, then mechanical ventilation is discontinued, and the patient is extubated. Inflation with a large tidal volume before extubation may prevent laryngospasm, which occasionally occurs during extubation. Intermittent mandatory ventilation (IMV) was first introduced as a technique to aid weaning from mechanical ventilation in adults. Despite the theoretical advantages, IMV has not been conclusively shown to be beneficial or superior to other methods of weaning. In infants, continuous flow through the ventilator circuit decreases the work of breathing and may aid in weaning. Weaning may be delayed due to slow resolution of the underlying disease process, decreased ventilatory drive, and ventilatory pump failure (Table 6–3). When muscle weakness is present, weaning should generally be slow, allowing sufficient time for muscle strength and endurance to be regained. Techniques for muscle training used in adults have not been studied in children. Ventilatory requirements can be reduced by decreasing CO_2 production through reduced excess caloric intake. Muscle loading may occur during IMV due to patient asynchrony and increase the work of breathing; prolonged asynchrony can result in muscle fatigue. In patients who have been ventilated for a prolonged period, a tracheostomy can aid the weaning process by decreasing airway resistance, dead space, and the work of breathing. In these patients, tracheostomy increases patient comfort and allows better interaction between the patient and caregivers. *Pressure-support ventilation* is a form of assisted ventilation in which the ventilator assists the patient's spontaneous effort with a mechanical breath with a preset pressure limit. Pressure support has been

Table 6–3. CAUSES OF WEANING FAILURE

Slow resolution of underlying disease	Inspiratory muscle loading
Persistent atelectasis	Asynchrony with ventilator
Pulmonary edema	Muscle injury or disease
Lower airway obstruction	Phrenic nerve injury
Ineffective ventilation	Increased work of breathing
Decreased ventilatory drive	Abdominal distension
Sedation	Lower airway obstruction
Brainstem dysfunction	Circulatory failure
Metabolic alkalosis	Fever
Ventilator pump failure	Metabolic acidosis
Muscle weakness	Other system disease
Prolonged paralysis	Circulatory failure
Malnutrition	Multiple organ system failure
Fatigue from excessive work	

mainly used to wean patients from mechanical ventilation. Although theoretically this method of weaning is attractive, its benefit in the weaning process has not been established in infants and children. A relative contraindication for the use of pressure-support ventilation is a very high baseline spontaneous respiratory rate. There is a finite lag time involved from the initiation of a breath to the sensing of this effort and the subsequent delivery of a mechancial breath. In infants breathing at a relatively fast rate (50 to 60 breaths/min), this lag time may be too long, resulting in asynchrony between the patient and the ventilator.

HIGH-FREQUENCY VENTILATION

High-frequency ventilation refers to methods of ventilation characterized by supraphysiologic ventilatory frequencies and low tidal volumes (less than or equal to physiologic dead space). *High-frequency positive-pressure ventilation* refers to ventilation with a tidal volume of 3 to 4 mL/kg at a frequency of 60 to 100 breaths/min with a ventilator with a small internal dead space, low internal compliance, and minimal compression of gases. *High-frequency jet ventilation* refers to delivery of inspiratory gases at a very high velocity through a jet injector introduced into the endotracheal tube, usually at rates of 100 to 400 breaths/min, with inspiratory times of 20% to 30% of the duty cycle. *High-frequency oscillatory ventilation* refers to ventilation at frequencies of 900 to 3600 breaths/min, with alternating positive and negative pressure produced with a piston pump or diaphragm. Mechanisms involved in gas transport during high-frequency ventilation include accelerated axial dispersion; increased collateral flow through pores of Kohn; intersegmental gas mixing, or "pendelluft" phenomenon; Taylor dispersion; asymmetric gas flow profiles; and gas mixing within the airway due to nonlinear pressure-diameter relationship of the bronchi.

The theoretic advantage of high-frequency ventilation is the ability to ventilate effectively at low airway pressures. High-frequency ventilation has been found to be very useful in the operating room for use in airway surgery, where airway movement has to be reduced to a minimum. Studies of the use of high-frequency ventilation in premature infants with idiopathic respiratory distress syndrome have shown improvement in gas exchange with lower airway pressures and amelioration of interstitial emphysema. A large multicenter trial of high-frequency oscillation did not show any advantage over conventional mechanical ventilation in premature newborns with idiopathic respiratory distress syndrome. A more recent study demonstrated that newborn infants with respiratory distress syndrome treated with high-frequency oscillation had a decreased incidence of chronic lung disease. Although the role of high-frequency ventilation in pediatric respiratory failure is unclear, recent studies suggest that high-frequency ventilation may be useful in the management of acute respiratory failure.

BIBLIOGRAPHY

Kirby RR, Smith RA, Desautels DA: Mechanical Ventilation. New York, Churchill Livingstone, 1985.
McPherson SP: Respiratory Therapy Equipment. St. Louis, CV Mosby, 1985.
Nichols DG, Rogers MC: Developmental physiology of the respiratory system. *In* Rogers MC (ed): The Textbook of Pediatric Intensive Care. Baltimore, Williams & Wilkins, 1987, pp 83–112.
Nunn JF (ed): Nunn's Applied Respiratory Physiology. Oxford, UK, Butterworth-Heinemann Ltd., 1993.
Venkataraman ST, Orr RA: Mechanical ventilation. *In* Fuhrman BP, Zimmerman JJ (eds): Pediatric Critical Care. St. Louis, CV Mosby, 1992, pp 519–543.
Venkataraman ST, Saville A, Wiltsie D, Frank J, Boig CW Jr: Pediatric respiratory care. *In* Dantzker DR, MacIntyre NR, Bakow ED (eds): Comprehensive Respiratory Care. Philadelphia, WB Saunders, 1994, pp 1004–1032.

6.3 Acute Upper Airway Obstruction

JONATHAN B. KRONICK, MD, PhD, FRCPC, FAAP

Acute upper airway obstruction in children is a potentially life-threatening emergency that must be promptly and effectively managed. In this chapter, we focus on the general principles underlying the pathophysiology, differential diagnosis, and management of severe upper airway obstruction in children. Selected disorders are discussed either because they are common (e.g., croup, foreign body aspiration) or because of the necessity of prompt recognition and treatment to avoid significant morbidity or mortality (e.g., supraglottitis).

Definition

Acute upper airway obstruction includes any disorder that *compromises the caliber of the child's upper airway,* including disease processes affecting the nasal or oral pharynx, larynx, and the extrathoracic and upper intrathoracic tracheas. Obstructive disorders involving the lower airways are discussed in another chapter (Chapter 6.4).

Pathophysiology

Just as the unique characteristics of the child's upper airway must be considered when securing the airway (see Chap. 2), these anatomic differences also predispose the child's upper airway to obstruction. The smaller the airway, the more prone it is to obstruction, whether by external compression, an intramural process, or intraluminal material such as mucus or a foreign body. Because the intraluminal area available for gas flow is inversely related to the *fourth* power of the radius of the cylinder, a relatively *small decrease in the radius of a small airway causes significantly more narrowing* than the same amount of narrowing in a larger airway (Fig. 6–7).

The child forced to breathe against the increased resistance of an obstructed upper airway must generate a larger negative intrapleural pressure to overcome the obstruction and achieve adequate ventilation. Compared with that of the adult, the *more compliant chest wall* of the child causes intercostal and sternal retractions and decreased effectiveness of chest wall movement. The intrathoracic airways tend to expand on inspiration, whereas the extrathoracic airways tend to expand on exhalation. Conversely, the extrathoracic airway tends to narrow on inspiration, especially when there is a large gradient between the intrapleural pressure and atmospheric pressure (Fig. 6–8). Thus, extrathoracic upper airway obstruction tends to result in *symptoms that are preferentially found during inspiration,*

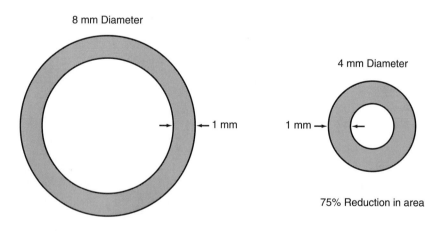

Figure 6–7. One millimeter of edema decreases the area available for gas flow by 75% in a small (4 mm) airway but by only 44% in a large (8 mm) airway because the area is proportional to the fourth power of the radius.

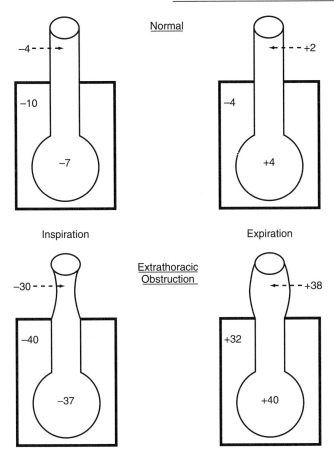

Figure 6–8. Extrathoracic upper airway obstruction worsens on inspiration *(bottom left)*. Numbers indicate pressure in mm Hg with the assumption that atmospheric pressure is 0. Box represents the thoracic cage; cylinder, the airway; and circle, the lungs. *Top,* Normal situation; *bottom,* effect of extrathoracic obstruction. Note the increased intrathoracic pressures required to overcome the obstruction.

whereas lower airway obstruction tends to preferentially affect expiration (e.g., asthma and bronchiolitis). With either upper or lower airway obstruction, the child's attempts to take larger tidal volumes tend to worsen the obstruction and may result in increased symptoms (e.g., stridor or wheeze). This phenomenon underlies the importance of *avoiding stress* in the child with severe airway obstruction.

Differential Diagnosis

There are many disorders that may compromise the child's upper airway. A useful classification of these disorders involves characterizing the disease process

Table 6–4. CLASSIFICATION OF SUPRAGLOTTIC UPPER AIRWAY OBSTRUCTION
IN CHILDREN

Disease	Comment/Example
Noninfectious	
Foreign body	Especially in toddlers
Trauma, burns	May primarily affect the airway
Allergic	Anaphylaxis, angioneurotic edema
Laryngomalacia	Onset in infancy of noisy breathing
Neoplasia	Hemangioma
Malformation	Cystic hygroma, thyroglossal duct cyst
Infectious	
Abscess	Peritonsillar, retropharyngeal, often trismus
Mononucleosis	May respond to steroids
Supraglottitis	Decreasing incidence with immunization
Diphtheria	Rare unless not immunized

by whether the disease is *infectious* or *noninfectious* and whether it primarily
affects the airway *above the glottis* or *below the glottis* (Tables 6–4 and 6–5).
Infectious disorders are the most common cause of airway obstruction in children,
with croup (laryngotracheobronchitis) being the most frequent cause of acute upper
airway obstruction. Supraglottitis, which includes epiglottitis, appears to occur
much less frequently since the introduction of *Haemophilus influenzae* vaccine.
Other organisms may also cause supraglottitis, so even complete immunization of
the pediatric population will not prevent all cases of supraglottitis. A number of
the disease processes (Tables 6–4 and 6–5) may affect both the supraglottic
and the subglottic airway (e.g., foreign body aspiration, trauma, burns, allergic
reactions).

Table 6–5. CLASSIFICATION OF SUBGLOTTIC UPPER AIRWAY OBSTRUCTION
IN CHILDREN

Disease	Comment/Example
Noninfectious	
Foreign body	Especially in toddlers
Trauma, burns	May primarily affect the airway
Allergic	Anaphylaxis, angioneurotic edema
Neoplasia	Hemangioma
Malformation	Tracheal stenosis
Tracheomalacia	May mimic lower airway obstruction
Acquired	Subglottic stenosis 2° to previous airway manipulation
Infectious	
Croup	Common, usually mild
Bacterial tracheitis	Easily confused with croup and supraglottitis

General Principles

CLINICAL EVALUATION

When confronted with a child with upper airway obstruction, the first step is to assess the severity to determine whether immediate airway intervention is required. *Rapid assessment of the severity* of the obstruction includes assessment of the heart rate, respiratory rate, stridor, retractions, color, air entry, and level of consciousness (Table 6–6). Children must be frequently reassessed as upper airway diseases may progress rapidly.

The child with severe airway obstruction must receive urgent intervention regardless of the underlying etiology (Fig. 6–9).

INVESTIGATIONS

Few investigations are indicated in children presenting with acute severe airway obstruction. Children without life-threatening airway obstruction may require radiographs of the soft tissues of the neck and/or chest. In croup syndromes, the anterior/posterior radiograph reveals loss of shouldering of the airway lucency known as the *steeple* or *rat tail sign*. In contrast, children with supraglottitis generally have a normal anteroposterior soft tissue radiograph of the neck; however, the lateral view reveals ballooning of the pharyngeal airway and thickening of the aryepiglottic folds and/or an enlarged epiglottitis *(thumb sign)*. In croup

Table 6–6. RAPID ASSESSMENT OF SEVERITY OF AIRWAY OBSTRUCTION

Respiratory rate	Generally increases as obstruction worsens
	Severe obstruction, the rate may decrease in the exhausted child: high risk of apnea
Heart rate	Generally increases as obstruction worsens
	May decrease in severe hypoxemia, especially in infants
Stridor	Caused by turbulent air flow in obstructed airway
	Disease dependent (+ + + in croup; ± in supraglottitis)
	Generally increases as obstruction worsens
	May decrease as exhaustion supervenes in severe obstruction or if very diminished gas flow
Retractions	Includes use of accessory muscles, intercostal and sternal retractions, and tracheal tug
	Tends to increase as severity of obstruction worsens
	May decrease with exhaustion in severe obstruction
Color	Absence of cyanosis does not exclude hypoxemia
	Cyanosis indicates significant hypoxemia and likely severe obstruction
Auscultation (air entry)	Breath sound intensity correlates inversely with the severity of obstruction
	Beware of the "silent chest"
Behavior	The happy, consolable child is unlikely to have severe obstruction
	Agitation equates to hypoxemia until proved otherwise
	Obtundation equates impending respiratory failure

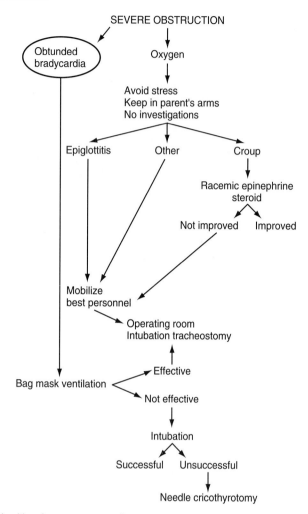

Figure 6–9. Algorithm for management of severe upper airway obstruction. All children should be admitted to the pediatric intensive care unit once the airway is secured.

syndromes, other than ballooning of the pharynx, the lateral view of the neck is usually normal. Selected patients with airway obstruction may require laryngoscopy or bronchoscopy for diagnostic and/or therapeutic purposes. Children with bacterial tracheitis or supraglottitis require bacterial cultures of the airway and blood; whereas children with typical viral or spasmodic croup should not have bacterial cultures unless their presentation is atypical or they are immunocompromised.

Management

GENERAL PRINCIPLES

Severe Obstruction. The child with severe life-threatening airway obstruction needs urgent management by the most skilled personnel available (see Fig. 6–9). While attempting to avoid stressing the child, *100% oxygen should be administered* and the awake child should ideally receive an *inhalational anesthetic* in the operating room. After establishment of deep anesthesia, the airway should be secured through either *endotracheal intubation* or tracheostomy. In many centers, both an anesthesiologist and a surgeon are available, and in all centers the most skilled personnel should be summoned urgently. Bronchoscopy may be advantageous in establishing the airway. The endotracheal tube should be one-half to one size smaller than would normally be inserted in a child of that age or size. Neuromuscular blockade to facilitate intubation should be avoided in children with upper airway obstruction.

The child in extremis due to severe upper airway obstruction should initially receive *bag-and-mask ventilation with 100% oxygen.* High airway pressures are essential to even partially overcome the obstruction. Therefore, the mask must have a perfect seal, and depending on the system being used, the high-pressure pop-off value may have to be disabled. The vast majority of children with severe life-threatening airway obstruction can be sufficiently oxygenated to prevent bradycardia and cardiac arrest with the use of *appropriate* bag-and-mask ventilation. In the rare situation in which bag-and-mask ventilation is inadequate and intubation is not possible, transtracheal catheter insertion or emergency tracheostomy must be performed. Unless one is experienced with performing a tracheostomy, transtracheal needle cricothyrotomy is recommended. The highest flow of 100% oxygen that can be delivered through the catheter is then administered. Periodically, the system must be disconnected to allow exhalation to occur. The child should then have the airway secured in a more permanent manner (intubation or tracheostomy) as soon as possible.

Specific Disease Processes

CROUP (LARYNGOTRACHEOBRONCHITIS)

Clinical Features. Croup is a common viral infection affecting the subglottic area, the narrowest part of the pediatric airway. Most children do not progress to severe obstruction. Croup tends to be worse in the young child or the child with underlying airway compromise (e.g., subglottic stenosis, airway hemangioma, tracheomalacia) and is characterized by a prodrome of low-grade fever and coryza, followed by stridor and a *barking "seal-like" cough* that is virtually pathognomonic. Retractions are prominent, and the child does not prefer any particular posture. Viral croup tends to progress over 2 to 3 days and to be worse in the evenings. Children generally *do not appear toxic.* Children with severe croup who are more than 3 years old may have underlying airway pathology that has been brought to clinical attention due to a supervening viral infection.

Spasmodic croup, which probably is an allergic phenomenon, comes on very rapidly and usually is not associated with an upper respiratory tract infection but otherwise is virtually indistinguishable clinically from viral croup.

Etiology
Viral
    parainfluenza (frequent)
    adenovirus (infrequent)
    influenza (infrequent)
    measles (especially during epidemics)

Management
Mild disease, outpatient treatment
Significant disease (stridor at rest), hospitalization and supportive care that includes
    hydration and oxygen
Severe disease, pediatric intensive care unit admission
    General treatment
        nothing by mouth
        IV rate at maintenance
        FIO_2 to keep SpO_2 at $\geq 95\%$
    Monitoring
        pulse oximetry
        ECG and respiratory
    Medication
        nebulized racemic epinephrine (works transiently by local vasoconstriction)
            <1 year, 0.25 mL/dose q 30–60 min PRN
            >1 year, 0.50 mL/dose q 30–60 min PRN
        steroids
            inhaled budesonide, 1000 μg/dose q4h
            systemic dexamethasone, 0.5 mg/kg IV q6h
        antibiotics are not indicated unless secondary bacterial infection occurs
    Intubation indication
        exhaustion
        increased requirement for or decreased effect of racemic epinephrine
    Extubate
        when leak around endotracheal tube is <20 cm H_2O positive pressure

SUPRAGLOTTITIS

Clinical Features. Supraglottitis or epiglottitis is an infectious cellulitis of the supraglottic structures, including the aryepiglottic folds, arytenoids, and epiglottis. Onset is usually *rapid over 3 to 6 hours* and includes high fever, drooling, and a preference for the tripod position. There usually is significant sore throat, and the child refuses to drink or swallow. The child often appears frightened and toxic. Stridor and cough are uncommon. The voice tends to be muffled, whereas in croup the voice tends to be hoarse.

Etiology
Haemophilus influenzae
Streptococcus
Staphylococcus aureus
Moraxella catarrhalis
Rarely viral

Management
General
  suspicion of supraglottitis
    avoid stress
    administer oxygen
    admit to operating room **stat** for inhalational anesthetic; supraglottitis must
      be confirmed or excluded
  supraglottitis confirmed
    intubate or perform tracheostomy
    culture supraglottic area and blood
    admit to pediatric intensive care unit
    nothing by mouth
    IV rate at maintenance
Monitoring
  SpO_2
  $TcPCO_2$, ECG, and respirations
Medication
  broad-spectrum antibiotics, pending cultures (e.g., cefuroxime: 100–150 mg/
    kg/day divided q6h)
  restrain and sedate the patient to prevent self-extubation
Extubate
  when supraglottic swelling is resolved (inspect daily by nasopharyngoscopy)
    and leak around endotracheal tube is <20 cm H_2O positive pressure.

BACTERIAL TRACHEITIS

Clinical Features. Bacterial tracheitis (pseudomembranous croup) *shares similarities with both viral croup and supraglottitis.* Affected children often begin their illness with an upper respiratory tract infection and, occasionally, classic viral croup. Secondary bacterial infection of the subglottic region results in high fever, toxicity, and the production of purulent sputum. The course may be prolonged and heralded by the rapid onset of high fever and clinical deterioration. The diagnosis is often made at the time of laryngoscopy when *purulent secretions* are aspirated from the upper trachea or, occasionally, as a result of a lateral neck radiograph that reveals the wall of the upper trachea to have an irregular appearance due to accumulation of inflammatory material within the lumen.

Etiology
Staphylococcus aureus
Moraxella catarrhalis
Haemophilus influenzae
Streptococcus

Management
   Admit to pediatric intensive care unit
   General
      diagnosis often made at time of laryngoscopy/intubation (+ + + purulent
         secretions in trachea)
      intubation and culture of tracheal aspirate and blood
      mechanical ventilation (usually required)
      vigorous tracheal toilet
      nothing by mouth and IV rate at maintenance
   Monitor
      SpO_2, $TcPco_2$, ECG, respiration, and blood gases if ventilated
   Medication
      broad-spectrum antibiotics, pending cultures (e.g., cefuroxime: 100 to 150
         mg/kg/day divided q6h)
      sedate and restrain the patient to prevent self-extubation
   Extubation
      when airway secretions decrease and a leak around endotracheal tube is <20
         cm H_2O positive pressure.

OTHER DISEASES

   Foreign body aspiration is particularly common in toddlers. Foreign body
aspiration may occur remotely from the time of presentation. Delayed presentation
is most common when the foreign body is lodged in the lower airway rather than
the upper airway. A foreign body should be considered in the differential diagnosis
of all children with respiratory distress that is not clearly associated with an
infectious process or other obvious etiology. A suspected foreign body below the
glottis requires urgent bronchoscopy for removal.
   As indicated (see Tables 6–4 and 6–5), a wide variety of disorders may
present acutely with upper airway obstruction. Evaluation of airway patency is the
first priority in the management of the child with *trauma* and is discussed in
Chapter 4. Fifty percent of children with a *hemangioma* affecting the airway have
cutaneous hemangiomas. Other neoplastic disorders may present with the gradual
onset of progressive airway obstruction, whereas *congenital malformations* of the
airway often present early in infancy or with an otherwise trivial airway infection.
Airway obstruction due to *allergic* phenomena is often accompanied by urticaria,
hypotension, and lower airway obstruction.
   Airway obstruction occurring soon after extubation in the pediatric intensive
care unit is often due to mural edema in the subglottic region but occasionally
may also be due to failure of the child to adequately clear secretions or to vocal
cord injury.
   Management. Management of the wide variety of additional disorders that
may obstruct the child's upper airway must be individualized by the specific
etiology. Many of the neoplastic and structural disorders require bronchoscopy for
diagnosis. Treatment may include not only insertion of an airway but also specific
surgical therapies.

Prognosis

The prognosis of upper airway obstruction in children is primarily dependent on two factors: the etiology and the effectiveness of treatment. Because hypoxemia is an inevitable consequence of inadequately treated severe airway obstruction, all children with upper airway disease have the potential risk of hypoxic end organ injury, particularly brain injury. Most children with treatable causes of upper airway obstruction should have a good outcome if treatment is provided in a timely manner.

BIBLIOGRAPHY

Kilham H, Gillis J, Benjamin B: Severe upper airway obstruction. Pediatr Clin North Am 34:1–14, 1987.
Landau LI, Geelhoed GC: Aerosolized steroids for croup. N Engl J Med 331:322–323, 1994.
Manning SC, Ridenour B, Brown OE, Squires J: Measles: an epidemic of upper airway obstruction. Otolaryngol Head Neck Surg 105:415–418, 1991.

6.4 Lower Airway Disease

NARENDRA C. SINGH, BSc, MB, BS, FRCPC, FAAP
YVES OUELLETTE, MD, PhD, FRCPC
PHILIP JOCHELSON, MD
MARK K. WEDEL, MD, JD, FACP

Respiratory failure is defined as the inability of the respiratory system to maintain adequate gas exchange, resulting in hypoxemia and hypercarbia. Diseases of the lower airway account for a significant number of patients with this condition and are responsible for a large proportion of pediatric critical care admissions. Lower airway pathology is often characterized by obstruction resulting from secretions, airway edema, and bronchoconstriction. The major conditions characterized by these pathophysiologic changes are bronchiolitis, asthma, pneumonia, and adult respiratory distress syndrome (ARDS).

Pathophysiology

A number of anatomic and physiologic factors unique to children are responsible for an increase in lower airway disease (Table 6–7). When a disease state is superimposed on these intrinsic factors, the final common pathway of respiratory failure results from increased edema, secretions, and bronchospasm. The resultant

Table 6–7. LOWER AIRWAY ANATOMIC AND PHYSIOLOGIC DIFFERENCES BETWEEN THE INFANT AND THE ADULT AND CLINICAL IMPLICATIONS

Lower Airway Characteristics	Clinical Implications
Respiratory pump	
Underdevelopment of chemical and neuronal control	Periodic breathing and apnea
↓ Chest wall compliance	↑ Lung collapse
↓ Fatigue resistance muscle fibers	↑ Respiratory muscle fatigue
Pulmonary circulation	
Underdeveloped with increased musculature	↑ Pulmonary artery pressures
Airway and lungs	
Smaller airway (resistance ∞ $1/r^4$, r = radius)	↑ Airway obstruction
Weak cartilaginous support	Compression of trachea during forced expiration
Alveolar surface area Infant: 2.8 m^2 8 yr: 32 m^2 Adult: 75 m^2	Early respiratory failure with loss of alveolar mass
Collateral ventilation (not developed <8 yr)	↑ Lung collapse
Adult FRC>>>CC, Infant FRC>CC	↑ Lung collapse
↓ Airway elasticity	↑ Lung collapse
↓ Alveolar surfactant and elasticity	↑ Lung collapse

FRC, functional residual capacity; CC, closing capacity.

effect is often ventilation/perfusion (V̇/Q̇) mismatch and hypoxia. Depending on the disease state, one or more of these factors may predominate.

Bronchiolitis

Bronchiolitis is an acute inflammatory disease characterized by small airway obstruction. Although other viruses (e.g., adenovirus, influenza, parainfluenza) may be the causative agent, the name *respiratory syncytial virus* (RSV) is used almost synonymously with bronchiolitis. RSV is the most common respiratory pathogen in early childhood, accounting for 50% to 90% of cases of bronchiolitis and 5% to 40% of cases of pneumonia. The peak incidence occurs at 2 to 5 months. The mortality is usually low, although in the high-risk group (e.g., immunocompromised, congenital heart disease, bronchopulmonary dysplasia [BPD] pulmonary hypertension, prematurity), mortality increases significantly.

PATHOPHYSIOLOGY

Infants are at greater risk for developing bronchiolitis due to an underdeveloped immune system, high airway resistance, and a lack of previous exposure

(Fig. 6–10). *Hypoxia* is the primary abnormality of gas exchange. The moderate hypoxia seen in a majority of cases is likely due to V̇/Q mismatch; however, in severe hypoxemia, right-to-left intrapulmonary shunting may account for the high oxygen requirement. Most patients are able to compensate for the increase in dead space by increasing minute ventilation; however, hypercarbia usually results from respiratory muscle fatigue and a fall in minute ventilation.

CLINICAL MANIFESTATIONS

The severity of the clinical presentation often depends on the age of the child, size of the inoculum, immune status, and presence of certain risk factors. There often is a history of exposure, followed by *cough, sneezing, rhinorrhea,* and a *low-grade fever.* The child gradually progresses to significant respiratory distress characterized by tachypnea, retractions, and wheezing. Infants may present with *apnea* without significant respiratory symptoms. Findings on physical examination demonstrate profuse rhinorrhea, tachypnea, cyanosis, and use of accessory muscles. Auscultation demonstrates diffuse wheezes and rales with prolonged expiration.

DIAGNOSIS

Diagnosis can be suspected based on (1) seasonal presentation (November through March), (2) age of <2 years, (3) characteristic clinical presentation, (4) chest radiography showing hyperinflation in the majority of patients (however, peribronchial thickening is seen in 50% of cases), and (5) identification through the use of rapid diagnostic testing (immunofluorescent staining of infected epithelial cells and direct fluorescent antibody or enzyme-linked immunosorbent assay [ELISA] for viral antigens).

MANAGEMENT

As with all critically ill pediatric patients, a rapid assessment of the airway, adequacy of ventilation, and hemodynamic evaluation is required. Very close

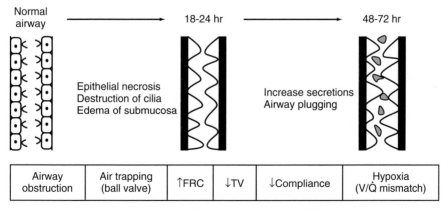

Figure 6–10. Pathophysiology of bronchiolitis.

observation for apnea is essential, especially in infants <6 months old. *Hospitalization* should be considered for patients <6 months old with increased respiratory rate and apnea and for all patients with moderate-to-severe distress. Patients with moderate-to-severe stress and high oxygen requirements should be considered for *intensive care unit (ICU) admission,* as should patients presenting with apnea.

General

Oxygen should be given and titrated with pulse oximetry to keep SaO_2 at >92% to 95%. The patients should be kept NPO because intubation may be necessary. An IV line should be inserted, and maintenance fluids should be started.

Monitoring

Cardiorespiratory monitoring should be initiated to observe for periodic breathing and apnea. Pulse oximetry is used to titrate the FIO_2 to keep the SaO_2 at >92% to 95%. Transcutaneous CO_2 monitoring may assist in evaluating the adequacy of ventilation. Blood gas analysis should be performed to evaluate $PaCO_2$ and pH to determine whether the child is compensating or requires assisted ventilation.

Medication

Salbutamol (0.03 to 0.1 mL/kg; maximum, 1 mL) administered via nebulization may be beneficial in some patients. If there is clinical improvement, then depending on the severity of the disease process, the interval can vary from 1 to 4 hours. Some infants will not respond, and therefore the drug should be discontinued.

Antibiotics are not recommended routinely; however, if there is uncertainty regarding the diagnosis, especially in the presence of pulmonary infiltrates, antibiotics should be considered. Between 6 months and 5 years of age, *Cefuroxime* (75 to 150 mg/kg/day divided every 8 hours) is recommended. *Steroids* have no place in the acute management of patients with bronchiolitis. *Ribavirin* should be considered in treatment of the high-risk patients early in the disease process. The most recent recommendations by the American Academy of Pediatrics support this practice (Table 6–8).

Intubation and Mechanical Ventilation

There are no absolute criteria for intubation; most patients do not require intubation. Patients with RSV bronchiolitis should be considered for *intubation* if they have recurrent apnea and impending respiratory failure (e.g., lethargy, signs of fatigue, cyanosis on oxygen, $PaCO_2$ >65 mm Hg). Although there are no contraindications to any drugs during intubation, morphine should be avoided due to the histamine-releasing property. Recommended drugs are *atropine, ketamine,* and *succinylcholine.* Ketamine is used for sedation and has the added benefit of bronchodilating properties.

Due to the large quantity of secretions and the persistent air trapping, positive

Table 6–8. RIBAVIRIN RECOMMENDATIONS

The intent of the new recommendation is to allow practitioners to decide whether ribavirin therapy is appropriate by taking into account the particular clinical situation and the practitioner's own preferences. Recommendations may be modified as new information becomes available. Ribavirin aerosol therapy may be considered in the following list of selected infants and young children at high risk for serious RSV disease.

- Those with complicated congenital heart disease (including PH) and those with bronchopulmonary dysplasia, cystic fibrosis, and other chronic lung disease. Previously healthy premature infants (<37 weeks' gestational age) and those <6 weeks old are also at greater risk for severe RSV illness but less so than patients with underlying disease.
- Those with underlying immunosuppressive diseases or therapy (e.g., those with acquired immunodeficiency syndrome, severe combined immunodeficiency disease, or organ transplantation) who have high mortality and/or prolonged RSV illness. Immunocompromised children were excluded from analysis in the two recent studies.
- Those who are severely ill with or without mechanical ventilation. Because the severity of illness is often difficult to judge clinically in infants with RSV infection, useful guidelines include blood gas measurements and the infant's response to other therapies.
- Hospitalized patients who may be at increased risk of progressing from a mild to a more complicated course because they are younger than 6 weeks or have an underlying condition, such as multiple congenital anomalies or certain neurologic or metabolic diseases (e.g., cerebral palsy or myasthenia gravis).

pressure ventilation can often pose a challenge. *Limiting the positive end-expiratory pressure (PEEP)* is recommended due to the high functional residual capacity (FRC). Consideration should be given to high-frequency oscillation in an attempt to limit the barotrauma. Because some high-risk patients, such as infants with BPD, have a high pulmonary artery pressure (PAP), consideration should be given to administer nitric oxide to lower the PAP. Evaluation of the use of liquid ventilation is under way in a multicenter study of acute pediatric lung injury, including RSV bronchiolitis. This is a multicentre, randomized, controlled study of the safety and efficacy of partial liquid ventilation with AF0141 (sterile perflubron) in children with acute parenchymal lung injury (Alliance Pharmaceutical Corp, San Diego).

OUTCOME

Although the mortality is in general <1%, the mortality for high-risk patients is ≥20% to 30%. Because the majority of these patients have nosocomial infections, it is necessary to curb the spread, identify and isolate infected patients, and monitor and treat high-risk patients sooner.

Bacterial Pneumonias

Pneumonia is an acute inflammation of the lungs resulting from the invasion and replication of an infectious agent. Pneumonias may be broadly defined as *community acquired* and *nosocomial pneumonias*.

ETIOLOGY

The vast majority of the community acquired pneumonias have a nonbacterial origin; only 10% to 15% are of bacterial origin. The organisms responsible for the community acquired pneumonias are often age dependent (Table 6–9). Respiratory tract infections make up 15% to 30% of nosocomial infections in admissions to the pediatric ICU, accounting for 2% to 3% of all pediatric ICU admissions.

PATHOPHYSIOLOGY

Nosocomial pneumonias may result from any one of four mechanisms: hematogenous, aspiration, direct inoculation or aerosolization, and contiguous spread.

The pediatric ICU patient is an ideal candidate for the development of nosocomial pneumonia due to (1) predisposing conditions (e.g., nutritional status, chronic lung disease), (2) immunocompromise, (3) increased aspiration (e.g., gastroesophageal reflux, altered level of consciousness, decreased cough and gag), and (4) bacterial colonization (antibiotic use).

Endotracheal intubation predisposes to sinusitis, acts as a foreign body, impairs cough and swallowing, alters oral flora, and impairs ciliary function, all of which predispose the intubated child to the development of pneumonia.

In severe disease, there is significant volume loss and reduced pulmonary compliance. Significant changes can occur in vital capacity (VC) and total lung volume (TLV) depending on the severity of the alveolitis. $\dot{V}/Q$ mismatch occurs as a result of regional changes in blood flow, decreased parenchymal compliance, and airflow obstruction due to inflammation.

CLINICAL MANIFESTATIONS

Community acquired bacterial pneumonias are often preceded by an upper respiratory tract infection that has failed to resolve. The signs may vary depending on the age of the child and the responsible pathogen. Complaints include high

Table 6–9. ETIOLOGY OF BACTERIAL PNEUMONIA

	Community Acquired Pneumonia		Nosocomial Pneumonia*
Neonate		Group B *Streptococcus*	*Pseudomonas*
		E. coli	*S. Aureus*
		Other enterics	*Klebsiella*
		S. Aureus	*Enterobacter* sp.
1–3 mo		S. Pneumoniae	*Candida* sp.
		H. Influenzae B	
4 mo to 5 yr		S. Pneumoniae	
		H. Influenzae B	
>5 yr		M. Pneumoniae	
		S. Pneumoniae	

*National Nosocomial Infection Surveillance, 1984.

fever, chills, headache, cough, irritability, and restlessness. Patients with basal pneumonias may have abdominal complaints, including nausea, vomiting, pain, and diarrhea. It is not uncommon for a child with a basal pneumonia to present with an acute abdomen. Physical examination can include nasal flaring, cyanosis or pallor, retraction, tachypnea, decreased breath sounds, and fine crackling.

The clinical manifestation of *nosocomial pneumonias* are often less specific. It is essential for the clinician to have a high index of suspicion in intubated and ventilated pediatric patients. Although this list is not definitive, patients with the following should be considered for further evaluation: increased sputum production and purulence, fever, increased oxygen and ventilatory requirement, and deterioration in the recovery phase of a viral pneumonia.

DIAGNOSIS

Community acquired bacterial pneumonias should be suspected in a child who deteriorates after showing signs of improvement from an acute viral infection. The distinction needs to be made between a viral and bacterial pneumonia. The child with a viral pneumonia generally has a low-grade fever and is nontoxic. The *white blood cell (WBC) count* will be higher in bacterial pneumonias with a significant left shift. The *chest radiography* in viral pneumonias (RSV) is often hyperinflated with diffuse patchy infiltrates, whereas in a bacterial pneumonia, there are often areas of consolidation. Blood cultures are positive in only 3% to 20% of cases.

Nosocomial pneumonias are often difficult to diagnose because an increase in sputum, fever, and infiltrates on chest radiograph may be as the result of other disease processes. Differentiating colonization from pneumonia in the intubated patient also poses a significant problem; nosocomial pneumonias are misdiagnosed in 30% of cases.

Endotracheal aspirates are often used to support the diagnosis of pneumonias; however, due to contamination and colonization, this method has a low sensitivity and specificity. Other methods have been proposed; *bronchoalveolar lavage* is used increasingly because it is safe and reliable and isolated lung segments can be lavaged. It is imperative that the overall clinical condition of the child be examined before hematologic, microbiologic, and radiologic evidence is interpreted.

MANAGEMENT

Most patients with bacterial pneumonia can be discharged home on antibiotics. Patients should be *considered for admission* if he or she is in moderate-to-severe distress, requires oxygen, is <6 months, or is not tolerating oral intake.

Few patients with community acquired bacterial pneumonia require ICU admission because with early diagnosis and appropriate treatment they will respond.

General

A rapid evaluation of the ABC should be done. Patients in moderate-to-severe distress should be considered for oxygen, which should be titrated by pulse oximetry to keep the SaO_2 at >92% to 95%. The patient in severe distress should be kept NPO because intubation may be necessary. An IV line should be inserted in patients with moderate-to-severe distress to provide antibiotics and adequate hydration.

Monitoring

A cardiorespiratory monitor is necessary for patients in moderate-to-severe distress. Other monitoring includes pulse oximetry, capillary or arterial blood gas analysis (for moderate-to-severe distress), and electrolytes (if patient is vomiting).

Specific Therapy

An *antipyretic (acetaminophen)* should be administered for fever (15 mg/kg every 3 to 4 hours). The use of *antibiotics* is based on the patient's age, the severity of the condition, and whether the child can tolerate oral intake. For recommended antibiotics, see Table 6–10.

NOSOCOMIAL PNEUMONIA

Supportive care, including adequate hydration, antipyretic therapy, chest physiotherapy, frequent suctioning, and ventilatory support are required. Antibiotic use should be based on the nosocomial organisms commonly found in the individual ICUs and the patient's sensitivity to antibiotics.

Status Asthmaticus

Asthma is defined as a diffuse pulmonary disease characterized by hyperreactivity of the trachea and bronchi, causing generalized narrowing of the airway in response to certain nonspecific stimuli. *Status asthmaticus* is a life-threatening form of asthma characterized by unresponsiveness to the usual adrenergic drugs, resulting in respiratory failure. Asthma is the most common chronic illness in children. It is the leading cause of school absenteeism and accounts for 27 million physician visits annually. Although the mortality rate appears to be increasing, most of these deaths are preventable.

Table 6–10. SUGGESTED ANTIBIOTICS FOR ORAL AND INTRAVENOUS USE

Age	Oral	Intravenous
<3 mo		Ampicillin/cefotaxime
3–6 mo		Cefuroxime
6 mo to 5 yr	Amoxicillin/ampicillin/cefaclor	Cefuroxime
>5 yr	Erythromycin	Erythromycin

PATHOPHYSIOLOGY

The pathophysiologic events of status asthmaticus is summarized in Figure 6–11. The hallmark is an *increase in airway resistance*. This results in *hyperinflation* with V̇/Q mismatch. With an increase in dead space, there is a compensatory increase in minute ventilation, resulting in a fall in $Paco_2$ in the initial state. With increased work of breathing and deterioration in the compensatory mechanism, CO_2 production exceeds elimination, resulting in hypercarbia. If unchecked, the increasing hypoxia, hypercarbia, and acidosis will result in cardiovascular and cardiopulmonary failure.

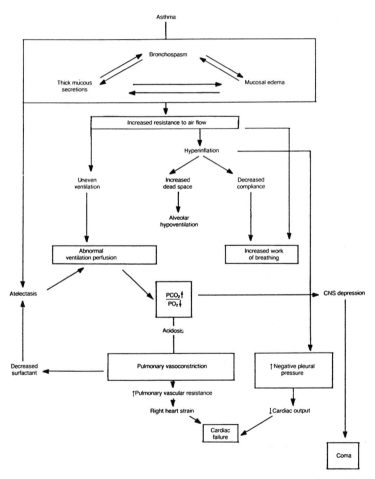

Figure 6–11. Pathophysiologic events in status asthmaticus, $Pco_2 = Paco_2$; $Po_2 = Pao_2$. (Modified from Siegel SC: Bronchial asthma. In Kelly C (ed): Practice of Pediatrics. Hagerstown, MD, Harper & Row, 1974, Chap 63, p 163.)

CLINICAL MANIFESTATIONS

Before embarking on a thorough history and physical examination, a brief evaluation of the patient to determine the degree of respiratory distress and adequacy of oxygenation is suggested. Most asthmatic attacks are preceded by an upper respiratory tract infection. Although the presentation varies with age, cough, dyspnea, and wheezing are the major clinical features. In some children, the attack may be characterized by progressive dyspnea, whereas others may present with intractable coughing. The degree of wheezing often does not correlate with the severity of the attack. However, absence of wheezing in a child with respiratory distress is indicative of severe disease. Along with signs of respiratory distress, pulsus paradoxus of >10 to 15 mm Hg indicates severe obstruction.

DIAGNOSIS

A history of asthma or recurrent hospital visits is usually obtained. In younger children, the possibility of bronchiolitis or foreign body should be considered, especially with a first attack. A chest radiograph will demonstrate hyperinflation. Spirometry is not practical in younger children and in patients in severe distress.

MANAGEMENT (Fig. 6–12)

General

A rapid evaluation of the ABC should be done. Oxygen by mask should be administered to keep SaO_2 at >92% to 95%. Patients should be kept NPO because intubation may be necessary and in the younger patients aspiration may occur. An IV line should be inserted for adequate hydration and maintenance fluids.

Monitoring

A cardiorespiratory monitor should be used to evaluate the heart and respiration rates. Pulse oximetry should be used to titrate FIO_2 to keep SaO_2 at >92% to 95%. Transcutaneous CO_2 monitoring may assist in evaluating adequacy of ventilation. A blood gas analysis should be done to determine the adequacy of ventilation and degree of compensation. A low $PaCO_2$ suggests that the child is able to compensate with an increase in minute ventilation. A normal or high $PaCO_2$ suggests that there is loss of compensation and the patient should be closely monitored and evaluated for escalation of pharmacotherapy or mechanical ventilation. Patients who fail to improve or have an acute deterioration should be considered for a portable *chest radiograph*. This should be evaluated for consolidation, collapse, pneumothorax, or foreign body. *Serum electrolyte* analysis should be done because both inhaled and intravenous β-adrenergic agents cause hypokalemia due to both an intracellular shift and an increase in urinary losses. Theophylline also causes an increase in urinary loss of potassium. An increase in potassium in the maintenance fluids as well as frequent monitoring may be necessary.

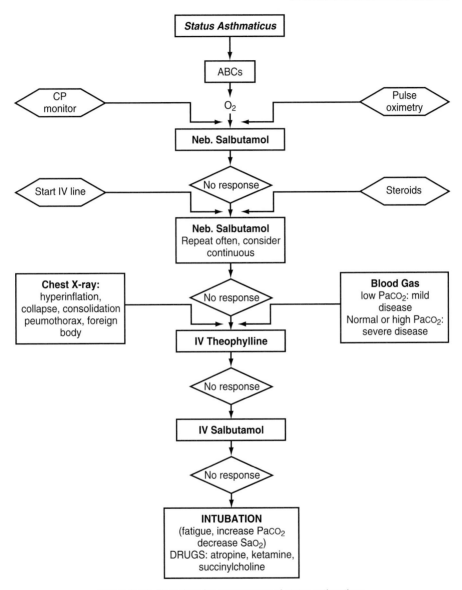

Figure 6–12. Flow chart for management of status asthmaticus.

Criteria for Intensive Care Unit Admission

Because the level of training of staff (e.g., nursing staff, house staff, respiratory therapists) and availability of equipment may vary among institutions, the criteria for ICU admission may be variable. Patients should be considered for ICU admission if there is a history of previous ICU admissions, frequent use of bronchodilators (every hour), failure to respond to standard therapy, physical signs of impending respiratory failure (e.g., cyanosis, altered level of consciousness, pulsus paradoxus of >10 to 15 mm Hg, use of accessory muscles), oxygen requirement of $>50\%$ to 60% to keep Sao_2 at $>90\%$, chest radiographic evidence of a pneumothorax or pneumomediastinum, or blood gas with a normal or high $Paco_2$.

Specific Therapy

Agonists

Nebulized. β_2-Receptor stimulation results in bronchodilation. Additional effects include an increase in diaphragmatic contractility and enhanced mucociliary clearance. These agents are the mainstay of therapy for management of acute asthma. *Salbutamol,* which is the most frequently used agent, should be nebulized in a dose of 0.03 to 0.1 mL/kg (maximum, 1 mL/dose). It can be administered *as frequently as is required,* including by continuous nebulization. Patients should be monitored for anxiety, tremor, nausea, vomiting, and tachycardia. As an alternative, *nebulized terbutaline* can be used.

Intravenous. When the patient fails to respond to repeated nebulized salbutamol, steroids, and, often, a trial of intravenous theophylline, intravenous *salbutamol* is used (loading dose of 10 µg/kg IV over 10 minutes followed by an infusion at 0.2 to 4 µg/kg/min; maximum, 10 µg/kg/min). The patient's hemodynamic function and serum electrolytes should be monitored closely. Intravenous *terbutaline* has also been used successfully (loading dose of 10 µg/kg over 30 minutes followed by an infusion at 0.1 µg/kg/min; increase by 0.1 µg/kg/min every 30 minutes if needed to a maximum of 4 µg/kg/min). *Isoproterenol* has also been used as a continuous infusion (0.05 to 0.1 µg/kg/min; maximum, 2 µg/kg/min); however, in view of the higher incidence of cardiovascular side effects, salbutamol or terbutaline are preferred.

Theophylline

Although the β_2-agonists have replaced theophylline in the acute management of asthma, there continues to be a limited role for theophylline in the treatment of status asthmaticus. *Theophylline* should be considered for use in the emergency department when patients do not respond to treatment with nebulized β_2-agonists. If patients respond to intravenous theophylline, they can often be cared for on a pediatric ward; once treatment with an intravenous β_2-agonist is started, in most institutions, the patient is admitted to the ICU. Theophylline is administered in a loading dose of 5 to 6 mg/kg slowly followed by an infusion at 1 mg/kg/hr. Theophylline levels should be carefully monitored along with clinical evidence of complications (e.g., tachycardia, nausea, vomiting, tremors, and seizures).

Corticosteroids

Steroids have been demonstrated to benefit asthmatics due to the anti-inflammatory properties. Recent studies show that steroids improve Pao_2 and lung function, reduce the duration and severity of bronchospasm, and reduce the need for hospitalization if started early; steroids should be used early in the management of status asthmaticus (hydrocortisone [5 mg/kg q6h] or methylprednisone [1 to 2 mg/kg IV q6h]).

Anticholinergic Agents

Stimulation (e.g., by dust or cold) of cholinergic receptors in the airway can result in reflex bronchoconstriction. Inhaled *ipratropium bromide* concurrent with a β_2-agonist has been shown to produce improvement in lung function compared with the use of a β_2-agonist alone. The nebulized dose is 0.5 to 1 mL (125 to 250 μg) diluted in 2 mL of normal saline.

Magnesium Sulfate

There have only been case reports on the use of magnesium sulfate in children with acute asthma. The exact mechanisms by which magnesium sulfate causes bronchodilation are unclear; however, it is thought to counteract calcium-mediated smooth muscle contraction through its interaction with calcium homeostasis. Magnesium sulfate is not currently used routinely at all institutions. The recommended dose is 30 to 70 mg/kg over 20 to 30 minutes. Side effects include hypotension, bradycardia, flushing, malaise, and a transient sensation of facial warmth.

Intubation and Mechanical Ventilation

From 20% to 30% of pediatric ICU admissions for status asthmaticus require mechanical ventilation. Because the morbidity associated with mechanical ventilation is high, all efforts are made to avoid mechanical ventilation. *Indications* for intubation include patient fatigue, $Paco_2$ rising and >50 to 60 mm Hg, Sao_2 <90% in 100% O_2, complications of asthma (pneumothorax, pneumomediastinum), and failure despite maximum pharmacotherapy.

The principle for the use of *intubation drugs* should be that (1) the physician should be comfortable with the use of the drugs and (2) the drugs should cause no harm to the patient. Premedication with atropine (0.01 to 0.02 mg/kg) to blunt vagal stimulation should be followed by the administration of a sedative. Narcotics have the theoretical disadvantage of histamine release, and therefore benzodiazepines (e.g., midazolam, diazepam) should be considered. In view of its bronchodilator property, ketamine (1 to 2 mg/kg) is the ideal sedative. Most patients also require a paralyzing agent (1 to 2 mg/kg succinylcholine).

Mechanical ventilation of an asthmatic can be a tremendous challenge. Patients should be *volume ventilated* to ensure sufficient alveolar ventilation during periods of changing airway resistance. Because the phase of expiration in asthmatics is prolonged, the respiratory rate and inspiratory time should be adjusted to *allow for sufficient exhalation.* This limits air trapping, "auto-PEEP," and the possibility of a pneumothorax. PEEP should be routinely avoided due to its effect on elevating FRC, although PEEP may be required in some patients to decrease airway closure during expiration and allow alveolar emptying.

Numerous investigators have examined controlled hypoventilation in adults in an attempt to limit the degree of barotrauma. This *permissive hypercarbia* has been demonstrated to be safe in adults and should be considered in the pediatric patient who is not responding to conventional ventilation in which high pressures are required.

Sedation/Paralysis

Most patients will require continuous sedation and paralysis during mechanical ventilation to facilitate ventilator synchronization. Midazolam infusion should be considered; however, in very severe cases, ketamine infusion (1 to 2 mg/kg/hr) with the added bronchodilator properties could be beneficial. Agents commonly used for paralysis include pancuronium or vecuronium.

OUTCOME

Deaths from asthma often occur out of the hospital, often in children who are steroid dependent and poorly compliant. Mild asthmatics may also experience a sudden severe bronchospastic attack, resulting in cardiac arrest. In-hospital deaths are very uncommon and are often secondary to out-of-hospital cardiac arrests.

Adult Respiratory Distress Syndrome

Adult respiratory distress syndrome (ARDS) is a clinical syndrome of acute respiratory failure characterized by (1) respiratory distress with hypoxemia, intrapulmonary shunting, and decreased lung compliance; (2) radiologic evidence of diffuse pulmonary infiltrates; (3) absence of heart failure, and (4) a precipitating pulmonary or nonpulmonary event. It is estimated that 1% of admissions to the pediatric cardiac care unit are as a result of ARDS. The mortality rate has been reported to be as high as 60%.

PATHOPHYSIOLOGY

Sepsis, trauma, pneumonia, near-drowning, aspiration, and cardiopulmonary arrest are common conditions that initiate a chain of events resulting in acute alveolar damage. Although significant advances have been made in the understanding of the cellular pathophysiology related to ARDS, the exact mechanism leading to alveolar damage is unknown. A simplified view of this dynamic process is provided in Figure 6–13.

CLINICAL MANIFESTATIONS AND DIAGNOSIS

It is important that the clinician recognizes patients who are at increased risk for ARDS so that early diagnosis and management can be initiated; *risk* for ARDS includes sepsis, trauma, near-drowning, aspiration, shock, pneumonia, and burns. Patients will gradually exhibit signs and symptoms of *respiratory distress*. The patient will have increasing cyanosis and tachypnea with diffuse rales or ausculta-

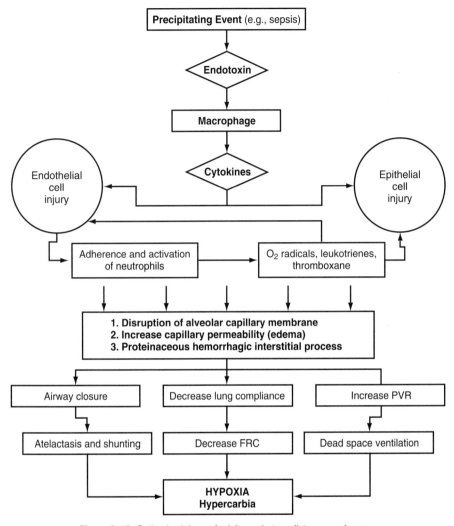

Figure 6–13. Pathophysiology of adult respiratory distress syndrome.

tion. The *chest radiograph* may be normal initially but may gradually progress to pulmonary edema without cardiomegaly.

MANAGEMENT

Although management should be focused on the precipitating factors (e.g., sepsis), the chain of events have already been put in motion in the development of significant lung disease. The primary form of therapy for ARDS is *supportive care*.

General

Oxygen should be administered to keep the SaO_2 at >92% to 95%. Most patients with ARDS will require intubation and mechanical ventilation. These patients are often intubated and ventilated for other reasons (e.g., aspiration or sepsis) and then subsequently develop ARDS.

A *nasogastric tube* should be inserted to decompress the stomach. If patients are kept NPO, consideration should be given to the use of *ranitidine*.

Patients with ARDS require *central vascular access* for monitoring and drug administration. *Fluids* should be restricted to 80% maintenance in view of the pulmonary edema.

For *sedation, midazolam* or a narcotic (by continuous infusion) should be instituted. Depending on the severity of the illness and the degree of ventilatory support, a paralyzing agent (*vecuronium* or *pancuronium*) should be considered.

Monitoring

Monitoring should include cardiorespiratory monitoring; pulse oximetry, to keep SaO_2 at >92% to 95% if possible; CO_2 monitoring, transcutaneously or by the end-tidal method to provide a continuous recording of the adequacy of ventilation; central venous monitoring, to monitor central venous pressure and intravascular volume; radial arterial line, for continuous blood pressure monitoring; echocardiography, to rule out left ventricular failure or congestive heart failure; Swan-Ganz monitoring, for patients requiring significant ventilatory support with high PEEP to provide evidence of left ventricular failure and allow the clinician to define more objectively the "optimal PEEP" (to maximize oxygenation and avoid adverse effects of PEEP); chest radiograph, initially to aid in the diagnosis and at least daily to monitor the progress of the disease and monitor for complications (e.g., pneumothorax); and blood gas analysis, as often as required (with noninvasive monitoring, the frequency could be decreased significantly).

Mechanical Ventilation

It is recommended that patients should receive high tidal volumes (12 to 15 mL/kg), a prolonged inspiratory time, and a slow respiratory rate. This allows for a more uniform distribution of ventilation while limiting the peak airway pressure. *PEEP* continues to be the mainstay of treatment for improvement of oxygenation. PEEP works by stinting open, fluid-filled alveoli and recruiting collapsed lung segments. This results in a decrease in intrapulmonary shunting and a decrease in dead space ventilation, resulting in improvement in oxygenation and ventilation.

The following are suggested guidelines for the use of PEEP:

- High PEEP should not be used prophylactically.
- Rule out cardiac dysfunction.
- Ensure adequate intravascular volume because patients may become hypotensive.
- Begin at 4 to 5 cm H_2O and increase in increments of 3 to 5 cm H_2O until FIO_2 is <60%.

- With incremental increase in PEEP, the following should be frequently evaluated: FIO_2, vital signs, cardiac output, and O_2 delivery, if possible.
- Be prepared to begin inotropic support if the cardiac output falls and does not respond to volume. Decrease PEEP if the cardiac output does not respond.

Novel Therapy

Surfactant. Surfactant therapy has been introduced in some centers as adjunctive therapy if there is failure of conventional ventilation. Few studies have evaluated this form of therapy; however, those patients who did benefit were administered surfactant early (within 48 to 72 hours) in the disease process, before the onset of irreversible changes.

Nitric Oxide. Patients with ARDS have an increase in pulmonary vascular resistance and PAP and significant $\dot{V}/\dot{Q}$ mismatch. In a few studies, nitric oxide has been shown to decrease the pulmonary vascular resistance and improve oxygenation. It is postulated that nitric oxide dilates the pulmonary capillary around the ventilated alveoli, thereby shunting blood away from the unventilated alveoli and consequently improving oxygenation (see Chapter 6.1).

High-Frequency Oscillation. (See Chapter 6.2, Mechanical Ventilation)

Liquid Ventilation. An exciting new ventilator strategy that is undergoing clinical testing is liquid ventilation with perflubron. Liquid ventilation can be done in one of two ways: as partial liquid ventilation or as total liquid ventilation. Partial liquid ventilation is a simple process in which the lungs are filled to a functional residual capacity (FRC) with perflubron and the physician then ventilates the patient with gas tidal volumes using a standard conventional mechanical ventilator. Total, or tidal, liquid ventilation involves the liquid replacement of all gas in the lung as well as in the ventilator. This form of ventilation is more complex, principally due to fluid mechanics.

Perflubron is the only medical-grade perflurocarbon currently available for clinical use and a number of unique physical characteristics make it ideal for liquid ventilation (Table 6–11).

These physical characteristics provide a number of potential clinical benefits, including improved surface tension and pulmonary compliance, lavage, and mobili-

Table 6–11. PHYSICAL CHARACTERISTICS OF PFC

Oxygen	53 mL/100 cc
Carbon dioxide	210 mL/100 37°C and 760 mm Hg
Low surface tension	18 dynes/cm
High density	1.92 g/mL
Positive spreading coefficient	+2.7 dynes/cm
Vapor pressure	1 mm Hg

PFC is colorless, odorless, insoluble in water, immiscible with body fluids, nontoxic, biochemically inert, and chemically stable.

zation of alveolar debris, as well as the ability of perflubron to spread to the nondependent portion of the lungs. The net result is a more optimal lung volume, more homogeneous ventilatory pattern, improved gas exchange, reduced airway pressures, and the potential to mitigate ventilator-induced volutrauma, barotrauma, and oxygen toxicity.

Perflubron is not metabolized by the body but instead leaves the lung through evaporation. This evaporative process is affected by several items, including the vapor pressure of perflubron, minute ventilation, and body temperature.

Preclinical studies have been conducted in a wide variety of animal species, acute lung injury models, and lung sizes. The data from these studies indicate improvements in both gas exchange and pulmonary mechanics. At least one of these studies has tied these changes to an improvement in survival.

Preliminary data from a number of ongoing preclinical investigations have demonstrated the anti-inflammatory properties of perflubron. The mechanisms for this anti-inflammatory effect has not been fully elucidated; however, there are data to suggest both a direct anti-inflammatory effect and a mechanical or barrier effect. The physical properties of perflubron as a dense, immiscible alveolar-filling liquid may prevent the alveolar leak that is so characteristic of the inflammatory cascade.

Perflubron may also prevent nosocomial infection. This may be due to the barrier effect as well as to the fact that bacteria cannot survive for an extended period in perflubron due to the absence of the nutrients required for bacterial growth. Perflubron is very stable and is not inhibited by proteinaceous debris. As the result of the high density, the potential to shunt blood to the nondependent portion of the lung may improve V/Q mismatch. There also is some preliminary evidence to suggest the mitigation of oxygen toxicity.

Initial studies were conducted in adult, pediatric, and neonatal patients on extracorporeal life support (ECLS). Subsequent studies have been conducted in patients who were not receiving ECLS, including premature neonates with hyaline membrane disease and pediatric and adult patients with ARDS. Although these studies were nonrandomized safety studies, preliminary data revealed physiologic improvements in both gas exchange and pulmonary mechanics.

Those studies also showed that partial liquid ventilation with perflubron is clinically well tolerated. Adverse effects that have been considered to possibly be related to the use of perflubron include those frequently seen in these patient populations (e.g., pneumothorax and desaturations due to mucus plugging). Larger studies will be necessary to further assess the significance of these observations. Long-term follow-up (>1 year) has been conducted in a number of neonatal, pediatric, and adult patients with no evidence to suggest any long-term adverse consequences. The higher-than-expected survival rates, together with the above-mentioned safety information, indicate an acceptable safety profile for the intended patient populations, and as a result, large, prospective, randomized, controlled clinical studies are under way in the United States and Canada.

OUTCOME

The mortality from pediatric ARDS continues to be high despite a better understanding of the pathophysiology and more sophisticated technology. Most deaths in patients with ARDS do not have a respiratory cause but rather are due to the triggering event (e.g., sepsis) or multiorgan system failure.

BIBLIOGRAPHY

Andrews CP, Coalson JJ, Smith JD, Johanson WG: Diagnosis of nosocomial bacterial pneumonia in acute, diffuse lung injury. Chest 80:254, 1981.

Chantarojanasiri T, Nichols DG, Rogers MC: Lower airway disease: bronchiolitis and asthma. *In* Rogers MC (ed): Textbook of Pediatric Intensive Care. Baltimore, Williams & Wilkins, 1987, p. 211.

Committee on Infectious Diseases, 1995 to 1996: Reassessment of the indications for ribavirin therapy in respiratory syncytial virus infections. Pediatrics 97:1, 1996.

Donowitz LG: High risk of nosocomial infection in the pediatric critical care patient. Crit Care Med 14:26, 1986.

Eigen H, Gerberding KM: Lower airway disease. *In* Holbrook PR (ed): Textbook of Pediatric Critical Care. Philadelphia, WB Saunders, 1993, p. 517.

Horan TC, White JW, Jarvis WR, et al: Nosocomial infection surveillance, 1984. Centers Dis Control Surveillance Sum 35:17SS, 1986.

Mudge GH, Wriner IM: Water, salt, and ions. *In* Gilman AG, et al (eds): Goodman & Gilman's The Pharmacological Basis of Therapeutics, ed 8. New York, McGraw-Hill, 1990, p. 704.

Reisman J, Galdes-Sebalt M, Kazim F, et al: Frequent administration by inhalation of salbutamol and ipratropium bromide in the initial management of severe acute asthma in children. J Allergy Clin Immunol 81:16, 1988.

Rice TB, Torres A: Pneumonitis and interstitial disease. *In* Fuhrman BP, Zimmerman JJ (eds): Pediatric Critical Care. St. Louis, Mosby-Year Book, 1991, p. 465.

Sarma VJ: Use of ketamine in acute severe asthma. Acta Anaesthesiol Scand 36:106, 1992.

Skoner DP, Fischer TJ, Gormley C, et al: Pediatric predictive index for hospitalization in acute asthma. Ann Emerg Med 16:25, 1987.

6.5 Extracorporeal Membrane Oxygenation

HEIDI J. DALTON, MD

Extracorporeal membrane oxygenation (ECMO) is a modified form of cardio-pulmonary bypass that can support the cardiac and pulmonary functions of patients with severe, presumably reversible, cardiac or pulmonary dysfunction.

Who Is a Candidate?

ECMO has been applied to patients ranging in age from neonatal to adult (usually <60 years old).

GENERAL RECOMMENDATIONS FOR EXTRACORPOREAL MEMBRANE OXYGENATION PATIENTS

General guidelines include the following: gestation of >36 weeks, birthweight of >2 kg, no uncorrectable coagulopathy, absence of severe neurologic dysfunction or severe chromosomal abnormality (trisomy 21 patients have received ECMO), presumed reversible cardiac or pulmonary dysfunction, absence of multiorgan failure for >24 to 48 hours, mechanical ventilation for no greater than 7–10 days before ECMO, and no underlying lethal disease (immunocompromised patients and patients with solid organ or bone marrow transplant are usually excluded from ECMO rescue).

CRITERIA FOR EXTRACORPOREAL MEMBRANE OXYGENATION (ALL AGES)

Other criteria include failure of other available therapies (e.g., surfactant, high-frequency ventilation, inhaled nitric oxide, permissive hypercapnia, and liquid ventilation), oxygenation index (OI) of >40 (or persistently in the range of 25 to 40 and increasing), Pao_2/FIO_2 of <150 mm Hg (normal Pao_2/FIO_2 at FIO_2 21% and Pao_2 100 = 476), persistent air leaks, mean airway pressure of >18 to 20 cm H_2O, peak inspiratory pressure of >35 to 40 cm H_2O, and alveolar-arterial oxygenation difference (A-aDO$_2$) of >610 × 8 hours or >645 × 4 hours (*neonates*) or of >475 for >6 hours (*infants and children*).

For cardiac patients, criteria include severe, presumably reversible cardiac dysfunction despite fluid resuscitation and inotropic support. A majority of cardiac ECMO is performed in the postoperative period after repair of congenital heart defects. Patients with myocarditis or pretransplantation or post-transplantation heart patients are also supported.

DURATION OF EXTRACORPOREAL MEMBRANE OXYGENATION

The duration for neonates is persistent pulmonary hypertension of the newborn (PPHN), 3 to 7 days and congenital diaphragmatic hernia (CDH), 7 to 14 days. For pediatric or adult patients, the usual duration is 2 to 3 weeks, but successful runs of >6 weeks' duration have been reported.

When to stop ECMO is determined by complications that require removal from ECMO (e.g., severe bleeding, persistent infection, neurologic damage) or determination that recovery of cardiac or pulmonary function will not occur.

In cardiac patients, if there is no recovery of cardiac function by 3 days of ECMO, then recovery is not likely. Consider listing the patient to undergo heart transplantation or discuss withdrawal of support at a maximum of 5 to 7 days.

Common Indicators of Lung Injury

ALVEOLAR-TO-ARTERIAL OXYGENATION DIFFERENCE

The alveolar to arterial oxygenation difference (A-aDO$_2$) is calculated as the following:

$$PaO_2 \text{ (expected)} = FIO_2 \text{ (barometric pressure} = \text{water vapor pressure)} - PaCO_2/RQ$$

where the respiratory quotient (RQ) of 0.8 is often assumed to be 1 and is omitted from the calculation. The A-aDO$_2$ would be the observed PaO$_2$ subtracted from the expected PaO$_2$.

- Example: For a sick neonate at sea level, PaO$_2$ = 40 mm Hg, PaCO$_2$ = 50 mm Hg, and FIO$_2$ = 100% A-aDO$_2$ = [1.0 (760 − 47) − 50] − 40 = 623 mm Hg.
- Example: For a normal adult at sea level, PaO$_2$ = 100 mm Hg, PaCO$_2$ = 40 mm Hg, breathing room air, the A-aDO$_2$ = [0.21 (760 − 47) − 40] − 100 = 9.7 mm Hg.

OXYGENATION INDEX

The oxygen index (OI) is calculated as the following:

$$(\text{Mean airway pressure} \times FIO_2)/PaO_2$$

- Example: Mean airway pressure = 20 mm Hg, FIO$_2$ = 100%, and PaO$_2$ = 50 mm Hg, so OI = (20 × 100)/50 = 40.

If the OI is <25, the patient should have a good outcome. If the OI is 25 to 40, the chance of death is 50%; however, the trend of the OI is most important in this group. If the OI continues to be in the 30s for >4 hours, then the patient is likely to get worse. If the OI is >40, the chance of death is >80%. If the OI remains at >40, the physician should strongly consider ECMO rescue.

The OI takes into account the amount of mean airway pressure and FIO$_2$ used to obtain a certain PaO2 response and thus may be a better indicator than is the A-aDO$_2$ of how "sick" the patient is. It is excellent for determining a trend over time.

Types of Extracorporeal Membrane Oxygenation

VENOARTERIAL

Advantages

Support of Cardiac and Pulmonary Functions. Increase in the drainage to the ECMO circuit provides more well-oxygenated blood to return to the patient; decrease in the flow to the ECMO circuit allows more blood to enter the native pulmonary circuit. In patients with severe respiratory disease whose lungs heal and who are able to effectively exchange gas, as ECMO flow is decreased, adequate oxygenation and CO$_2$ removal are noted.

Excellent Oxygenation and CO$_2$ Elimination. Oxygenation is controlled by the proportion of blood bypassed into ECMO circuit. "If the O's are low, increase the flow."

CO$_2$ removal is controlled by the amount of gas sweeping through the oxygenator to remove CO$_2$ from the blood. Usually, about 80% support of cardiac output by ECMO is sufficient for adequate circulatory and gas exchange. Initial flow goals are 100 to 120 mL/kg/min for neonates, 70 to 90 mL/kg/min for older children, and 70 mL/kg/min for adults.

Usually One Surgical Site Is Needed. In venoarterial access for neonates and small children, the right common carotid artery into the arch of the aorta and the right internal jugular vein to right atrium sites are used.

In large children and adults, for arterial access, the right common carotid artery into the arch of the aorta and the femoral artery to the iliac or descending aorta sites are used. The axillary or subclavian artery is rarely used. For venous access, the right internal jugular vein to the right atrium and the femoral vein to the interior vena cava/right atrium junction sites are used. The subclavian to the right atrium site is rarely used.

Disadvantages

Ligation (or perhaps repair at decannulation) of a major artery is required. Carotid ligation or repair has a potential risk for stroke. Also, debris, clots, and air returning from the ECMO circuit go directly into the arterial circulation and may cause brain damage.

With the femoral artery, adequate oxygenation to the brain must be ensured. Follow the patient's neurologic status with the use of a pulse oximeter on the ear or nose and measurement of venous oxygen saturation in superior vena cava or jugular bulb. If the femoral artery is used for return from ECMO circuit, remember that arterial ECMO flow will mix with aortic flow from the left ventricle; oxygenation will be determined by the mix of these two flows. Saturation will not be 100% except in arterial circuit distal to ECMO flow return (i.e., lower extremities). Under most conditions, oxygen saturations of >80% will be noted in upper body and provide adequate oxygen delivery.

The improper positioning of the aortic cannula can lead to intimal damage and aneurysm formation, aortic valve damage, or coronary artery ischemia.

VENOVENOUS

Venovenous ECMO maintains the normal flow of blood through the body. Venous drainage usually occurs via the right atrium to the ECMO circuit and then back to the patient via another venous site. This is used primarily in neonates and in older children and adults. It requires adequate native cardiac function to provide circulatory support.

Advantages

Venovenous ECMO maintains the normal flow of blood through body; the debris, clots, and air return to the venous circulation and is trapped in the lungs. Well-oxygenated blood flow to the pulmonary artery (possibly decreasing pulmonary vascular resistance) occurs. No arterial ligation or repair is needed. Excellent CO_2 removal occurs, even at a low flow.

Disadvantages

Venovenous ECMO requires adequate cardiac function to provide support and often requires two surgical sites. Malpositioning of venous cannulas can lead to excessive recirculation of oxygenated blood in the ECMO circuit and poor support to the patient. Only 30% to 50% of total cardiac output support can be provided. Lower Pao_2 and arterial saturations must be acceptable (normally, >85% arterial saturation cannot be obtained). If adequate oxygen delivery is maintained, the patient will have venous saturation of >70%, no acidosis, and good perfusion.

Sites. For neonates, a double-lumen single cannula (14F only) is available. It should be placed via the right internal jugular vein into the superior vena cava/right atrial junction; drainage occurs via the proximal lumen, and reinfusion occurs via the distal lumen.

For older children and adults, drainage usually occurs via the right internal jugular vein to the superior vena cava/right atrium junction. Reinfusion occurs via the saphenous/femoral vein to the inferior vena cava/right atrial junction. The bilateral saphenous/femoral veins may also be used for drainage and return. Percutaneous cannulation sets are available in kits with cannulas of sizes 15F to 21F.

Starting Extracorporeal Membrane Oxygenation

YOUR ROLE DURING CANNULATION

- *Be there to watch the patient!* Often, the cannulating physician is too busy to watch the patient's vital signs and keep them stable during the procedure.
- Have dosages calculated and code medications ready.
- Have a designated IV access line available to give medications/fluids during cannulation.
- Have volume ready (e.g., blood, albumin, and so on).
- Be sure patient has recently received a dose of a paralytic/analgesic agent before beginning the procedure.
- Check calcium and potassium levels and pH of primed circuit blood; severe hypocalcemia, hyperkalemia, or acidosis may cause the patient to arrest once ECMO is instituted. Additional calcium or bicarbonate may be added to the circuit to adjust electrolytes and the metabolic state of blood.
- Check $Paco_2$ and Pao_2 of primed circuit blood before ECMO; if the patient has high $Paco_2$ before ECMO, check to ensure that $Paco_2$ in circuit prime is also high to prevent a rapid fall in $Paco_2$ on initiation of ECMO, leading to severe changes in brain blood flow.
- Check activated clotting time (ACT) for patient before ECMO. Normal ACT is 80 to 120 seconds. For cannulation, ACT is usually >300 seconds. Maintenance ACT on ECMO is 180 to 220 seconds (can drop to 160 to 180 if bleeding is a problem). If patient has disseminated intravascular coagulopathy or coagulopathy before ECMO, the initial loading dose of heparin may be adjusted to <100 units/kg. If cannulation is difficult and prolonged, remember to recheck patient ACT to see whether additional heparin is required.

- Have radiographic equipment accessible when cannulation is complete to take an immediate film to check cannula placement.
- Assign someone to go to radiology and bring back the film immediately. Do not let the surgeon leave until cannula placement is checked.

WHAT TO DO DURING EARLY PHASE OF EXTRACORPOREAL MEMBRANE OXYGENATION

1. Vasodilation secondary to complement activation is frequent and may require rapid volume expansion to obtain adequate ECMO flow. Have extra packed red blood cells, whole blood, fresh frozen plasma (FFP), and albumin on hand. Platelet aggregation in the circuit also occurs, so have platelets available to administer.
2. The venous saturation monitor may be the best indicator to follow during initiation of ECMO. Follow it to determine when adequate flow has been achieved. Normal venous saturation is 70% to 75%.
3. Obtain preoxygenation and postoxygenation arterial blood gases to ensure that membrane oxygenator is functioning adequately and that ECMO flow is sufficient for the patient's oxygen delivery requirements.
4. Begin turning ventilator settings down to target levels.
5. If using venovenous ECMO, reduce ventilator settings slowly. If using venoarterial ECMO, you may reduce ventilator settings more quickly.
6. Check electrolyte levels, calcium, complete blood count (with platelet count), and prothrombin and partial thromboplastin times within the first 2 hours of ECMO. Replace platelets if <100,000. Consider FFP if partial thromboplastin time is >150 seconds (try to keep it between 60 and 150).
7. Discontinue inotropic drips once ECMO is begun if blood pressure is stable or high (be careful when doing this if patient is on venovenous ECMO).
8. Write new orders for ECMO:

- Emergency ventilator settings for patient if ECMO has to be emergently stopped (should be posted at bedside).
- Order platelet counts q6–12h. Keep platelets at >100,000 (>150,000 if bleeding).
- Watch electrolytes; usually patients need less sodium and more potassium (possible secondary hypoaldosteronism from altered kidney flow).
- Check prothrombin and partial thromboplastin times and fibrinogen daily. If partial thromboplastin time is >150, consider FFP. If fibrinogen is low, consider the use of cryoprecipitate.
- Be aware of what parameters are desired for Pao_2, $Paco_2$, ACTs, and venous saturation (usually ECMO specialists have a sheet of parameters that physicians fill out daily; specialists adjust ECMO flow, gas concentrations. and heparin drip to maintain parameters within accepted ranges).
8. Omit heparin in other drips and lines.
9. Do not perform needlesticks or invasive procedures without meticulous attention to hemostasis (patient is fully heparinized) and checking with the attending first.

Patient Management

VENTILATOR SETTINGS

Neonates and Pediatric Patients to ≈1 Year of Age. High PEEP (10 to 14 cm H_2O) may maintain FRC and shorten length of ECMO run. Restrict peak inflating pressure (PIP) to <25 to 30 cm H_2O. Rate should be 10 bpm. The use of a jet or an oscillator can also maintain lung volume without as much barotrauma. In neonates, total collapse of lungs can be allowed to seal air leaks (patient placed on continuous positive airway pressure [CPAP] or T-piece alone). Most air leaks seal within 48 hours of such treatment.

Older Pediatric and Adult Patients. High PEEP recommended (15 to 20 cm H_2O may be required). A good rule of thumb is to place ventilator settings so that mean airway pressure is approximately two thirds of that of the last pre-ECMO ventilator setting. Maintain PIP at <30 to 35 cm H_2O, even if this means using high PEEP. Expect the tidal volume that is obtained to be small due to small delta P. Use 6 to 10 breaths/min. Allowing the patient to wake up and breathe spontaneously is helpful; use pressure support to augment lung recruitment. If patient 30 kg, a jet or an oscillator may be useful.

Chest physiotherapy in the form of vibration, suctioning, and lavage is helpful to remove secretions. Bronchoscopy also is beneficial. Leaving the patient awake and using pressure support ventilation may also improve lung recruitment. Measurement of exhaled tidal volume and expired CO_2 is helpful; an increase in tidal volume and expired CO_2 may indicate recovery of viable lung tissue. Reexpansion of collapsed lungs may be very difficult and may require very high levels of PIP and PEEP and hand-ventilation. We have tried the use of a jet or an oscillator to improve lung recruitment with variable success.

MEDICATIONS

Sedation. Remember that continuous infusions may build up in fat stores and that some drug is lost via membrane (or hemofilter if in use). However, bolus drugs are not as efficient for nursing care. Commonly used medications include lorazepam (Ativan) (0.1–0.2 mg/kg PRN; high-dose infusion can lead to propylene glycol toxicity), midazolam (0.1–0.2 mg/kg; frequently requires escalating dose; long-term infusion is reported to give neurologic abnormalities; will be off patent soon; now is more expensive but the most popular agent used in the intensive care unit), diazepam (Valium) (0.1–0.2 mg/kg; cheap and effective; a bolus is preferred but not often popular with nursing staff), and other drugs, such as phenobarbital and pentobarbital.

Analgesics. Morphine (0.1 to 0.5 mg/kg) is usually infused; remember that it can build up in fat stores. Doses required over time are often much higher than expected. Fentanyl (1–50 μg/kg/hr) is usually infused; remember that tachyphylaxis occurs and the dose needs to be increased. This is more expensive than morphine.

Paralytics. It is best to let the patient wake up and move (some) and breathe on his or her own. This also allows good neurologic monitoring. In Europe, patients are awake, eat, watch TV, and do schoolwork. Maintenance of cannula position and safety is the only true restriction to movement. If needed, pancuronium bromide, vecuronium, atracurium, or metocurine iodide can be used. Remember that long-term neuropathy can occur, especially if the patient is also receiving steroids.

Antibiotics. To treat what is known is the best course but hard to follow. Broad-spectrum antibiotics may lead to resistant pathologic bacteria or fungus. If an antibiotic must be used to prevent cannula infection, cefazolin sodium is recommended. For fungal infections, if there is a positive blood culture from the circuit for fungus, you can try cutting out and replacing the circuit, but a fungal blood infection in a patient on ECMO is usually lethal.

NUTRITION

Nutrition is one of most important keys to success. We try to use enteral nutrition as soon as it is tolerated. Nasoduodenal (ND) placement may be necessary if nasogastric feedings are not tolerated. Also, a gut motility agent, such as metoclopramide monohydrochloride monohydrate or cisapride, can be used. Maintain adequate calories with hyperalimentation and lipids. Follow carbohydrate load and the nutritionist's advice for proper formula. If fluid administration with adequate nutrition needs is too great, consider hemofiltration to remove excess fluids. If the patient is unable to tolerate enteral feedings, administer an H_2-blocker or antacid to prevent stress ulcerations. The use of low-dose infusions into gut at even 2 to 5 mL/hr may help maintain mucosal integrity and prevent bacterial translocation.

ANTICOAGULATION

ACTs are still used primarily to adjust heparin level. Daily prothrombin and partial thromboplastin times and fibrinogen level can guide replacement of factors and help prevent bleeding. We give FFP to keep partial thromboplastin at <150 seconds and to keep fibrinogen at >150. In cases of severe bleeding, heparin has been discontinued for >12 hours at flows of 5 liters, and no clotting was observed. In patients with a high likelihood of bleeding, aminocaproic acid has been helpful. Load with 100 mg/kg over 20 minutes and run drip at 10 to 15 mg/kg/hr. Usually, the aminocaproic acid drip is discontinued in 2 to 3 days. Often, increased circuit clotting occurs with aminocaproic acid use. In anecdotal reports, other agents, such as aprotonin, vasopressin, and estrogen, have also been helpful.

WEANING

Venoarterial

The traditional method of weaning is to set a goal Pao_2 or Svo_2 and to decrease ECMO flow rate by 20 to 50 mL/hr or every few hours (may drop flows faster if desired). For patients <10 kg, "idling" flow is considered to be 250 mL/min. For larger patients, minimal flows of 500 mL/min are recommended to prevent clotting or stagnant flow in circuit. When a patient is at <50% of ECMO support, ventilator settings may need to be increased to provide support.

Typical ventilator settings for a neonate are FIO_2 of <50%, PIP of <30 cm H_2O, PEEP of 5 to 10 cm H_2O, and intermittent mandatory ventilation (IMV) of 20 to 35 breaths/min. A jet ventilator and an oscillator may also be used to wean off ECMO. Patients will have to be returned to conventional ventilation at some point.

Settings for pediatric patients are FIO_2 of <50%, PIP of <35 cm H_2O, PEEP of 5 to 10 cm H_2O, and IMV of 20 of 30 breaths/min. Mean airway pressure is <15 cm H_2O. A jet or an oscillator can also be used to wean off ECMO.

For adults, settings are PIP of <35 cm H_2O, PEEP of 5 to 10 cm H_2O, IMV of 15 to 25 breaths/min, and FIO_2 of <60%. Mean airway pressure is <18 cm H_2O. Adults and older patients may benefit from tracheotomy while on ECMO to improve pulmonary toilet.

Note that in large patients and adults, clamping off the cannula for trial should include flushing and filling them with heparin. However, reinstitution of ECMO, or "flashing," cannula may still send showers of emboli to patient. Be sure to maintain anticoagulated status during trial and probably for several hours after decannulation to prevent thrombus formation.

Venovenous

When the patient is ready for trial, increase the vent settings to desired post-ECMO level and then cap off the oxygenator. Cease the gas flow to the membrane, and cap the gas outlet port. No gas exchange across membrane will occur, and the patient must do all of the "work" on his or her own. Follow the blood gases; if the gases are acceptable and the patient is hemodynamically stable, consider decannulation. Remember that if the gas to the membrane is off for long, the gas phase of the membrane envelope will collapse and will need to be reopened if ECMO is reinstituted. Sometimes, membranes will get stagnant areas in them during the period of capping off and may not be as efficient when ECMO is reinstituted.

Basic Troubleshooting

POOR SYSTEMIC OXYGENATION AND OXYGEN DELIVERY

Too Little Flow

Venous pressure is increased by volume administration.

Hazard. Increased volume may lead to volume overload, edema, and impaired healing of pulmonary tissue. Increased circulating volume may lead to increased blood flow into pulmonary circuit, thus increasing the amount of desaturated blood and lowering oxygen delivery (see Fluid Overload).

Improper Placement of Drainage Cannula. Cardiac ECHO may be helpful to determine the exact placement of cannula. In larger patients, a transesophageal ECHO may provide more accurate information.

Increase Gravity Drainage. Raise the height of the patient above the pump; you can use shock blocks under the legs of the bed. We have also placed air mattresses under the patient and inflated them to increase height. The most important determinant of venous drainage remains adequate venous pressure and cannula/circuit drainage size.

Wrong-Size Cannula or Circuit. Cannulas can handle only a limited amount of flow. Additional drainage cannulas (in a separate site) or larger venous drainage tubing may be needed. Remember that increased venous drainage may help increase flow, but you must monitor the inlet/outlet pressures of the oxygenator to determine when the recommended pressure and flow for oxygenator are reached; the chances of oxygenator failure or circuit rupture are higher at very high flows and pressures.

Fluid Overload

Systemic oxygenation is determined by a mixture of well-saturated blood returning from ECMO circuit and that returning from the patient's lungs and ejected from the left ventricle (presumably poorly saturated in bad respiratory failure); increased blood flow through the native heart/lung circuit will reduce systemic oxygen saturation. *Remember that the venous saturation and overall patient status are more important in determining adequate oxygen delivery than is PaO_2 or measured oxygen saturation.*

Example. Flow via native lungs with severe respiratory failure and low ventilator settings will not saturate blood much more than with the venous saturation with which they are perfused. If venous saturation is 70%, the blood returning from the lungs may be only 75% saturated.

Flow from ECMO circuit is 100% saturated on return to patient.

If 50% flow is to circuit and 50% is through the lungs, total oxygen saturation will be (75% + 100%)/2, or 87.5%.

To increase the saturation of blood, flow into the circuit must be increased (assuming that the lungs cannot contribute further) or the total circulating volume must be decreased to thus reduce the amount going through the lungs. This can be done with diuretics, fluid restriction, and hemofiltration. Remember that if the circulating volume is decreased too much, oxygen consumption will increase and venous saturation will fall (indicating too little oxygen delivery) or the ECMO circuit flow may not be able to be maintained at the current level. A falling venous oxygen saturation may indicate that too little circulating volume is available to handle the needs of the tissue.

Failing Oxygenator

If the oxygenator is unable to exchange gas, the blood that is leaving the oxygenator may not be 100% saturated. Increase the FIO_2 to membranes, and recheck preoxygenation and postoxygenation blood gases. A decrease in the postoxygenation PaO_2 value of ≥ 100 may indicate the need for a new oxygenator. Increasing the sweep gas flow will remove water vapor build up and improve oxygenation.

Increased Metabolic Rate and Oxygen Delivery Need

If increased flow fails to benefit the patient with increased metabolic rate and oxygen delivery need, cool the patient (approximately 35°C), increase sedation, induce paralysis, and/or transfuse with packed red blood cells (if hematocrit is <40).

As a last resort, if adequate oxygenation cannot be maintained with ECMO circuit manipulations and decreasing oxygen consumption, FIO_2 to lungs or ventilator settings may need to be increased to obtain any beneficial contribution by the lungs. Remember that the goal of ECMO is to use the least-toxic ventilator settings possible to provide optimal healing of pulmonary tissue.

Carbon Dioxide Retention

Failing Oxygenator. If the patient's PCO_2 is high, try increasing sweep gas flow through oxygenator. Recheck preoxygenation and postoxygenation blood gases after sweep gas is elevated for 15 to 30 minutes and see whether CO_2 removal is enhanced. If PCO_2 is still elevated or the difference between premembrane and postmembrane PCO_2 values is small, consider changing the oxygenator. Also consider changing the oxygenator to one that is a larger size if PCO_2 values are always higher than expected. In large patients, the use of two oxygenators will increase membrane surface area to enhance gas exchange.

Increased CO_2 Production. Follow maneuvers to decrease metabolic rate: cooling patient, sedation, and paralysis. Decreasing carbohydrate load in enteral or hyperalimentation preparations may also be helpful.

CO_2 Still Too High. Remember that permissive hypercarbia is not life threatening. Accept higher $PaCO_2$, and give bicarbonate if pH <7.20. You may also have to increase ventilator settings if the situation is severe. Sometimes, the use of a high-frequency ventilator (e.g., jet, oscillator) is helpful in such patients to achieve some gas exchange without inducing additional barotrauma.

Common Catastrophes

LOSS OF VENOUS RETURN TO CIRCUIT

Problem. Patient has low venous blood volume.
Solution. Administer fluids if the patient is hypovolemic; consider inotropy if heart failure is evident.

Problem. There is a kinked cannula or venous return line.
Solution. Relieve the kink or obstruction.

Problem. The right atrium collapsed due to pneumothorax, pneumopericardium, or pericardial tamponade.
Solution. Immediately administer volume to improve venous return and maintain some ECMO flow.

Final. Correct the underlying cause (place chest tube, drain tamponade, and so on). When performing a procedure on a heparinized ECMO patient, be meticulous about hemostasis. Insertion of a needle into the chest to relieve presumed pneumothorax is not recommended; it may lead to profuse bleeding if a vessel is hit.

CIRCUIT RUPTURE

1. *Call for help!*
2. Clamp patient off circuit immediately (usually already done by ECMO technician).
3. Place patient on emergency ventilator settings.
4. Give volume and code medications as needed.
5. Ensure that no air is in circuit once fixed before returning patient to ECMO.

ACCIDENTAL DECANNULATION

1. Hold pressure on site.
2. Call for help (usually surgical).
3. Give volume and code medications as needed.
4. Place patient on emergency ventilator settings.
5. Try to maintain ECMO circuit flow through bridge to prevent circuit from clotting during recannulation.

BIBLIOGRAPHY

Dalton HJ, Fuhrman BP, Siewers RD, del Nido P, Thompson AE: Extracorporeal membrane oxygenation for cardiac rescue in children with severe myocardial dysfunction. Crit Care Med 21:1020–1028, 1993.

Dalton HJ, Thompson AE: Extracorporeal membrane oxygenation (ECMO). *In* Fuhrman B, Zimmerman J (eds): Pediatric Critical Care. St. Louis, Mosby-Year Book, 1991.

Fuhrman BP, Dalton HJ: Progress in pediatric extracorporeal membrane oxygenation. Crit Care Clin 8:191–202, 1992.

Morton AB, Dalton HJ, Thompson AE, et al: Extracorporeal membrane oxygenation for pediatric respiratory failure: five-year experience at the University of Pittsburgh. Crit Care Med 22:1659, 1994.

6.6 Use of Nitric Oxide in Pulmonary Hypertension

NARENDRA C. SINGH, BSc, MB, BS, FRCPC, FAAP
CATHERINE BURKE-TREMBLAY, RRT
JOHN B. GORDON, MD, CM

Nitric oxide (NO) is a potent dilator of vascular smooth muscle that likely represents an important endothelium-derived relaxing factor (EDRF). Recent interest has focused on inhaled NO as a pulmonary vasodilator. This chapter provides a comprehensive overview of the issues surrounding the safe and effective use of NO in the clinical setting, the pathophysiology and limitations of current therapy in pulmonary hypertension (PH), the use of NO as a "selective pulmonary vasodilator," and a safe and effective delivery system for NO in the clinical setting.

Pulmonary Hypertension: General Approach and Limitations of Current Therapy

PATHOPHYSIOLOGY

PH, with its attendant morbidity and mortality, is a common end result of several diseases ranging from acute respiratory failure to congenital heart disease. In adults, PH is defined as a mean pulmonary artery pressure (PAP) of >25 mm Hg. However, *this definition is of little use in pediatric patients* because the normal mean PAP changes with age. Furthermore, simply measuring mean PAP provides little information concerning the etiology of PH. Therefore, the diagnosis and management of neonatal and pediatric PH are better approached by applying Ohm's law to the pulmonary circuit. Ohm's Law states that $Q = \Delta P/R$ (Q is blood flow, ΔP is pressure difference between two ends of a vessel and R is resistance to flow). Although this may be simplistic, it can be readily appreciated from this formula that mean PAP may be elevated due to increased pulmonary blood flow (e.g., large left-to-right shunting with congenital heart disease), increased downstream pressure (e.g., mitral stenosis), or increased pulmonary vascular resistance (PVR). The two former causes are relatively uncommon and are generally the purview of the cardiovascular surgeon. Various factors may increase PVR. *Poiseuille's law* states (among other things) that resistance to flow of a fluid through a tube varies inversely with the fourth power of the radius of the tube (see Fig. 6–7, Chapter 6.3). Thus, the most important factor causing an increase in PVR is a decrease in the inner diameter of small resistance arteries. This decrease in diameter can be relatively fixed, such as occurs with advanced vascular remodeling in primary PH. Therapy in this case is often limited to lung transplantation. The decrease in diameter can also be due to active vasoconstriction, typically seen in patients with increased arterial muscularization and/or diminished endogenous modulator activity. Medical management aimed at improving pulmonary blood flow is the mainstay of therapy for PH in this situation.

STANDARD THERAPY FOR PULMONARY HYPERTENSION

The initial treatment of PH includes sedation, optimization of cardiac function, and the reversal of hypoxemia. If mechanical ventilation is required, *sedation* is increased to minimize adrenergic output, and muscle relaxation is often initiated. The *Pao_2 is maintained at >100 mm Hg,* particularly if this can be achieved without inducing O_2 toxicity. In addition, treatment of the disease that precipitated the increase in PVR is initiated. However, despite these measures, PVR frequently remains increased, necessitating the institution of vasodilator therapy.

Alkalosis therapy has been widely used in the treatment of neonatal and pediatric PH over the past 15 to 20 years. This is based on studies showing that hypocarbic or metabolic alkalosis (pH 7.50 to 7.60) causes acute pulmonary vasodilation in both animals and humans. However, hyperventilation may result in significant barotrauma; hypocarbia may significantly decrease cerebral blood flow; and alkalosis has recently been shown to enhance pulmonary vascular reactivity in some animal models. Thus, some groups have suggested that alkalosis may not be the ideal first-line therapy for PH. Furthermore, even when alkalosis therapy is used, PVR often remains high or subsequently increases, necessitating other interventions.

Several *intravenous vasodilators* have been used over the years in the acute management of PH. Of these, sodium nitroprusside and prostacyclin exemplify many of the advantages and disadvantages of the intravenous vasodilators. On the positive side, both are potent vasodilators with short half-lives, making it possible to titrate them to effect. In addition, their modes of action are relatively well known. Prostacyclin acts on the vascular smooth muscle by stimulating adenylate cyclase and possibly by increasing guanylate cyclase activity and K^+ channel opening. Sodium nitroprusside is an endothelium-independent vasodilator that also stimulates guanylate cyclase activity in vascular smooth muscle and may increase K^+ channel opening (see below). However, on the negative side, both of these agents also cause systemic vasodilation and impair hypoxic pulmonary vasoconstriction. Thus, infusion of either may result in significant systemic hypotension and worsened ventilation/perfusion matching with profound hypoxemia. Thus, a "selective" pulmonary vasodilator for use in the treatment of PH has long been sought.

NITRIC OXIDE

In 1980, Furchgott and Zawadzki coined the term "endothelium-derived relaxing factor" when they reported that acetylcholine caused relaxation of aortic rings and strips when the endothelium was intact but not after it had been removed. In the 1980s, several groups demonstrated that this *EDRF was NO* or a very similar compound. Endothelium-derived NO (EDNO) has subsequently been shown to be a potent modulator of pulmonary vasoconstriction due to hypoxia, sepsis, and other pressor stimuli. The mechanism of EDNO activity has been fairly well described. Various stimuli (e.g., the endothelium-dependent vasodilators histamine and bradykinin, shear stress, and others) can increase constitutive NO synthase activity within the endothelial cell. This NO synthase catalyzes the Ca^{2+}-dependent conversion of L-arginine to L-citrulline and EDNO. EDNO then traverses from the endothelium to the adjoining vascular smooth muscle, where in the presence of Ca^{2+}, it enhances guanylate cyclase activity, resulting in increased cyclic GMP (cGMP). cGMP then induces vascular relaxation through relatively poorly understood mechanisms (Fig. 6–14).

Because NO is readily bound to and inactivated by hemoglobin, the vascular response to EDNO is very localized, and exogenous NO has little vasodilator properties when administered intravenously. This property of NO led Zapol and colleagues to investigate the potential use of inhaled NO in the treatment of PH. It was hypothesized that inhaled NO would traverse the alveolar epithelium to the vascular smooth muscle, thus inducing vascular relaxation, and any NO that got beyond the vascular smooth muscle and endothelium to the bloodstream would quickly be inactivated. Indeed, they and others found in various animal models that inhaled NO markedly attenuated pulmonary vasoconstriction induced by hypoxia or sepsis without altering systemic blood pressure. Several groups have subsequently shown that inhaled NO in concentrations as low as <6 to 20 parts per million (ppm) reduced PVR in infants, children, and adults. Furthermore, because inhaled NO is delivered only to ventilated blood vessels, it improves rather than worsens ventilation/perfusion matching. Thus, inhaled NO has been termed a "selective" pulmonary vasodilator.

CLINICAL APPLICATIONS

Indications

Inhaled NO has been demonstrated to be a potent selective pulmonary vasodilator in some patients with *PH*. The greatest benefit so far has been seen in

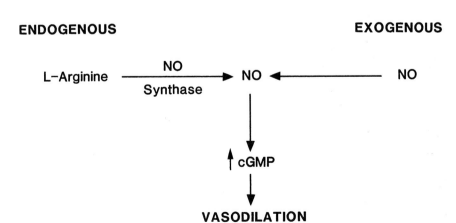

Figure 6–14. Endogenous and exogenous mechanisms of NO activity.

neonates with PH of various etiologies (sepsis, muconium aspiration, and so on). Also, NO is being evaluated and shows great promise in the perioperative period in patients with *congenital heart disease* and PH. There have also been reports of some benefit in patients with *adult respiratory distress syndrome.*

Equipment

The first goal in designing a delivery system for NO delivery is to make it easy to use, reliable, and safe. This portion of the chapter focuses on analyzers, circuits, and scavenger systems.

Analyzers:

Inhaled NO can be measured by two methods: chemiluminescence and electrochemical detection.

The *chemiluminescence analyzer* works on the principle that NO reacts with ozone, thereby generating photons that are then detected and expressed as a concentration in ppm. The chemiluminescence method is the accepted gold standard for NO measurement; however, it was designed for industrial use and is expensive and bulky and has a high noise level. With the *electrochemical analyzer*, NO reacts with water, resulting in the generation of an electrical current that is expressed as a concentration in ppm. The electrochemical analyzers are compact, relatively inexpensive, and noise free. It is imperative that regardless of the analyzer chosen for clinical use, alarms are present to allow safe delivery of NO. *The ideal analyzer is small, easy to operate and calibrate, and has alarms.* It should be unaffected by water vapor and FIO_2 and should give precise and continuous readings.

Circuit:

It is necessary to develop safe, accurate, and adaptable systems to deliver NO to patients with PH. There are two methods for the delivery of NO (Figs. 6–15 and 6–16). Purified NO in concentrations of 450 to 1000 ppm, with balanced nitrogen, is available in patient delivery tanks. A double-stage stainless steel regulator with a silicone O ring between the tank and the regulator is attached to the cylinder. A stainless steel flowmeter designed for use with NO is attached to the regulator. Figure 6–15 illustrates how the NO/nitrogen tank connects to the inlet on one side of the blender and is balanced on the other side by a 50 psi wall O2 source. From the blender outlet, a high-pressure hose attaches to the high-pressure inlet of the ventilator. Variations in the patient's minute ventilation and compressible volume in the circuit make this an alternative selection for larger patients. One potential problem with this system is the fact that at low concentrations of NO (10 to 20 ppm) and at FIO_2 of 0.21, small changes in the nitric blender can result in marked changes in NO concentration. Figure 6–16 illustrates that the NO/nitrogen blend is connected to the inspiratory limb of the ventilator circuit via a T connector. This simplified delivery reduces the time that NO is exposed in the circuit with O_2, with a consequent reduction in NO_2 production.

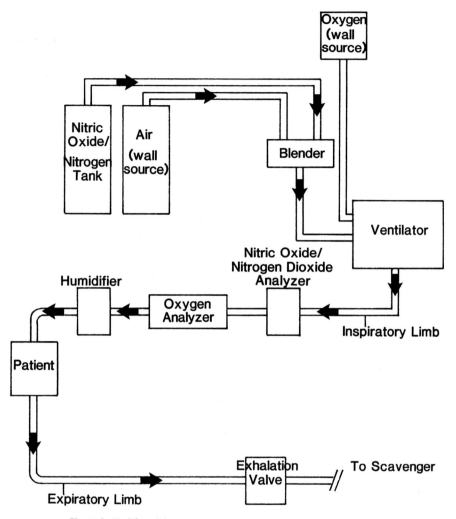

Figure 6–15. NO tank is connected to the inlet on one side of the blender.

Scavenger

An effective expiratory gas scavenger is necessary to prevent NO and NO_2 from being released into the ambient air. A concentration of NO and NO_2 may be detected in expired gas, in part from contamination of the expiratory circuit by inspired gas and endogenous protection. The scavenging system acts as a capacitor from which the gas can be removed by a wall vacuum.

Exhaled gas is collected through an open-ended coaxial circuit, which is connected to the exhalation port, via a 22-mm connector. The fresh-gas flow portion of the coaxial circuit is connected to a vacuum regulator. A continuous

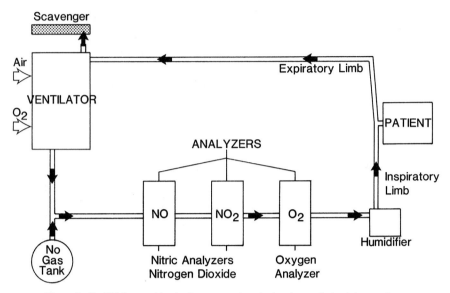

Figure 6–16. NO/nitrogen blender is connected to the inspiratory limb of the ventilator.

vacuum source is set at enough negative pressure to render a zero concentration of NO_2 and NO when analyzed. To monitor the effectiveness of the scavenger system, NO must be periodically measured from either the open end of the expiratory port or in the room at any time during its use. The NO scavenger system is shown in Figure 6–17. Regardless of the delivery system chosen by the clinician, it is imperative that the exhaled gases be scavenged.

Patient Care While on Nitric Oxide

Table 6–12 suggests a concentration at which to begin and action to be taken if the desired O_2 saturation is not attained. NO may be weaned to a minimal level if an optimal saturation is attained and there is no significant evidence of right-to-left shifting. NO may be weaned off from 1 to 5 ppm after evidence of some reversal of the disease process or evidence of methemoglobinemia of >5%. It is not uncommon for neonates to be exquisitely sensitive to even 1 ppm, therefore necessitating resumption of NO.

Limitations, Toxicity, and Monitoring (Table 6–13)

Although several studies have shown that inhaled NO can attenuate pulmonary vasoconstriction without inducing hypotension or worsening oxygenation, the drug is not a panacea. Some patients exhibit a marked and gratifying improvement; however, *others do not seem to respond at all.* The current success rates with the use of inhaled NO in infants and children ranges from 20% to >80%. Several factors that may reduce the effects of inhaled NO have been suggested. For

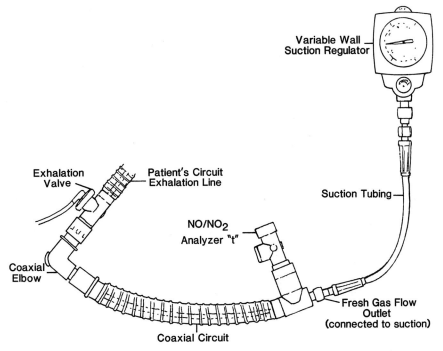

Figure 6–17. NO scavenger system.

Table 6–12. NITRIC OXIDE DELIVERY

	Dose of Nitric Oxide (ppm)	Action
Start NO	Initially, 20 ppm for 4 hr to a maximum of 40 ppm	Increase NO if: ↓ Sao$_2$ <90% ↑ Difference in preductal and postductal saturation of >5–10% Two-dimensional echocardiography demonstrating shunt at patent ductus arteriosus
While on NO	Lowest possible ppm to maintain saturation >95%	Wean NO if: Preductal and postductal Sao$_2$ ≥95% There is no demonstrated preductal or postductal saturation difference There is no demonstrated shunt at the PDA
Weaning from NO	Low dose, 1–5 ppm, and eventually 0	Discontinue if: OI <12–15 *or* Methemoglobin (2–5%)

Table 6–13. MONITORING NITRIC OXIDE

Monitoring	Rationale	Corrective Action
NO_2	Results from the reaction between NO and O_2	Monitor NO_2 levels continuously If levels rise, increase scavenger suctioning pressure, or consider lowering NO level
Methemoglobinemia: NO has affinity for haemoglobin that is 1500 times greater than that of CO_2	Intravascular binding of NO to hemoglobin. Leads to: Inadequate O_2 delivery Hypoxia or death in high levels	Monitor methemoglobin levels using cooximeter q15min initially and then q4h

example, severe pulmonary edema or hemorrhage may limit delivery of the inhaled NO to alveoli. In addition, the very feature that makes inhaled NO a selective pulmonary vasodilator (i.e., rapid inactivation by hemoglobin) may limit the efficacy of the drug if the site of vasoconstriction lies within large pulmonary veins downstream from the alveoli. It is essential that multicentered trials be undertaken to identify factors that influence both the efficacy and toxicity of inhaled NO.

NO is a relatively unstable free radical that is rapidly converted to NO_2 in the presence of O_2. NO_2 is a major component of acid rain and in high concentrations can cause *significant lung damage*. NO is therefore stored in N_2 and mixed with O_2 immediately before delivery to minimize NO_2 formation. Furthermore, both NO and NO_2 concentrations must be monitored when it is administered clinically. Levels of NO_2 of <2 ppm are generally considered to be safe. The other major potential toxicity of NO is methemoglobin formation due to the reduction of hemoglobin when it binds NO. This has rarely proved to be a problem in clinical practice. Nevertheless, frequent methemoglobin levels should be measured, and if methemoglobin levels exceed 5%, the concentration of NO should be reduced. In patients with deficiencies of reducing enzymes (e.g., glucose-6-phosphate dehydrogenase), the need to use NO should be seriously weighed against the potential risks. Finally, it should be noted that NO may *prolong bleeding time* and the long-term consequences of inhaled NO therapy on lung growth and development are unknown.

Future Directions

Although inhaled NO is clearly useful in the treatment of PH in some patients, it is not always effective, and the delivery and monitoring can be somewhat cumbersome with the present technology. Thus, the search for the perfect pulmonary vasodilator continues. Current efforts include the combination of a selective cGMP phosphodiesterase inhibitor with inhaled NO to achieve a greater or more-sustained dilator response to low concentrations of inhaled NO. In addition, the potentially increased selectivity of inhaled prostacyclin is being investigated by several groups. Regardless of which of these new "selective" pulmonary vasodilators is used, we must all pay careful attention to potential adverse effects. Remember, *primum non nocere.*

BIBLIOGRAPHY

Chatburn R, Lough M: Handbook of Respiratory Care. St. Louis, Year-Book Medical Publishers, 1990.

Dhillon JS, Singh NC, Johnson CC, Burke-Tremblay C, Dvali L, Kronick JB: Comparison of the accuracy of nitric oxide (NO) measurement: three electrochemical analyzers (ECA) versus the chemiluminescence analyzer (CLA). Crit Care Med 23:A191, 1995.

Frostell C, Fratacci MD, Wain JC, Jones R, Zapol WM: Inhaled nitric oxide: a selective pulmonary vasodilator reversing hypoxic pulmonary vasoconstriction. Circulation 83:2038, 1991.

Furchgott RF, Zawadzki JV: The obligatory role of endothelial cells in relaxation of arterial smooth muscle by acetylcholine. Nature 288:373–376, 1980.

Kinsella JP, Neish SR, Shaffer E, et al: Low-dose inhalational nitric oxide in persistent pulmonary hypertension of the newborn. Lancet 2:819, 1992.

Lonnqvist PA, Winberg P, Lundell B, Sellden H, Olsson GL: Inhaled nitric oxide in neonates and children with pulmonary hypetension. Acta Paediatr 83:1132, 1994.

Moncada S, Palmer RMJ, Higgs EA: Nitric oxide: physiology, pathophysiology, and pharmacology. Pharmacol Rev 43:109, 1991.

Pepke-Zaba J, Higenbottam TW, Dinh-Xuan AT, Stone D, Wallwork J: Inhaled nitric oxide as a cause of selective pulmonary vasodilatation in pulmonary hypertension. Lancet 2:1173, 1991.

Rich GF, Murphy GD, Roos CM, Johns RA: Inhaled nitric oxide: selective pulmonary vasodilation in cardiac surgery patients. Anesthesiology 78:1028, 1993.

Sellden H, Winberg P, Gustafsson LE, Lundell B, Book K, Frostell CG: Inhalation of nitric oxide reduced pulmonary hypertension after cardiac surgery in a 3.2 kg infant. Anesthesiology 73:577, 1993.

Snow DJ, Gray SJ, Ghosh S, et al: Inhaled nitric oxide in patients with normal and increased pulmonary vascular resistance after cardiac surgery. Br J Anaesth 72:185, 1994.

7

Cardiovascular

7.1 Cardiovascular Monitoring

SAMI D. SHEMIE, MD, CM, FRCPC

The primary function of the cardiovascular system is to transport oxygen. Cardiocirculatory failure is characterized by an inadequate delivery of oxygen to meet metabolic demand. Because oxygen delivery depends on oxygen content and cardiac output, the aim of cardiovascular monitoring is to identify changes in cardiac output. Direct and accurate measurements of cardiac output are routinely difficult, so indirect parameters (Table 7–1) must be relied on to monitor the pediatric patient. Table 7–2 highlights invasive and noninvasive methods of cardiovascular assessment, which ultimately have three purposes:

1. To identify the presence and severity of a cardiovascular problem
2. To monitor the evolution and response to therapy
3. To determine the underlying nature of the cardiovascular disease

Treatment is directed toward improving flow, i.e., cardiac output, to improve oxygen delivery.

Physical Examination

Physical findings reflect physiologic responses to a decrease in cardiac output and dysfunction of the end organs that rely on adequate perfusion.

- Cardiovascular: tachycardia, hypotension (age adjusted)
- Vascular: peripheral pulses (low volume, rapid pulse)
  - Initially, distal pulses are most affected.
  - In determination of pulse volume with positive pressure ventilation, a decrease may indicate impaired preload and an increase may indicate impaired contractility.
- Central nervous system: irritability, decreased level of consciousness

Table 7–1. HEMODYNAMIC ASSESSMENTS

Preload	Central venous pressure, pulmonary capillary wedge pressure, atrial pressure, ventricular end-diastolic pressure, echocardiographic end-diastolic ventricular dimension
Contractility/stroke volume	Arterial pulse pressure, stroke work index, echocardiographic ejection fraction
Afterload	Arterial diastolic pressure, systemic/pulmonary vascular resistance, echocardiographic ventricular wall stress

- Skin: cool extremities, pallor, decreased capillary refill, mottling, cyanosis
- Renal: oliguria (<0.5 mL/kg/hr), fluid retention
- Temperature: core (esophageal, rectal, tympanic); peripheral (skin) gradient >5C° indicates hypoperfusion
- General: hydration status; peripheral edema, hepatomegaly, ascites may indicate elevated central venous pressure

Laboratory Investigations

- Arterial blood gases: hypoxemia, acidosis
- Mixed venous oxygen saturations (MVo_2): index of increased cellular oxygen extraction due to reduced oxygen delivery. MVo_2 <40% indicates that the limits of compensation are being reached. Measurements may be made intermittently or continuously (intravascular fiberoptic catheter) and ideally in the pulmonary artery in the absence of intracardiac left-to-right shunt. Alternative sites (right atrium, vena cava) may be used; however, the MVo_2 and arteriovenous oxygen difference may be a less reliable reflection of the absolute cardiac output but can be used serially
- Serum lactate: serial measurements reflect anaerobic metabolism due to reduced oxygen delivery
- Blood urea nitrogen and creatinine: renal function indexes

Table 7–2. TYPES OF CARDIOVASCULAR MONITORING

	Noninvasive	Invasive
	Physical examination	Intra-arterial pressure
	Laboratory evaluation	Central venous pressure
	Pulse oximetry	Pulmonary arterial pressure
	Echocardiography	Direct atrial pressure
	Radiography	Pulmonary wedge pressure
		Cardiac output
		Cardiac catheterization

Respiratory Evaluation

- Oxygenation: arterial blood gases, pulse oximetry (oxygen saturation, excellent correlation to Pao_2 from range of 60% to 100%), transcutaneous Po_2
- Ventilation: arterial blood gases, end-tidal CO_2 (reliable in the absence of endotracheal tube leak), respiratory rate

Chest Radiography

- Cardiac size: cardiothoracic ratio of >0.6 in infants and of >0.5 in children indicates cardiomegaly
- Pulmonary vasculature:
  - ☐ Increased pulmonary artery flow: enlarged central pulmonary artery with peripheral plethora
  - ☐ Increased capillary/venous pressures: pulmonary edema

Electrocardiography

Continuous ECG monitoring is mandatory; it primarily yields information about heart rate. Abnormal rhythms should be recorded from multiple leads to avoid incorrect diagnosis. Twelve-lead ECG must be evaluated for details of rhythm, axis, electrical intervals (PR, QRS, QT_c), chamber size, and ischemic injury patterns (ST segments, T waves). The relationship of the P wave to the QRS complex must be established to determine the presence of a sinus mechanism and atrioventricular synchrony. If the P wave is difficult to identify, esophageal electrodes or recording from epicardial atrial electrodes placed at the time of cardiac surgery is essential.

Echocardiography

Echocardiography is the most complete noninvasive assessment of cardiac structure and function. There are three basic techniques:

- *M-mode:* a single linear ultrasound beam
  - ☐ Indices of contractility: shortening fraction, ejection fraction
  - ☐ Wall thickness
  - ☐ Chamber size
- *Two-dimensional echocardiography:* tomographic views along different axes of heart and great vessels
  - ☐ Precise anatomy
  - ☐ Chamber and vessel size
  - ☐ Valve size and patency
- *Doppler/color Doppler:* a reflected echocardiographic wave frequency that is changed by the direction and velocity of blood flow. With color flow

Doppler, red indicates toward the transducer and blue indicates away from the transducer.
  □ Blood flow: velocity, location, direction, for example, valve regurgitation, intracardiac shunts

Arterial Blood Pressure

Arterial blood pressure is an indirect measurement of perfusion as dictated by the equation:

$$Q = \Delta P/R$$

where Q is blood flow (cardiac output), ΔP is mean arteriovenous pressure gradient, and R is vascular resistance (Table 7–3).
Four parameters of arterial blood pressure must be considered:

- Systolic arterial pressure
- Diastolic pressure
- Pulse pressure (systolic minus diastolic pressure)
- Mean arterial pressure (diastolic pressure plus one third pulse pressure)

There are three noninvasive methods of measurement:

- *Auscultatory* (sphygmomanometer and stethoscope): not suitable for continuous monitoring, falsely elevated pressures seen with a small cuff
- *Oscillometric* (e.g., Dinamap): one tube to the cuff produces cuff inflation, and the other transmits sensed pressure to the transducer. Oscillations in the cuff applied around the arm are recorded, yielding systolic, mean, and diastolic pressures. Advantages are its automated frequency, independence of Korotkoff sounds, and greater accuracy than auscultation.
- *Doppler ultrasonic:* vascular turbulence in an artery distorted by the compression of a blood pressure cuff. Doppler sounds, unlike Korotkoff sounds, are generated when there is any movement of blood. There is increased

Table 7–3. ARTERIAL BLOOD PRESSURE MEASUREMENTS

Method	Advantages	Disadvantages
Auscultatory	Noninvasive	Noncontinuous, unreliable in shock
Oscillometric	Noninvasive, frequent measurements, automated	Noncontinuous
Doppler	Noninvasive, independent of Korotkoff sounds, most reliable noninvasive method in shock	Noncontinuous
Intra-arterial	Highest accuracy, continuous measurement, functions in circulatory collapse, blood sampling	Invasive, thrombosis, infection

reliability in patients with shock compared with conventional methods. It can be used serially and unobtrusively.

Invasive Intravascular Pressure Monitoring

Pressure may be continuously measured in a peripheral artery, central venous site, cardiac chamber, or pulmonary vascular site. A pressure-measuring device, that is, a transducer, is used and must be properly calibrated and dampened. It has the advantage of continuous measurements and trends and allows for blood sampling.

INTRA-ARTERIAL PRESSURE

Intra-arterial pressure is the only way to continuously measure blood pressure. Radial, dorsalis pedis, posterior tibialis, or femoral sites are preferred. Intra-arterial pressure continues to function during deterioration of the peripheral circulation. The normal arterial pulse contour has sharp upstroke during rapid ejection, followed by slow ejection and subsequent decrease. The dicrotic notch denotes the end of ejection and closure of the aortic valve. The subsequent decrease in arterial pressure to diastole is attributed to normal aortic runoff to the systemic vascular bed. As the pressure wave moves distally from the aorta, the systolic pressure increases and the diastolic decreases. Mean arterial pressure remains constant. Estimates can be made of cardiac output based on the quality of the arterial pulse contour. Low cardiac output syndromes may show a rapid ejection and a narrow pulse pressure. The area under the curve may be integrated to estimate cardiac output.

ATRIAL PRESSURE

Atrial pressure is an indirect measurement of ventricular preload, that is, ventricular end-diastolic volume. Pressure is measured as an index of volume, so it must be remembered that interpretation of these measurements depends on the compliance of the ventricle and normal functioning of the atrioventricular valve. Ventricular hypertrophy or atrioventricular valve stenosis may result in less ventricular filling for any given atrial pressure.

- Right atrial pressure
  - □ Directly measured via right atrial line inserted at the time of surgery
  - □ Indirectly measured via central venous pressure line
- Left atrial pressure
  - □ Directly measured via surgically placed left atrial pressure line
  - □ Indirectly measured via pulmonary capillary wedge pressure

Central venous, right atrial, pulmonary capillary wedge, and left atrial pressure recordings have three waves (Fig. 7–1):

1. a wave: atrial contraction, follows the P wave on the ECG

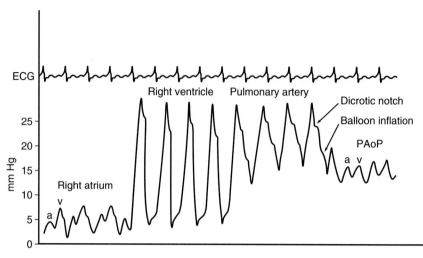

Figure 7–1. Representative recording of pressures as a Swan-Ganz catheter is inserted through the right side of the heart into the pulmonary artery (PA). The first waveform is a right atrial (RA) tracing with characteristic a and v waves. The right ventricular, PA, and PA wedge tracings follow in sequence. The pressures and waveforms shown here are normal. Note that the wedge tracing shows a and v waves transmitted from the left atrium. In addition, the wedge pressure (mean) is less than PA diastolic pressure. The wedge tracing is not always this distinct, but a very damped tracing or a mean wedge pressure greater than PA diastolic pressure usually indicates some mechanical problem in the system (e.g., air bubble in the connecting tubing, catheter tip "overwedged," balloon inflated over distal orifice, catheter tip in zone 1 or zone 2). In a patient with severe mitral regurgitation, the large transmitted left atrial v waves occasionally may cause the wedge tracing to resemble a PA tracing. In such a case, careful analysis of the waveforms and attention to where peak pressure occurs in relation to the ECG complex usually will avoid misinterpretation. (Redrawn from Matthay MA: Invasive hemodynamic monitoring in critically ill patients. Clin Chest Med 4:233, 1983.)

    2. v wave: ventricular contraction, timed with the closing of the atrioventricular valve

    3. c wave: isovolemic contraction, aortic/pulmonic and mitral/tricuspid valves are closed

With atrioventricular valve stenosis, atrial pressure will be elevated with a marked elevation in the a wave. Atrioventricular valve regurgitation causes increased atrial pressures with a large atrial v wave.

Pulmonary Artery Catheterization (Swan-Ganz)

A balloon-tipped flow-directed catheter is inserted into the pulmonary artery (see Fig. 7–1) to allow measurement of cardiac output (equipped with a thermistor); right atrial, pulmonary arterial, and pulmonary capillary wedge pressures; and mixed venous saturations (Table 7–4). The catheter tip should be positioned in West zone III, where pulmonary arterial pressure exceeds pulmonary alveolar

Table 7–4. VARIABLES DERIVED FROM PULMONARY ARTERY CATHETERIZATION

Variable	Formula	Normal Range
Hemodynamic		
Stroke index	$SI = CI/hr$	30–60 mL/m^2
Cardiac index	$CI = CO/BSA$	3.5–5.5 L/min/m^2
Systemic vascular resistance index	$SVRI = \dfrac{79.7 \, (MAP - CVP)}{CI}$	800–1600 dyne • sec/cm^5/m^2
Pulmonary vascular resistance index	$PVRI = \dfrac{79.9 \, (MPAP - PCWP)}{CI}$	80–240 dyne • sec/cm^5/m^2
Oxygen Transport		
Arterial oxygen content	$Cao_2 = (Hb)(1.34)(\% \, sat) + (Pao_2)(0.003)$	17–20 mL/dL
Mixed venous oxygen content	$Cvo_2 = (Hb)(1.34)(\% \, sat) + (Pvo_2)(0.003)$	12–15 mL/dL
Oxygen content difference	$a\text{-}vDO_2 = Cao_2 - Cvo_2$	3–5 mL/dL
Oxygen availability	$O_2 \, avail = Cao_2 \times CI \times 10$	550–650 mL/min/m^2
Oxygen consumption	$\dot{V}o_2 = CI \times a\text{-}vDO_2 \times 10$	120–200 mL/min/m^2

CO, cardiac output; BSA, body surface area; MAP, mean arterial pressure; CVP, central venous pressure; MPAP, mean pulmonary artery pressure; PCWP, pulmonary capillary wedge pressure; Hb, hemoglobin.

pressure. Pulmonary arterial diastolic pressure may accurately reflect left atrial pressure only when the pulmonary vascular resistance is normal.

Cardiac Output

Cardiac output may be measured in one of four ways (Table 7–5). The first three methods apply the principle of dilution of an indicator, i.e., oxygen, Cardio-Green, or cold fluid, respectively. The change in concentration of a substance over time is proportional to the volume of blood in which it is being diluted, i.e., flow.

Table 7–5. CARDIAC OUTPUT METHODS

Method	Equipment Required	Advantages	Disadvantages
Fick	Systemic arterial catheter, mixed venous catheter, spirometer/oximeter	Shunt detection	Cumbersome
Dye dilution	Systemic arterial catheter, central venous catheter	Shunt detection	Cumbersome
Thermodilution	Central venous catheter, pulmonary arterial catheter	No blood sampling, frequent repetition	Inaccurate with left-to-right shunts
Doppler	Pulmonary/aortic transducer	Noninvasive, no blood sampling	Inaccurate, operator dependent

In general, single absolute values may be difficult to interpret. Serial measurements are more appropriate and reflect relative changes in cardiac output and response to therapy.

Fick Principle. Cardiac output is proportional to oxygen consumption. Measurement of oxygen uptake and arteriovenous oxygen difference across the lungs determines pulmonary blood flow, which equals cardiac output.

$$CO = Vo_2/(Cao_2 - Cvo_2) \times 100$$

Measurement of oxygen consumption may be accomplished through analysis of expired gases. Alternatively, the arteriovenous oxygen difference may be assessed as an indirect indicator of cardiac output. Increased arteriovenous oxygen difference indicates increased oxygen extraction by the tissues and reflects reduced cardiac output.

Thermodilution. Thermodilution is the most frequently used form of cardiac output management in intensive care. Through a Swan-Ganz catheter, a measured volume of ice water or saline is injected into a chamber on the right side of the heart, and the temperature is measured in the most distal site (pulmonary artery). Adequate mixing of blood with the cold injectate occurs during passage of the mixture through two heart valves and one cardiac chamber. The injection is made via the proximal port of the pulmonary artery catheter, and the temperature change is monitored with the distal thermistor. Cardiac output curves are generated, and a computer is used to determine the difference between injectate and patient temperature; a temperature-time curve is integrated automatically.

Indocyanine Green Dye Dilution. A nontoxic indicator dye that may be injected into a peripheral or central venous system and sampled at any convenient arterial site. After injection, the blood is continually withdrawn from an arterial site into a photodensitometer, and the concentration of the indicator is measured. The curve reaches a peak and then decays exponentially. This is followed by a small secondary curve, which represents recirculation of the indicator dye. The down slope of the initial curve is extrapolated to zero to estimate carbon dioxide. In the presence of an intracardiac shunt, distortion of the curve occurs, which can be used to estimate the degree of shunting.

Echocardiography Doppler. The change in velocity of an ultrasonic beam is proportional to the velocity of blood flow. Cardiac output equals the mean velocity of systolic flow, the cardiac rate, and the cross-sectional area of the artery being measured. A transducing Doppler probe can be used to quantify the aortic blood flow, and the cross-sectional area of the aorta is determined with echocardiography. Concern exists regarding the accuracy of ultrasound measurements, and at present, it remains a technique used only for research purposes.

Cardiac Catheterization

Cardiac catheterization is a combined hemodynamic and angiographic procedure for diagnosis and therapy. Data derived include vascular and chamber pressures, cardiac output, vascular resistance, shunt fractions, and anatomic clarity (Fig. 7–2). (A detailed description of the technique and methods is beyond the scope of this report.)

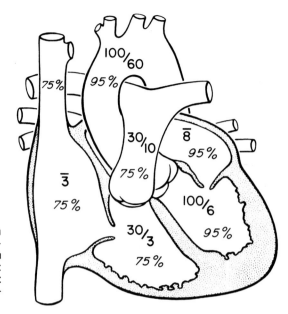

Figure 7–2. Catheterization data in the normal pediatric heart with pressure (mm Hg) and oxygen saturation (%). (From Ream AK, Fogdall RP: Acute Cardiovascular Management: Anesthesia and Intensive Care. Philadelphia, JB Lippincott, 1982.)

BIBLIOGRAPHY

Lake CL: Monitoring of the pediatric cardiac patient. *In* Lake CL (ed): Pediatric Cardiac Anesthesia. East Norwalk, CT, Appleton & Lange, 1993, pp. 83–118.

Martin GR, Holley DG: Cardiovascular monitoring and evaluation. *In* Holbrook PR (ed): Textbook of Pediatric Critical Care. Philadelphia, WB Saunders, 1993, pp. 259–278.

Moller JH: Assessment and monitoring of cardiovascular function. *In* Fuhrman BP, Zimmerman JJ (eds): Pediatric Critical Care. St. Louis, Mosby–Year Book, 1992, pp. 315–322.

7.2 Arrhythmias in the Pediatric Intensive Care Unit

MARC D. LeGRAS, BSc, MD, CM, FRCPC, FACC

The heterogeneous population of patients in a pediatric intensive care unit may have a wide variety of rhythm disturbances. Many of the arrhythmias, however, have a similar mechanism, which means that regardless of whether the patient is a neonate or teenager or is involved in a motor vehicle accident or status postcardiac surgery, the principles of arrhythmia recognition and management are virtually the same. Thus, with a disciplined approach of thinking about the arrhythmia rather than immediately treating it, rhythm disturbances can be overcome.

Definitions

Supraventricular Tachycardia. Supraventricular tachycardia (SVT) involves structures located above the bundle of His, that is, the atria, atrioventricular (AV) node, and/or His bundle. The term has replaced paroxysmal atrial tachycardia because the latter does not evoke the possibility of gradual-onset arrhythmias (ectopic tachycardia) or those not necessarily originating only in the atria (junctional ectopic tachycardia [JET]). Atrial fibrillation and atrial flutter are included in the list of SVTs because the term refers to a compilation of specific types of arrhythmias rather than a grouping by etiology. There is no specific heart rate criterion for the diagnosis of SVT but rather a sudden onset of a more rapid heart rate, or a heart rate displaying lack of physiologic variability with respirations or over time, or a rhythm with an abnormal P wave–to–QRS relationship.

Ventricular Arrhythmias. These arrhythmias originate below the His bundle, that is, in the ventricles. They are traditionally recognized as wide-complex arrhythmias. However, in neonates, a QRS duration of 80 milliseconds is outside the normal range of QRS duration and may represent a ventricular arrhythmia.

Bradycardia. Bradycardia is defined in relation to the established heart rate ranges for different age groups (infants, <90 bpm; adolescents, <60 bpm). Third-degree atrioventricular block or complete heart block (CHB) specifically refers to complete AV dissociation, in which the atrial rate is faster than the ventricular rate and there is no evidence of AV node conduction. In second-degree AV block, there is varying AV node conduction manifesting as nonconducted P waves or Wenckebach (progressive PR prolongation and then nonconducted P wave).

Pathophysiology

TACHYCARDIA

There are three main mechanisms of tachycardia: reentry (Fig. 7–3a), abnormal impulse formation (Fig. 7–3b), and triggered arrhythmias (rarely encountered in the pediatric clinical setting, with the exception of digoxin toxicity; these arrhythmias result from afterdepolarizations).

BRADYCARDIA

Most frequently, bradycardia results from nonconducted atrial extrasystoles, sinus node dysfunction after cardiac surgery, hypoxia, central nervous system injury, and antiarrhythmic drugs.

CHB and varying degrees of AV node dysfunction are acquired after cardiac surgery or may be congenital.

ABNORMAL IMPULSE FORMATION

REENTRY

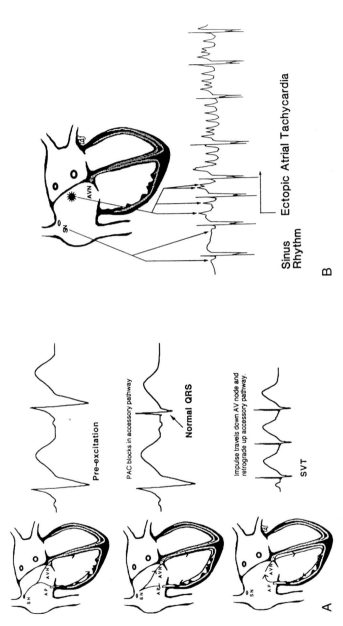

Figure 7-3. *A,* Reentry supraventricular tachycardia in a patient with preexcitation. Note the loss of the Δ wave during supraventricular tachycardia (SVT), which involves atrioventricular reentry. *B,* Ectopic atrial tachycardia spontaneously occurs after normal sinus rhythm. Note the "warm-up phenomenon," in which there is a gradual speeding up of the ectopic P wave during tachycardia initiation. (Courtesy of Cameron Finlay.)

Surgically acquired cases usually involve direct trauma to the AV node or specialized conducting bundles. Individuals with corrected transposition (AV and ventriculoarterial discordance, L-transposition of the great arteries) as well as left atrial isomerism (polysplenia syndrome) are at higher risk of surgically acquired CHB but may develop this spontaneously (≤2% per year).

Congenital CHB in the setting of a structurally normal heart is usually associated with maternal systemic lupus erythematosus or other autoimmune disease.

General Approach to Arrhythmias

1. Rule Out Hemodynamic Compromise

Hemodynamically Unstable. Electrical cardioversion is indicated in the presence of *tachycardia* (Fig. 7–4). Remember that the blood pressure is difficult to determine in the presence of a very rapid heart rate and that some chest discomfort and minor ST-segment changes are common and do not necessarily indicate the level of hemodynamic compromise. A reduced level of consciousness is a sure sign of hemodynamic compromise. When *bradycardia* is the cause, use *atropine* and/or *isoproterenol* while organizing emergency temporary pacing.

Hemodynamically Stable. There is time to carefully analyze the nature of the arrhythmia and start with conservative measures.

Electrical Cardioversion Technique. In infants and children, place the cardioversion paddles over the anterior and posterior chest—this is most efficient in this age group. For cardioversion, start with 0.5 J/kg; in defibrillation, start with 2 J/kg. Synchronize in all instances except for *defibrillation* (in cases of ventricular fibrillation or asystole). If the patient is receiving *digoxin,* a bolus of *lidocaine* before cardioversion is recommended. Cardioversion is not effective for atrial ectopic tachycardia (AET) or junctional tachycardia.

2. Obtain Historical Data

Enquire whether there was a sudden or gradual onset and determine the duration. Is there structural heart disease or a prior history of arrhythmias? Has there been recent surgery, central nervous system injury, or infection? Review medications, electrolytes, and evidence for sepsis.

3. Identify the Arrhythmia

Perform a 12-lead ECG. An ECG plus an understanding of the clinical setting is key to identifying the arrhythmia. Do not rely on a monitor rhythm strip; this rarely leads to the correct diagnosis. A 12-lead ECG within 1 hour of return to the intensive care unit is mandatory for patients who have undergone cardiac surgery to document the postoperative ECG appearance; this is valuable for comparison if a postoperative arrhythmia ensues.

Perform a three-lead rhythm strip during an acute intervention. This will

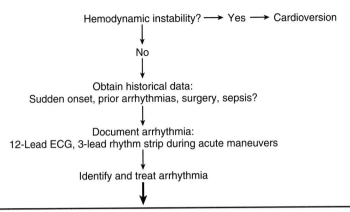

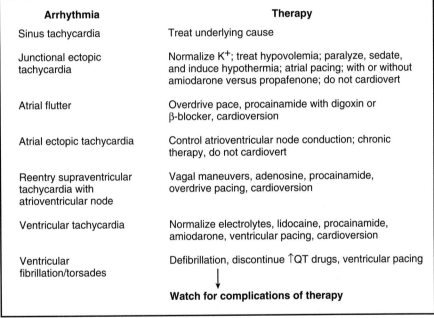

Figure 7–4. Approach to tachyarrhythmias.

help confirm or establish a diagnosis by demonstrating the mechanism of arrhythmia termination, and it will help in future therapeutic decisions.

Find the P waves. What is the relation of P waves to QRS? What is the QRS duration?

Tachycardia

- P waves precede QRS with 1:1 relationship: sinus tachycardia, AET, atrial flutter with 2:1 block

- Rapid P waves with variable AV node conduction: atrial flutter, AET
- P waves buried in QRS or immediately follow QRS: AV node or atrioventricular reentry
- No P waves, irregular rhythm: atrial fibrillation, chaotic atrial tachycardia
- AV dissociation: narrow QRS indicates JET, wide QRS indicates ventricular tachycardia
- Wide QRS: ventricular tachycardia; may be SVT if patient has preexisting bundle-branch block or rate-dependent bundle-branch block

Bradycardia
- P waves precede QRS with constant PR: sinus bradycardia
- P waves precede QRS with variable PR: Is there second-degree AV block or Wenckebach? Are the P waves truly being conducted?
- No relation between P waves and QRS: faster P rate indicates complete heart block and slower P rate indicates sinus bradycardia with escape rhythm
- P waves irregular, frequent pauses: blocked or nonconducted premature atrial contractions (PACs)

4. Treat the Arrhythmia and Watch for Complications of Therapy

The initial arrhythmia diagnosis may not be correct; therefore, reassess the situation if therapy is unsuccessful.

Antiarrhythmic agents (Table 7–6) may cause hypotension or new arrhythmias. Toxicity may develop more readily in infants or if elimination is abnormal. Monitor levels when feasible.

Be prepared to cardiovert in case the acute therapeutic intervention worsens the arrhythmia (see Fig. 7–4).

Management of Specific Arrhythmias

TACHYCARDIA

Sinus Tachycardia

If the sinus tachycardia is very rapid, it may be mistaken for other types of SVT.

Diagnosis. A 12-lead ECG demonstrates that the origin of the P wave is from the sinus node (positive I, II, or aVF; P axis 0° to 90°) and P waves precede QRS 1:1 (usually <200 bpm).

Differential Diagnosis. AET or atrial flutter with 2:1 block.

Therapy. Treat hypovolemia, fever, sepsis, pain, and anxiety and identify iatrogenic causes. Antiarrhythmic drug therapy is rarely indicated and may worsen the situation.

Reentry Supraventricular Tachycardia with the Atrioventricular Node as Part of the Circuit

This SVT includes atrioventricular node reentry (AVNRT) and both preexcited or concealed accessory pathways (AVRT) (Fig. 7–5; see Fig 7–3a). Structural heart

Table 7–6. ANTIARRHYTHMIC DRUGS

Class	Drug	Dose	Comment
IA	Procainamide IV	<1 yr: load 7 mg/kg >1 yr: load 10–15 mg/kg Infusion 40–80 μg/kg/min	Load: no faster than 0.5 mg/kg/min; enhances AV node conduction
IB	Lidocaine IV	Bolus 1 mg/kg q5min Infusion 15–50 μg/kg/min	Maximum bolus 3 mg/kg
IC	Propafenone IV	2 mg/kg over 90 min Infusion 4–7 μg/kg/min	Hypotension
II	Esmolol IV	0.5 mg/kg over 3 min Infusion 50–300 μg/kg/min	Hypotension
	Propranolol IV	0.02–0.1 mg/kg over 2 min	Hypotension; caution under age 2 yr
III	Amiodarone IV	Load 5 mg/kg over 30–60 min Infusion 5–15 μg/kg/min	Rapid loading dose may cause hypotension
	Sotalol PO	2–6 mg/kg/day ÷ BID	
IV	Verapamil IV	0.1–0.2 mg/kg over 2 min	Adenosine preferred; avoid under age 2 yr; hypotension, maximum 5 mg/dose
Other	Adenosine IV	0.1–0.25 mg/kg/dose	Rapid IV bolus and flush; caution with asthma
	Atropine IV	0.02 mg/kg/dose	Minimum 0.1 mg, maximum 0.6 mg per dose
	Bretylium IV	5 mg/kg/dose over 1 min	Hypotension, maximum total 30 mg/kg
	Digoxin IV	≥37 weeks–2 yr Digitalize: 12 μg/kg/dose IV q6h × 3 Maintenance: 3.5 μg/kg/dose IV q12h >2 yr Digitalize: 10 μg/kg/dose IV q6h × 3 Maintenance: 6 μg/kg/dose IV daily	Levels are increased with IC, III, IV Oral dose = IV dose × 1.4 IV dose = oral dose × 0.7
	Isoproterenol IV	0.1–1.0 μg/kg/min infusion	Titrate to desired effect

Important: renal or hepatic dysfunction as well as prematurity will affect metabolism and clearance of drugs. Drug levels should be determined when possible, and patients should be monitored for signs of toxicity or new arrhythmias.

disease in this setting is limited to Ebstein anomaly; approximately 15% of these patients have an accessory pathway. AVNRT is virtually nonexistent below 3 years of age but becomes a frequent cause of reentry SVT by adolescence.

Diagnosis. Sudden-onset regular narrow-complex tachycardia with retrograde P waves that immediately follow the preceding QRS complex with a 1:1 relationship.

Look carefully for the small indentation of the P wave buried after the QRS or in the T wave; lead-by-lead comparison with the patient's 12-lead ECG in sinus rhythm is very helpful. In AVNRT, P waves are often not seen because they are buried in the QRS complex.

III

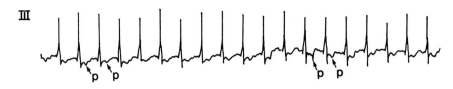

V₁

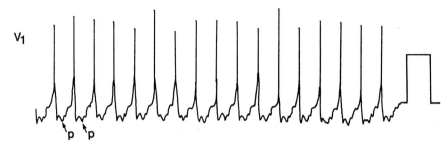

Figure 7–5. Reentry supraventricular tachycardia with the atrioventricular node as part of the circuit. Narrow-complex supraventricular tachycardia at 330 bpm with retrograde P waves visible immediately after the QRS complex. P, P waves. ECG of simultaneous leads III and V₁.

In patients with Wolff-Parkinson-White syndrome, the delta wave disappears, and there is a narrow QRS tachycardia in the majority of cases. Rarely, tachycardia involves impulses traveling anterograde down the accessory pathway and up the AV node; this must be distinguished from ventricular tachycardia.

Therapy. *Electrical cardioversion* for hemodynamic instability (0.5 J/kg).

Vagal maneuvers are best performed with forced Valsalva in older patients or the facial ice water application in younger children. *Facial ice water application* mimics the diving reflex and usually requires a seemingly inhumane application of a freezing ice water bag to the *entire* face and forehead with simultaneous airway/endotracheal tube occlusion for 15 to 45 seconds. When performed effectively, these maneuvers result in slowed AV node conduction and terminate reentry.

If vagal maneuvers are unsuccessful, the next step is pharmacologic and involves intravenous *adenosine*. Adenosine must be given as an intravenous bolus and is followed by a rapid hand-injected bolus of saline as centrally as possible because it is metabolized within seconds. Adenosine results in transient heart block; however, SVT may alternatively terminate with a PVC. Adenosine may worsen bronchospasm, requiring bronchodilators—consider alternatives in patients with severe asthma. Also proceed with caution in patients after heart transplant, in whom prolonged asystole may occur.

Intravenous verapamil is contraindicated in children <2 years of age and in patients receiving β-blockers. As a rule, acute use of intravenous verapamil has been replaced with intravenous adenosine.

If SVT recurs, does not respond to the above measures, or is difficult to differentiate from VT, an infusion of *procainamide* is indicated. After intravenous procainamide infusion, vagal and adenosine therapy may be more effective, and SVT may not recur.

Chronic therapy involves *digoxin*; β-blockers; and class IC, III, and IV drugs. In general, digoxin is not used in the presence of preexcitation.

Junctional Ectopic Tachycardia

JET is probably the most refractory and lethal of the postoperative arrhythmias because it does not respond to cardioversion, is difficult to treat medically, and results in the loss of AV synchrony in patients immediately after the most difficult of cardiac operations (Fig. 7–6).

The arrhythmia is most frequent in patients with preoperative and residual postoperative right ventricular hypertension. Extensive surgery near the AV node with structural or hypoxic damage is an important factor, as are postoperative fever and high levels of circulating catecholamines.

Diagnosis. Narrow QRS complex tachycardia with a rate of >120 bpm in the presence of AV dissociation; in this case, the ventricular rate is faster than the atrial rate.

Differential Diagnosis. Patients with the similar ECG findings with wide-complex tachycardia must be distinguished from those with ventricular tachycardia. In ventricular tachycardia, there will be a change in morphology compared with the immediate postoperative ECG before tachycardia. Also, capture beats from a conducted P wave will change the QRS morphology during ventricular tachycardia, and fusion beats may also be seen (these are QRS complexes intermediate between the usual QRS and a "ventricular" impulse). These fusion beats can be accomplished with atrial pacing, but spontaneously occurring sinus capture beats are equally diagnostic.

Therapy. If JET is treated early, antiarrhythmic drugs can often be avoided.

1. Treat hypovolemia and fever.
2. Correct hypokalemia to 4.0 to 5.0 mmol/L within 1 to 2 hours.
3. Patients should be paralyzed, sedated, and cooled to 35°C esophageal (or rectal) before considering the use of drugs.
4. Inotropic drug doses should be reduced as much as possible.

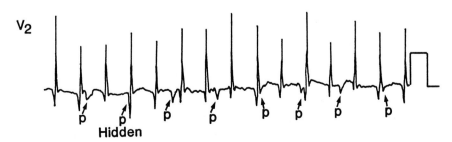

Figure 7–6. Junctional ectopic tachycardia. Note that there is a narrow-complex supraventricular tachycardia at 190 bpm with atrioventricular dissociation. P, P waves.

5. Once the tachycardia slows to <160 bpm, atrial pacing approximately 10 bpm faster than JET will not only provide atrioventricular synchrony but also may suppress JET (this is different from overdrive tachycardia termination).

6. *Start antiarrhythmic drugs* if the arrhythmia fails to respond to the previous measures or if it does not slow sufficiently to permit atrial pacing. *Amiodarone* is favored in the presence of unstable hemodynamics; the loading dose must be given slowly because it can lower the blood pressure if given rapidly. *Propafenone* is equally effective and is used when amiodarone is not available, if the patient is hemodynamically stable, or if the patient has not responded to amiodarone.

7. Cardioversion is ineffective for JET. Paired ventricular pacing is an impractical and dangerous maneuver, even by experts; repeat of loading doses of antiarrhythmic drugs is usually preferred.

8. Consider relieving residual right ventricular outflow tract obstruction. Extracorporeal membrane oxygenation may be useful if all else fails because JET tends to resolve over time.

JET usually resolves within 3 to 7 days, and therapies are removed in a reverse order to the above protocol. Long-term use of antiarrhythmic drugs is not indicated. Consultation with a cardiologist or electrophysiologist is essential throughout this clinical situation. (The management of congenital JET is different and is outside of the scope of this report.)

Atrial Flutter

Atrial flutter is increasingly common after the Fontan, Mustard, or Senning procedure (Fig. 7–7). It also occurs with long-standing mitral stenosis or other causes of atrial enlargement.

Diagnosis. This is the great masquerader in arrhythmias; suspect it when there is an elevated heart rate with minimal variation, especially if what appears to be a P wave is centered exactly between two QRS complexes. Ventricular rates of 150 bpm are suspicious.

Search all 12 leads of the ECG for flutter waves; these precede the QRS. Variable AV conduction is often seen. In atypical cases (late after cardiac surgery), flutter waves are not saw-toothed and may be more difficult to recognize.

Differential Diagnosis. AET (which may be seen in the same clinical setting) can also have variable AV conduction; sinus tachycardia or reentry SVT should also be considered. Adenosine may be used diagnostically to create variable AV conduction; this makes the flutter waves more obvious and demonstrates that the AV node is not involved.

Therapy. Beware of intracardiac thrombi in patients with dilated atria (e.g., mitral stenosis or post-Fontan) in long-standing incessant flutter; these patients may need anticoagulation before converting to sinus rhythm. Thrombi are sometimes visualized only with transesophageal echocardiography.

Atrial Pacing. If a patient has atrial pacing leads, overdrive pacing is frequently successful. This is performed for brief periods with higher pacing outputs starting 10% faster than the flutter rate.

Intravenous procainamide may terminate flutter, but this will not be immedi-

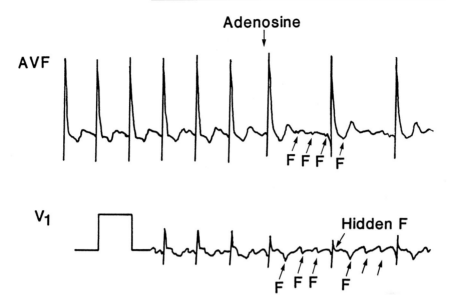

Figure 7–7. Atypical atrial flutter unmasked by intravenous adenosine. Adenosine is given intravenously in a patient who has undergone Fontan surgery. Adenosine causes reduced atrioventricular conduction of flutter waves, making these more visible. The flutter rate is 360 bpm with a ventricular rate of 180 bpm before adenosine. F, flutter waves.

ate. Procainamide should not be used without digoxin or β-blockers because it can enhance AV node conduction.

Electrical Cardioversion. Start with 0.25 J/kg and apply paddles front to back.

Chronic suppression is achieved with digoxin and *sotalol, propafenone, flecainide,* or *amiodarone.* Use caution in the presence of sinus node dysfunction; severe bradycardia and syncope may be precipitated in the absence of a pacemaker.

Atrial Ectopic Tachycardia

AET is frequently an incessant chronic arrhythmia that may result in reduced cardiac function (see Fig. 7–3b). This arrhythmia is not due to reentry; thus, it will not terminate with vagal maneuvers or cardioversion.

Diagnosis. AET is due to an ectopic pacemaker. Sometimes "warm up" and "cool down" are seen on ECG, which represent a speeding up and slowing down of the rhythm at the onset and termination, respectively. The P waves often have a morphology different from sinus and in most cases do not resemble flutter waves; there may also be variable AV conduction.

Differential Diagnosis. Sinus tachycardia, atrial flutter, chaotic atrial tachycardia.

Therapy. Acute measures revolve around reducing AV node conduction (esmolol or other β-blockers, digoxin) and starting chronic oral antiarrhythmic drugs (class IC or III). AET cannot be terminated by cardioversion or overdrive pacing.

Premature Ventricular Contractions

Isolated wide-complex beats may exhibit AV dissociation or fusion (a QRS morphology with the appearance of both a normal QRS and PVC).

Differential Diagnosis. PVCs must be differentiated from PACs with rate-dependent aberrancy. Patients who have frequent PACs as well as PVCs should be considered as having PACs only until proved otherwise, especially at younger ages.

Therapy. Therapy of PVCs is rarely indicated, although it is frequently tempting to suppress them. It is expected that arterial line output will transiently drop with PVCs, but overall, organ perfusion is most important. If PVCs are so frequent that they compromise end-organ perfusion and function, they should be treated with intravenous *lidocaine. Procainamide,* β*-blockers, or amiodarone* may be used if lidocaine is ineffective. Ventricular pacing may also suppress PVCs.

Ventricular Tachycardia

Ventricular tachycardia can occur after cardiac surgery, infarction (Kawasaki disease), myocarditis, or multiple myocardial hamartomas (infancy) (Fig. 7–8).

Diagnosis. Rapid wide QRS tachycardia (QRS duration greater than the upper limit for age: first year, <80 milliseconds; 1 to 10 years, <90 milliseconds; adolescents, <100 milliseconds). Other indications are a change in morphology from sinus rhythm, the presence of sinus capture beats with a different morphology, and fusion beats. Regarding AV dissociation, in younger patients, the retrograde conduction of the AV node is excellent, which may result in 1:1 retrograde P waves during ventricular tachycardia.

Differential Diagnosis. Similar arrhythmias of <120 bpm (or <10% faster than the underlying sinus rate) are termed accelerated ventricular rhythm; hemodynamically, they resemble ventricular pacing and have little clinical significance.

Start with the assumption that a wide-complex tachycardia is ventricular tachycardia, but attempt to differentiate it from JET with a wide QRS (pacing maneuvers discussed in "Junctional Ectopic Tachycardia" may be helpful), SVT with a wide QRS, or the rare patient with Wolff-Parkinson-White syndrome who conducts anterograde down the accessory pathway (rather than retrograde). The latter patient will have preexcitation on ECG, and the delta wave appearance will be identical in wide-complex tachycardia. Do not use the rate of tachycardia (i.e., 150 bpm indicates ventricular tachycardia); this is rarely helpful.

Therapy. *Electrical cardioversion* may be necessary, but ventricular tachycardia is often well tolerated hemodynamically. Start with 1 J/kg.

Treat hypoxia, hypotension, and electrolyte abnormalities.

Administer *intravenous lidocaine* as a bolus and maintenance dose. If this is ineffective, consider *procainamide* or *amiodarone.* Near-drowning patients with refractory arrhythmia may respond to *bretylium.*

Reassess potential drug toxicity daily, especially in the setting of hepatic and liver dysfunction, low cardiac output, or new arrhythmias. Reassess the need for antiarrhythmic agents daily in this situation.

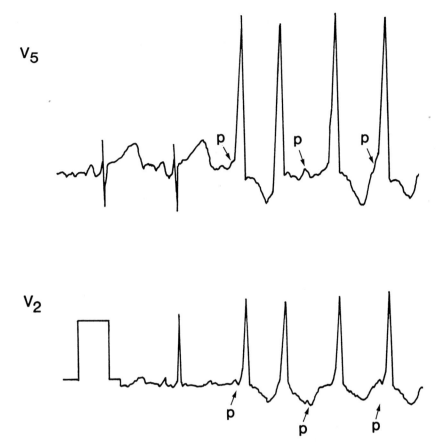

Figure 7–8. Ventricular tachycardia. Wide-complex tachycardia up to 220 bpm after sinus rhythm. Note change in QRS morphology from sinus and atrioventricular dissociation during ventricular tachycardia. P, P waves. The leads are simultaneous.

BRADYCARDIA

Postoperative Complete Heart Block

Postoperative CHB occurs most frequently with surgery involving ventricular septal defect closure or resection of tissues near the AV node (subaortic stenosis, ventricular septal defect enlargement) and frequently in patients with a predisposition to CHB such as corrected transposition or left atrial isomerism (polysplenia syndrome) (Fig. 7–9).

Diagnosis. On ECG or a *long* rhythm strip, there is atrioventricular dissociation in which the atrial rate is faster than the ventricular rate.

Differential Diagnosis. CHB is differentiated from an accelerated junction or ventricular rhythm because in CHB, the atrial rate is more rapid than the "escape"

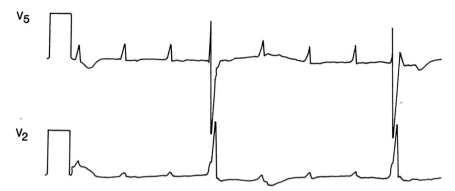

Figure 7–9. Complete atrioventricular block. Note atrioventricular dissociation and narrow-complex escape rhythm. P waves, 140 bpm; QRS, 40 bpm. No P waves are conducted. Leads are simultaneous.

rate, whereas in the latter two arrhythmias, the atrial rate slows or stops, giving rise to an escape rhythm; sometimes, lengthy rhythm strips are necessary to observe this.

The diagnosis of CHB should not be made in the presence of atrial silence (sinus arrest) without atrial pacing maneuvers to confirm lack of AV node conduction.

Concealed conduction (atrial fibrillation) and drug toxicity should be eliminated.

Patients who have AV node conduction that is inadequate to sustain adequate cardiac output or who are symptomatic should be treated as if they have CHB.

Therapy. *Ventricular pacing* with the use of temporary leads: epicardial, transvenous, and transesophageal. If pacing leads are not available, use *transcutaneous pacing* (Zoll) in the interim.

Temporary pacing techniques in which leads are easily displaced are not as reliable and require additional precautions and constant supervision.

Isoproterenol infusion may be used as a bridge between pacing techniques in an emergency but may not be effective.

In general, if acquired CHB or severe AV node dysfunction persists beyond 14 days, a permanent pacemaker should be implanted even if AV node conduction improves. This is because of the risk of late sudden-onset CHB and the ensuing risk of sudden death. However, if there is a poor underlying escape rhythm, many centers institute permanent pacing earlier than 14 days after surgery. (Postoperative pacing is discussed in another section.)

Bradycardia

Other than CHB and AV node dysfunction, the main causes of bradycardia involve sinus node dysfunction, blocked PACs, and iatrogenic causes (drugs). Blocked PACs are especially common in neonates; otherwise, look for central lines or other foreign objects causing PACs. Occasionally, hypoxia or increased intracranial pressure is implicated; rarely, hypothyroidism is a cause. Transient sinus arrest or bradycardia may also follow cardiac surgery; the sinus node extends from the posterior junction of the superior vena cava and right atrium down the posterolateral right atrium for ≤1.5 cm and thus can be damaged during cannulation or a number of atrial operations.

Diagnosis. An ECG with a long rhythm strip or a Holter monitor.

Therapy. Dictated more by symptoms than by rhythm. Underlying causes should first be corrected if possible.

Isoproterenol infusion (or possibly *theophylline* for sinus node dysfunction) or pacing is instituted.

MISCELLANEOUS ARRHYTHMIAS

Neonates may present with all forms of SVT except for AVNRT, which is rarely diagnosed before 3 years of age. Unique types of SVT include chaotic atrial tachycardia (CAT) and congenital JET. CAT has features of AET, atrial flutter, and atrial fibrillation and usually exhibits at least three different P-wave morphologies. As is the case in neonates with atrial flutter or frequent PACs, there usually is a structurally normal heart, and the natural history is toward gradual resolution in the first year of life. Therapy of CAT tends to be relatively conservative unless the patient is symptomatic. Digoxin and possibly class IC or III agents can be used. Congenital JET is rare and difficult to suppress and has considerable morbidity and mortality. Neonatal ventricular tachycardia is rare and may be due to myocardial hamartomas, myocarditis, or other myocardial abnormality. Large doses of amiodarone may be required. Surgical resection or cryoablation is successful.

Long QT syndrome (Fig. 7–10) should be ruled out in individuals with an unexplained *aborted sudden death* episode. There may be a history of recurrent syncope or "seizures" or frequent multiform ventricular arrhythmias. Affected persons may have inadvertently received a QT interval–prolonging drug or be susceptible to drug-induced QT prolongation. The family history may be positive (Jervell and Lange-Nielsen syndrome or Romano-Ward syndrome). Findings con-

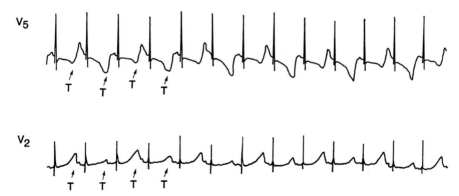

Figure 7–10. Prolonged QT interval and T wave alternans. Note the prolonged QT interval and alternating T-wave polarity (top) and alternating T-wave amplitude (bottom). The strips are simultaneous. T, T waves.

sist of QT prolongation (QT_c of >0.44), abnormal T-wave morphology, T-wave alternans or pause-dependent QT prolongation, or bizarre U waves. Most frequently, signs of *digoxin toxicity* consist of nausea and vomiting. Rhythm abnormalities include PVCs and, in more severe cases, sustained ventricular, junctional, or atrial tachycardia, or AV node dysfunction and significant bradycardia. Initial measures include stopping digoxin, obtaining immediate serum digoxin levels and electrolytes, and determining possible causes of digoxin toxicity. Digoxin immune Fab (Digibind) is used for severe toxicity, increasing hyperkalemia, or a potentially fatal ingestion.

BIBLIOGRAPHY

Fyler DC: Nadas' Pediatric Cardiology. Philadelphia, Hanley & Belfus, Inc., 1992.
Garson A Jr: The Electrocardiogram in Infants and Children: A Systematic Approach. Philadelphia, Lea & Febiger, 1983.
Gillette PC, Garson A Jr: Pediatric Arrhythmias: Electrophysiology and Pacing. Philadelphia, WB Saunders, 1990.
Park MK: How to Read Pediatric ECGs. Chicago, Year Book Medical Publishers, 1987.
Prystowsky EN, Klein GJ: Cardiac Arrhythmias: An Integrated Approach for the Clinician. New York, McGraw-Hill, 1994.

7.3 Cardiogenic Shock and Congestive Heart Failure in Infants and Children

BRADLEY P. FUHRMAN, MD
LYNN J. HERNAN, MD
MICHELE C. PAPO, MD, MPH

Cardiogenic shock is a clinical syndrome. It is a circulatory state in which the heart is unable to meet the demand of the body for perfusion and oxygen delivery. Cardiogenic shock is the most severe presentation of congestive heart failure (CHF) and represents absolute exhaustion of cardiac reserve.

Pathophysiology

Cardiogenic shock occurs when the cardiovascular system is either unable to compensate for an excessive workload or unable to perform normal work because of functional impairment. It often represents an abrupt destabilization of normal compensatory mechanisms. Some general causes of cardiogenic shock are listed in Table 7–7.

Coronary vascular occlusion, the most common cause of abrupt decompensation and cardiogenic shock in adults, is seldom a cause of cardiogenic shock in infants and children. Nevertheless, *myocardial ischemia is commonly the confounding variable on which outcome depends.* In general, CHF reduces stroke volume and diastolic blood pressure while elevating myocardial workload and oxygen demand. This may cause ischemia, which further reduces stroke volume and myocardial perfusion. This cycle, if allowed to proceed unchecked, may exhaust cardiac reserve and lead to cardiogenic shock.

For example, in the infant with a *congenital cardiac malformation,* CHF is often the direct result of ventricular volume overload of the heart. The infant with a ventricular septal defect, for example, may have so large a left-to-right shunt across the defect that only a small fraction of left ventricular inflow (left atrial return) is ejected to the aorta. *A 75% left-to-right shunt forces the left ventricle to pump four units of blood for every unit that enters the aorta.* In such a patient, the left ventricular volume load is massive. This requires an increase in left atrial pressure (preload) to achieve the requisite elevated left ventricular end-diastolic volume. Ultimately, the heart must hypertrophy to pump at this greater chamber circumference, making it less compliant and further increasing requisite preload. Pulmonary edema and respiratory symptoms may occur. Any demand for greater aortic flow will further elevate end-diastolic volume and left atrial pressure, thereby worsening the CHF. Conversely, an abrupt reduction in left atrial pressure, such as may occur during aggressive diuretic therapy, with diarrhea and dehydration, or after hemorrhage, may decrease stroke volume and cause cardiogenic shock.

Obstruction of a ventricle can cause CHF by exaggerating the ventricular work required to eject blood. When the metabolic cost of this work exceeds the potential of the coronary circulation to supply oxygen and substrate to the myocardium, coronary ischemia occurs. Critical aortic stenosis, for example, may present with heart failure in infancy. Myocardial ischemia may lead to endocardial fibroelastosis, subendocardial infarction, and loss of myocardial function. If cardiac reserve is exhausted, cardiogenic shock occurs. The infant with left ventricular

Table 7–7. PROCESSES CAUSING OR CONTRIBUTING TO CARDIOGENIC SHOCK

Mechanism	Example
Ventricular volume overload	Ventricular septal defect
Ventricular outflow obstruction	Aortic stenosis
Myocardial dysfunction	Myocarditis
Myocardial ischemia	Anomalous left coronary
Ventricular inflow restriction	Pericardial tamponade
Dysrhythmias	Paroxysmal atrial tachycardia
Anemia	Repetitive phlebotomy
Hypoxia	Transposition of great vessels
Systemic hypermetabolism	Fever

outflow tract obstruction who is faced with an abrupt demand for increased oxygen delivery to tissues, such as fever or intense crying, may deteriorate, develop myocardial ischemia, and progress to cardiogenic shock.

Ductus closure is another abrupt circulatory change that may precipitate cardiogenic shock. The infant with coarctation or interruption of the aortic arch may be subject to abrupt worsening of obstruction at the moment of ductus closure.

Muscle dysfunction may be a primary cause of CHF in infants and children. In cardiomyopathy or myocarditis, muscle function is impaired and contractility is reduced. Cardiogenic shock may be precipitated by any abrupt and excessive demand for myocardial work. Moreover, progressive myocardial dysfunction may impair the ability of the heart to meet even normal demand.

Primary myocardial ischemia can cause cardiogenic shock. In anomalous origin of the left coronary artery from the pulmonary artery, coronary perfusion pressure may be inadequate to support left ventricular work. This may precipitate infarction or cardiogenic shock or both.

Cardiac inflow restriction may also contribute to symptoms by elevating the preload required to fill even the normal ventricle, as in congenital or acquired mitral stenosis. In this situation, even minor increases in systemic oxygen demand or small decreases in cardiac filling time (associated with tachycardia) may inordinately elevate preload and precipitate pulmonary edema. Although seldom a cause of cardiogenic shock, restricted cardiac inflow may severely limit cardiac reserve. In pericardial tamponade, inflow restriction may severely limit cardiac reserve, and cardiogenic shock can occur.

Other causes of cardiogenic shock include dysrhythmias (fast or slow), profound anemia, severe hypoxia, and pathologic demand for oxygen delivery (e.g., thyrotoxicosis, pyrexia).

The above mechanisms may coexist and act synergistically to produce cardiac decompensation and, ultimately, cardiogenic shock.

Table 7–8 lists conditions that may cause cardiogenic shock in infants and children. This is not an exhaustive list but illustrates the diversity of conditions that may be associated with CHF in this age group.

Table 7–8. CONDITIONS THAT MAY CAUSE CARDIOGENIC SHOCK IN INFANTS AND CHILDREN

Congenital cardiac malformations
Congenital arteriovenous malformations
Anomalies of aortic arch
Endocardial fibroelastosis
Anomalous origin of left coronary artery
Cardiomyopathy
Myocarditis
Anemia
Congenital heart block
Tachyarrhythmias
Kawasaki syndrome
Endocarditis
Cardiac surgery

Clinical Presentation of Congestive Heart Failure

Because of the spectrum of decompensation encompassed by the term *congestive heart failure* and because of the age specificity of these manifestations, presenting findings are quite variable. In all age groups, heart failure implies cardiac enlargement, tachycardia, and tachypnea. In the neonate, because ventricular interdependence makes left and right heart failure virtually inseparable, hepatomegaly is virtually always present. Exercise intolerance may be manifest as dyspnea on exertion or as undue fatigue in the older child, or it may be manifest as feeding intolerance in the infant. Hypoxia may be a sign of pulmonary edema, in which case it is generally responsive to oxygen administration, or it may represent an associated aspect of congenital cardiac disease such as right-to-left shunting of blood or admixture of systemic and pulmonary venous return.

Clinical Presentation of Cardiogenic Shock

Cardiogenic shock is the superimposition of poor perfusion, diminished cardiac output, hypotension, and metabolic acidosis on the other manifestations of CHF. Metabolic acidosis, hypotension, poor perfusion, thready pulses, pallor, and diaphoresis are often presenting findings in ductus-dependent malformations such as coarctation, hypoplastic left heart syndrome, interruption of the aortic arch, and critical aortic stenosis. This presentation is the hallmark of vein of Galen aneurysm. Cardiogenic shock is also an occasional presenting picture in cardiomyopathy, anomalous origin of the left coronary artery, and myocarditis. In all age groups, sepsis may be accompanied by cardiogenic shock.

MANAGEMENT

The treatment of cardiogenic shock must begin with the same ABCs as resuscitation. The airway should be secured and mechanical ventilation be instituted to *reduce the work of respiratory muscles and ensure oxygenation.* Circulation must be supported as appropriate for the severity of the disorder.

The generalities of treatment are categorized in Table 7–9. In general, myocardial dysfunction is treated with drug therapy directed at enhancement of contractility. Cautious vascular volume expansion (preload augmentation of ventricular work with the use of the Frank-Starling mechanism) may improve cardiac output in the patient with cardiogenic shock and is a vital emergency measure. Once mechanical ventilation has been instituted, vascular volume expansion becomes relatively safe. Myocardial dysfunction will occasionally respond to afterload reduction, but in cardiogenic shock, afterload cannot be reduced until cardiac output has been restored. Relief of the underlying cause of ventricular overwork should be immediately planned in the patient with surgically treatable cardiogenic shock. Medical relief of overwork may be accomplished by reestablishing ductus patency in certain cardiac defects. In certain situations, diuresis may be the mainstay of decongestive therapy for CHF, but it usually plays little role in the treatment of cardiogenic

Table 7–9. TREATMENT OF CARDIOGENIC SHOCK IN INFANTS AND CHILDREN

Intubation and mechanical ventilation
Vascular volume expansion
Drugs that augment contractility
Digoxin
Catecholamines (dopamine, dobutamine, epinephrine, norepinephrine, isoproterenol)
Methylxanthines (theophylline)
Bipyridines (amrinone)
Myocardial workload reduction
Oxygen and positive end-expiratory pressure

shock. Oxygen therapy is effective insofar as it enhances arterial and myocardial oxygenation, relieves dyspnea, and reduces pulmonary vascular resistance.

Volume Expansion to Enhance Cardiac Output in Cardiogenic Shock

The infant or child with cardiogenic shock may, but does not always, exhaust his or her Starling mechanism reserve. Severe heart failure may interfere with oral fluid intake or may occur quite suddenly (as in ductus-dependent cardiac defects). This may interfere with the natural tendency of the body to expand vascular volume in the face of low cardiac output. The excessive use of diuretics may pose a similar problem. Volume expansion is, therefore, *a reasonable first line of treatment in cardiogenic shock unless preload is known to be adequate.*

Overzealous volume expansion can cause pulmonary edema or anasarca. It may produce myocardial edema that can interfere with diastolic function of the heart. Pulmonary edema in general responds to positive end-expiratory pressure. Anasarca is of little acute significance. An initial trial of volume expansion is, therefore, safe in the patient with cardiogenic shock.

Drugs That Enhance Myocardial Contractility

The general categories of inotropic agents are catecholamines, digitalis-like agents, and amrinone-like agents. Of these, the digitalis family has the longest tradition of use for cardiac inotropy.

Digoxin and related compounds inhibit activity of the membrane bound sodium-potassium ATPase. This raises intracellular sodium, which, in turn, slows the rate of exchange of intracellular calcium for extracellular sodium. The resultant rise in intracellular calcium augments contractility. This inotropic effect is not accompanied by tachycardia. In fact, digoxin is vagomimetic and slows the heart. This may be beneficial, as it lengthens diastole, allowing more time for cardiac filling. In the critical care setting, digoxin has been used less since the introduction of continuous catecholamine infusions. The reasons for this are the relatively long half-life, predominant renal clearance, and propensity to cause cardiac dysrhythmias of digoxin. This propensity of digoxin is exaggerated by hypokalemia. Diuretics, which may cause potassium depletion, add to this potential hazard of digoxin therapy.

Catecholamines act through the adrenergic receptor complex. These receptors are present in myocardium and in vascular and bronchial smooth muscle. Adrenergic receptors differ in their receptor specificity and in their regulatory proteins.

The distribution of receptors is a primary determinant of the effect of an agonist. For example, D_1 receptors, which are stimulated by dopamine, are found primarily in kidney, viscera, and coronary arteries. When stimulated, they cause renal, splanchnic, and coronary blood flow to rise, yet they have no detectable effect on skin perfusion because they are not present in skin.

Another determinant of agonist effect is relative potency at each kind of receptor (Table 7–10). For example, norepinephrine is a potent α-agonist and a weak β-agonist. Its effect is therefore predominantly to constrict systemic arterioles. It is a mild inotrope. Dopamine stimulates D_1 receptors at low, intermediate, and high doses, $β_1$ receptors at intermediate and high doses, and $α_1$ receptors only at high doses.

When an inotropic agent causes the heart to pump more blood at constant aortic pressure (a desired effect), cardiac workload is increased. This requires augmentation of oxygen delivery to the myocardium. For this reason, *catecholamine use may be associated with myocardial ischemia, even in nonischemic cardiac disease.*

All of the commonly used catecholamines, epinephrine, norepinephrine, dopamine, dobutamine, and isoproterenol, cause tachycardia. As the heart rate rises, diastole shortens proportionally more than does systole. This can interfere with cardiac filling, thereby diminishing stroke volume.

Catecholamines Are Intrinsically Arrhythmogenic. *Methylxanthines* (e.g., theophylline) and bipyridines (e.g., amrinone) augment contractility by elevating intracellular cyclic AMP but via mechanisms that are independent of the adrenergic receptor. Amrinone and its cogeners inhibit activity of phosphodiesterase III, which degrades only cyclic AMP. *Amrinone* raises intracellular calcium, is a positive inotrope, and is a systemic vasodilator. This combination of inotropic activity and afterload reduction may have special value in cardiogenic shock and in situations in which myocardial workload should not be excessively increased.

Treatment of Congestive Heart Failure by Reducing Cardiac Work. The burden of the heart, to meet the need of the body for systemic oxygen and substrate delivery while supporting its own metabolic requirements, can represent a conflict

Table 7–10. ADRENERGIC RECEPTORS

Receptor	Action	Order of Efficacy
$α_1$	Vasoconstriction	Epinephrine > norepinephrine isoproterenol
$β_1$	Inotropic, chronotropic	Isoproterenol, epinephrine, dobutamine > dopamine > norepinephrine
$β_2$	Vasodilation and bronchodilation	Isoproterenol > epinephrine > dobutamine > dopamine > norepinephrine
D	Vasodilation (renal)	Dopamine

of interest. In cardiogenic shock, when the heart is unable to bear this burden, forcing it to perform heroics will often cause myocardial necrosis. Other measures that are useful in infants and children focus on reducing cardiac work, to allow the pump to recover. This is of special importance after cardiac operations, when the heart has been injured by myocardial incision, put at risk of air embolism by opening the heart, and subjected to coronary ischemia followed by reperfusion with blood. Several of these measures are listed in Table 7–11.

Foremost among them is mechanical ventilation with oxygen, coupled with sedation and, as appropriate, neuromuscular blockade. *Mechanical ventilation alleviates the work of breathing,* which may be substantial if there is pulmonary edema or lung dysfunction. It protects the patient from risk of respiratory arrest when narcotics are used to relieve pain. Oxygen should be used to relieve arterial desaturation, as desaturation wastes a fraction of the cardiac output; desaturated blood carries oxygen inefficiently. Positive end-expiratory pressure is often used to alleviate arterial desaturation in the patient with pulmonary edema. Sedation, pain relief, and neuromuscular blockade limit endogenous catecholamine secretion, reduce sympathetic vasoconstriction to pain, and prevent patient movement, which contributes to circulatory demand.

Prevention of fever reduces metabolic demand that must be satisfied by activity of the heart. It also reduces heart rate, facilitates cardiac filling in diastole, and prevents or treats junctional ectopic tachycardia.

DEVICES TO SUPPORT THE FAILING HEART

Aortic balloon counterpulsion is possible in very small children but becomes increasingly challenging as catheter size declines, heart rate rises, or myocardial function worsens. Arrhythmias interfere with this modality.

Infants and children, like adults, can be supported with the use of extracorporeal devices if they experience temporary or permanent myocardial devastation. Extracorporeal membrane oxygenation (ECMO) has been shown to be useful as a method of cardiac rescue after repair of congenital cardiac malformations. Some postoperative patients are unable to support their circulation despite an adequate repair, and they develop cardiogenic shock. Although ECMO raises afterload in this setting by restoring adequate blood pressure, it relieves the heart of the burden

Table 7–11. MODALITIES USED TO REDUCE MYOCARDIAL WORK IN CARDIOGENIC SHOCK

Mechanical ventilation
Sedation
Pain relief
Neuromuscular blockade
Temperature control
Pharmacologic afterload reduction
Aortic balloon counterpulsion
Extracorporeal membrane oxygenation, ECLS, LVAD, RVAD

ECLS, extracorporeal life support; LVAD, left ventricular assist device; RVAD, right ventricular assist device.

of supporting the entire circulation. At the same time, it raises coronary artery diastolic pressure. It therefore "rests" both right and left ventricles. When it is used to rest the heart, it must be remembered that the left ventricle may be unable to eject at the higher afterload afforded by the extracorporeal pump. In this setting, left atrial return (flow through the ductus arteriosus, bronchial flow, residual antegrade flow across the pulmonary valve) may pool on the left side of the heart. Pressure could, in theory, rise in the left ventricle and atrium, until it equaled aortic diastolic pressure. When this occurs to a clinically important degree, pulmonary edema develops. This scenario can be prevented by "venting" the left atrium to the venous return of the ECMO circuit, by administration of inotropic agents, or by atrial septectomy in selected patients. ECMO has also been used with success in patients with myocarditis.

Other devices, such as left ventricular assist device and right ventricular assist device, can be used to move atrial return to the appropriate great cardiac vessel, completely or partially bypassing one ventricle. This does not require a membrane oxygenator and does not require systemic heparinization. In most infants and children, however, cardiogenic shock is a biventricular problem.

Summary

Cardiogenic shock is a lethal, unstable situation. Its presence implies inadequate myocardial reserve. It requires prompt stabilization at all ages.

BIBLIOGRAPHY

Dalton HJ, Siewers RD, Ruhrman BP, et al: Extracorporeal membrane oxygenation for cardiac rescue following surgery for congenital heart disease. Crit Care Med 21:1020, 1993.

Fuhrman BP: Regional circulation. *In* Fuhrman BP, Shoemaker WC (eds): Critical Care: State of the Art, Vol. 10. Anaheim, Society of Critical Care Medicine, 1989, pp. 338–339.

Fuhrman BP, Papo MC: Critical care after surgery for congenital cardiac disease. *In* Fuhrman BP, Zimmerman JJ (eds): Pediatric Critical Care. St. Louis, Mosby–Year Book, 1992, pp. 345–358.

Gaasch WH, Levine JH, Quinones MA, et al: Left ventricular compliance: mechanisms and clinical implications. Am J Cardiol 38:645, 1976.

Kubler W, Katz AM: Mechanisms of early pump failure in the ischemic heart: possible role of ATP depletion and inorganic phosphate accumulation. Am J Cardiol 40:467, 1977.

Notterman DA: Pharmacology of the cardiovascular system. *In* Fuhrman BP, Zimmerman JJ (eds): Pediatric Critical Care. St. Louis, Mosby–Year Book, 1992, pp. 323–338.

Takahashi M, Lurie P: Abnormalities and diseases of the coronary vessels. *In* Adams FH, Emmanouilides GC (eds): Moss' Heart Disease in Infants, Children and Adolescents, 3rd ed. Baltimore, Williams & Wilkins, 1989, pp. 630–635.

Talner NS: Heart failure. *In* Adams FH, Emmanouilides GC (eds): Moss' Heart Disease in Infants, Children and Adolescents, 3rd ed. Baltimore, Williams & Wilkins, 1989, pp. 890–911.

Rockley CE, Edwards JE, Karp RE: Mitral valve disease. *In* Hurst JW, Schlant RL, Rockley CE, et al (eds): The Heart, 7th ed. New York, McGraw-Hill, 1989.

7.4 Postoperative Cardiac Care for Congenital Heart Disease

MICHELE C. PAPO, MD, MPH
LYNN J. HERNAN, MD
BRADLEY P. FUHRMAN, MD

Postoperative care for the child after surgical correction for congenital heart disease is divided into two phases: the initial phase involves *supporting the myocardium* to prevent secondary injury to the heart and other organs, and the second phase involves the *weaning of external support* as the myocardium and other organs recover from the stress of surgery and cardiopulmonary bypass. Numerous factors dictate the course of the postoperative recovery period after surgical repair of congenital heart disease (Table 7–12).

Table 7–12. FACTORS DICTATING POSTOPERATIVE CARDIAC CARE FOR CONGENITAL HEART DISEASE

Congenital Heart Lesion	*Preoperative clinical status*
Cyanotic congenital heart disease	Metabolic/nutritional status
Ebstein's anomaly	Cardiopulmonary function
Tricuspid atresia	Infectious status
Single ventricle with pulmonary atresia	Immunologic status
Tetralogy of Fallot	Renal function
Truncus arteriosus	Neurologic function
Pulmonary atresia	Associated malformations/chromosomal
Atrioventricular septal defect	anomalies
Total anomalous pulmonary venous	Coagulation status
return	
D-Transposition of the great arteries	*Operative course*
Acyanotic congenital heart disease	Duration of cardiopulmonary bypass
Patent ductus arteriosus	Hypothermic circulatory arrest
Ventricular septal defect	Duration of aortic cross clamping
Atrial septal defect	Type of operative repair performed
Coarctation of the aorta	Ability to wean off cardiopulmonary bypass
Hypoplastic left ventricle	Level of support required off
Mitral atresia/stenosis	cardiopulmonary bypass
Aortic stenosis	
Interrupted aortic arch	
Anomalous coronary artery	

Pathophysiology

The heart is a resilient organ that can undergo the stress of cardiopulmonary bypass and transient periods of ischemia with full functional recovery. *Poor preoperative clinical status* before surgery can complicate the postoperative course and increase morbidity and mortality, even after a simple palliative procedure. Surgery is a stress, and therefore optimizing clinical status before surgery can aid in reducing postoperative morbidity. Children with cyanotic heart lesions are prone to increased fibrinolysis and bleeding after surgery, which can complicate their hospital course. During surgery, the duration of cardiopulmonary bypass, type of surgical repair, and ability to be weaned off bypass are important factors that affect the level of monitoring and cardiopulmonary support that will be required in the pediatric intensive care unit. *Cardiopulmonary bypass* causes leukocyte migration and the release of toxic mediators (e.g., thromboxanes, prostaglandins, leukotrienes, free radicals) that damage the pulmonary capillary endothelium. The longer the bypass time, the greater is the likelihood of capillary leak and pulmonary edema. Pulmonary endothelial damage can exacerbate pulmonary hypertension in susceptible patients. The goals of postoperative cardiac care for the child with congenital heart disease are to optimize cardiopulmonary support through external monitoring and to provide adequate analgesia/anxiolysis, while the myocardium recovers from the stress of surgical correction.

Differential Diagnosis

Surgical repairs can be viewed as being palliative or corrective. *Palliative repairs* are procedures that "bridge" or "stage" patients for definitive repair. Table 7–13 lists both palliative and corrective surgical procedures that are associated with common heart lesions. *Corrective surgical repairs* do not usually leave patients with residual defects and are often associated with more complex surgical corrections (e.g., tetralogy of Fallot) and therefore require more rigorous support in the initial phase of postoperative cardiac care.

Management

The goals of postoperative cardiac care are to (1) prevent secondary injury to the myocardium and other organs and (2) assess the need for external monitoring and cardiopulmonary support.

PHASE I: PREVENTION OF SECONDARY INJURY TO THE MYOCARDIUM AND OTHER ORGANS

Respiratory Support

A. Assess patency of the airway
B. Assess adequacy of ventilation

Table 7–13. PALLIATIVE AND CORRECTIVE REPAIRS
FOR CONGENITAL HEART DISEASE

Palliative Repairs	*Indication*
Systemic to pulmonary shunts	Pulmonary atresia
Blalock-Taussig	
Potts	
Waterston	
Glenn	
Pulmonary artery banding	Single ventricle, VSD
Atrial septectomy	Transposition of the great vessels
Corrective Repairs	
Patent ductus arteriosus ligation	PDA
Closure of a septal defect	ASD, VSD, AV canal, TOF
Fontan procedure	Single ventricle, tricuspid atresia
Rastelli procedure	Truncus arteriosus, pulmonary atresia
Norwood procedure	Hypoplastic left heart syndrome
Arterial switch (Jatene procedure)	Transposition of the great vessels
Atrial switch	Transposition of the great vessels
Mustard procedure	
Senning procedure	
Coarctectomy	Coarctation of the aorta
Valve repair or replacement	AS/AI, PS/PI, TS/TI, MS/MI

VSD, ventricular septal defect; PDA, patent ductus arteriosus; ASD, atrial septal defect; AV canal, atrioventricular canal; TOF, Tetralogy of Fallot; aortic stenosis (AS) or regurgitation (AI); pulmonary stenosis (PS) or regurgitation (PI); tricuspid stenosis (TS) or regurgitation (TI); mitral stenosis (MS) or regurgitation (MI).

C. Obtain chest radiograph to assess lung inflation, endotracheal tube position, intravascular lines, drains, and pacing wire placement
D. Assess pulmonary function
  1. Noninvasive
    a. Pulse oximetry
    b. Capnography: end-tidal carbon dioxide
    c. Transcutaneous oxygen/carbon dioxide monitoring
  2. Invasive
    a. Arterial blood gases
    b. Mixed venous blood gases
E. Mechanical ventilation
  1. Maintain adequate functional residual capacity with tidal volumes between 10 and 15 mL/kg and positive end-expiratory pressure (PEEP) of 2 to 4 cm H_2O
  2. Adjust fractional inspired oxygen (FIO_2) to maintain adequate oxygenation (arterial oxygen tension [PaO_2] of 75 to 100 mm Hg) in acyanotic lesions
    a. FIO_2 can be decreased and PEEP increased to limit pulmonary blood flow
    b. A high FIO_2 is used in patients with pulmonary hypertension (FIO_2 to keep PaO_2 at >100 mm Hg)
  3. Minute ventilation

    a. Maintain adequate rate and tidal volume to keep arterial carbon dioxide tension ($Paco_2$) at 35 to 45 mm Hg

    b. Acute exacerbations of pulmonary hypertension are treated with increasing inspired oxygen and hyperventilation to a pH between 7.50 and 7.60

    c. Airway pressure

        (1) Mean airway pressure should be adequate to prevent atelectasis and maintain lung inflation at functional residual capacity. Peak inspiratory pressure should be limited to ≤35 cm H_2O

        (2) *Overinflation* of the lungs causes a decrease in venous return, increase in right ventricular afterload; overinflation should be avoided under conditions of restricted pulmonary blood flow (e.g., pulmonary atresia)

        (3) PEEP can be used to prevent small airway closure and is beneficial when ventilation/perfusion mismatch is the cause of intrapulmonary shunting and hypoxia

Cardiac Support

A. Assess hemodynamics

  1. Noninvasive monitoring

    a. Assess peripheral perfusion

    Pulses: quality of central versus peripheral pulses

    Temperature: core versus peripheral skin temperature (toe temperature)

    b. Cardiac examination: palpation and auscultation

    c. Chest radiograph to assess heart size, mediastinum, and line placement

    d. Echocardiogaphy: transthoracic or transesophageal

    e. Electrocardiogram (ECG): 12 lead

  2. Invasive monitoring

    a. Arterial line placement: arterial pressure monitoring

    b. Central venous line placement: right atrial pressure monitoring

    c. Swan-Ganz catheter placement: provides central venous, pulmonary artery, and pulmonary capillary wedge pressure monitoring; cardiac output can be assessed by thermodilution or mixed venous saturation

    d. Transthoracic vascular line placement: direct monitoring of pulmonary artery (PA), left atrial, and right atrial pressures

B. Assess metabolic status

  1. Obtain arterial blood gases and serum lactate level to rule out hypoxemia, hypercarbia, and metabolic acidosis

  2. Rule out electrolyte abnormalities and assess ionized calcium, blood sugar, and magnesium levels

  3. Assess oxygen-carrying capacity by obtaining hemoglobin and hematocrit

C. Assess adequacy of renal function and urine output

  1. Urine output of >25 mL/hr for an adolescent/adult or >0.5 to 1 mL/kg/hr for a child/infant

  2. Monitor blood urea nitrogen and creatinine and obtain urinalysis

D. Assess need for sedation and pain control

  1. Assess need for sedation, anxiolysis, and analgesia

  2. Assess mental status and neurologic function after surgery

The hallmarks of inadequate oxygen delivery and poor cardiac output are poor perfusion, hypotension, acidosis, decreased urine output, and altered mental status.

E. Management to optimize and support myocardial function
  1. Optimize preload
     a. Volume given in 5- to 10-mL/kg boluses to increase central venous or left atrial pressure to 10 to 15 mm Hg
     b. Volume can consist of blood, colloid, or crystalloid
     c. Patients with systemic-to-pulmonary artery shunts or status post-Fontan procedure may require high central venous pressures to maintain pulmonary perfusion (15 to 20 mm Hg); the transpulmonary pressure gradient determines pulmonary perfusion
  2. Contractility
     a. Inotropic support is instituted when preload has been optimized but low cardiac output persists
     b. Inotropes can be used to increase contractility (see Chapter 7.5, Cardiovascular Pharmacology)
     c. Inotropes increase myocardial oxygen consumption; therefore, these drugs are used until their side effects outweigh their benefit
     d. Maintain normal ionized calcium levels with calcium chloride ($CaCl_2$) (10 to 20 mg/kg IV; 500 mg maximum/dose; central access needed) or calcium gluconate (100 mg/kg; 500 mg maximum/dose). Calcium infusions are frequently used in patients with DiGeorge syndrome
     e. Atrioventricular pacing can be used to increase heart rate and thus augment cardiac output since stroke volume is relatively small in children compared with adults
     f. Cardiac assist devices and extracorporeal life support (extracorporeal membrane oxygenation) have been used when pharmacologic support fails to improve cardiac output
     g. Consider delaying sternal closure until myocardial edema and contractility improve for 24 to 48 hours
  3. Afterload
     a. Factors that increase pulmonary or systemic afterload (vasoconstriction) include hypoxia, hypercarbia, acidosis, hypothermia, and pain
     b. Use of regional or systemic vasodilators can reduce ventricular work and therefore augment cardiac output when preload and contractility have been optimized (e.g., nitric oxide [pulmonary circulation], nitroprusside, and nitroglycerin)
     c. Afterload reduction is contraindicated in patients with residual outflow obstruction and lesions that require adequate diastolic pressure, for example, idiopathic hypertrophic subaortic stenosis
     d. Adequate preload is needed when using afterload-reducing drugs to prevent hypotension due to venodilation or a loss of arterial tone
  4. Diastolic dysfunction
     a. A noncompliant heart has poor diastolic relaxation; therefore, cardiac filling and myocardial perfusion are compromised
     b. Poor diastolic function is manifested by a small heart on radiography,

high filling pressures (right or left atrial pressures or both), and clinical signs of low cardiac output

c. Drugs that improve myocardial relaxation include amrinone (phosphodiesterase F-III inhibitor) and dobutamine (β_2-adrenergic agonist)

d. Avoid inotropes that cause excessive tachycardia and reduce diastolic coronary perfusion time (i.e., isoproterenol)

e. Aortic counterpulsation can increase coronary perfusion pressure by increasing diastolic aortic pressure during diastole (balloon inflation) and therefore improving myocardial perfusion

Fluid and Nutritional Support

A. Assess whether fluids are adequate
   1. Assess peripheral perfusion (pulses and capillary filling time)
   2. Assess preload via central venous pressure or left atrial pressure or both
   3. Adequate urine output
   4. Obtain electrolytes, blood urea nitrogen, creatinine, urine specific gravity, and hemoglobin and hematocrit levels
   5. Assess ongoing fluid losses through drains and chest tubes
B. Management of fluid/nutritional support
   1. Fluids given in 5 to 10 mL/kg boluses, monitoring preload and urine output
   2. Maintenance fluids usually restricted (one-half to two-thirds maintenance first 24 to 48 hours with adequate dextrose to prevent hypoglycemia)
   3. Nutritional support in the form of enteral feedings or hyperalimentation should be started within 48 hours of surgery

Coagulation and Hematologic Support

A. Assess whether coagulation is adequate
   1. Obtain serial hemoglobin and hematocrit, prothrombin and partial thromboplastin times, platelet count, and fibrinogen level
   2. Assess amount of losses through drains and chest tubes
B. Management of coagulation and hematopoietic deficiencies
   1. Blood losses are replaced with whole blood or packed red blood cells
   2. Anormalities in prothrombin and partial thromboplastin times can be corrected with fresh frozen plasma and keeping platelet count at >100,000
   3. Low fibrinogen levels and other factor replacement can be corrected with cryoprecipitate
   4. Amicar (aminocaproic acid) if given preoperatively can decrease bleeding secondary to fibrinolysis (initial bolus of 75 to 100 mg/kg IV and then 15 to 30 mg/kg/hr by continuous infusion) (over 30–60 min)
   5. Assess activated clotting time and give protamine for anticoagulation related to high heparin level (protamine can have side effects, including hypotension, bronchospasm, and acute pulmonary hypertensive crisis)

6. If bleeding is >10 mL/kg/hr despite blood and replacement for coagulation deficiencies, consider surgical exploration for assessment of location of bleeding
7. Blood products should be cytomegalovirus-negative and irradiated for children suspected of having DiGeorge syndrome or known to be immunocompromised to prevent graft-versus-host disease

Renal Support

A. Assess renal perfusion
   1. Assess urine output (>0.5 to 1 mL/kg/hr or >25 mL/hr in adolescent)
   2. If there is renal impairment, follow urine and serum electrolytes, blood urea nitrogen, creatinine, urine specific gravity, and urine analysis
B. Management of inadequate urine output
   1. Optimize preload with fluid replacement
   2. Assess adequacy of cardiac output and need for inotropes
   3. When preload and cardiac output are optimized, consider small doses of loop (furosemide) or osmotic (mannitol) diuretic
   4. Enhance renal perfusion with dopamine (1 to 5 μg/kg/min)

Gastrointestinal Assessment

A. Assess splanchnic perfusion
   1. Perform clinical examination for hepatomegaly, splenomegaly, abdominal distention, and ileus
   2. Obtain liver function tests (AST, ALT, bilirubin, prothrombin time) to evaluate hepatic insufficiency
   3. Evaluate nasogastric drainage for amount of fluid, color, pH, and absence or presence of blood
B. Management to maintain adequate splanchnic perfusion
   1. Place nasogastric tube and drainage to low intermittent suction
   2. Use antacids, carafate, or H_2 blockers (e.g., cimetidine, ranitidine) to prevent gastric stress ulceration
   3. Institute early nutritional support via enteral feedings or hyperalimentation
   4. Postcoarctectomy syndrome (mesenteric arteritis) (see "Coarctation of the Aorta")

Infection Control

Management for prevention of nosocomial infection
   1. Antibiotics are started before surgery and continued for 24 to 48 hours after surgery with adequate coverage for staphylococci
   2. Treat culture-proven infections with appropriate antibiotics and avoid prolonged use of broad-spectrum antibiotics
   3. If possible, remove drains and central lines within 48 to 72 hours after surgery
   4. Prophylactic antibiotics should be used in children after repair of congenital heart disease (Dajani)

Central Nervous System and Sedation

Management of analgesia and anxiolysis
1. Analgesia can be provided by intravenous infusions of opiates
   a. Fentanyl (2 to 4 μg/kg/hr via continuous infusion or 1 to 2 μg/kg IV every 30 to 60 minutes)
   b. Morphine (0.1 to 0.2 mg/kg IV every 1 to 2 hours)
2. Anxiolysis is provided by benzodiazepines
   a. Diazepam (0.1 to 0.2 mg/kg IV every 1 to 2 hours)
   b. Midazolam (0.1 to 0.2 mg/kg IV every 1 to 2 hours or via continuous infusion of 0.1 to 0.2 mg/kg/hr)
   c. Lorazepam (0.05 to 0.1 mg/kg IV every 1 to 2 hours)
3. Avoid histamine-releasing drugs, which can cause vasodilation and promote hypotension in hemodynamically unstable patients (e.g., morphine)
4. Patient-controlled analgesia and regional blocks can promote analgesia after thoracotomy
5. Muscle relaxants can be used to promote ventilator synchrony

PHASE II: CRITERIA FOR WEANING OF EXTERNAL MONITORING AND CARDIOPULMONARY SUPPORT

Criteria for Weaning Cardiopulmonary Support

A. Hemodynamic stability
B. Inotropic support has been weaned to low doses
C. Metabolic abnormalities have been corrected
D. Nutrition has been optimized to achieve positive nitrogen balance
E. Neurologic function is intact, including appropriate mental status, cough, and gag
F. Normal respiratory function
   1. Normal arterial blood gases
   2. Acceptable lung compliance (0.5 to 1.0 mL/cm H_2O/kg)
   3. Ventilator settings have been weaned to extubation settings
      a. Inspired oxygen concentration of ≤0.50
      b. Low mechanical ventilator rate (<10 breaths/min)
      c. PEEP weaned to ≤5 cm H_2O
      d. Peak inspiratory pressure of ≤35 cm H_2O
   4. Negative inspiratory force of ≥30 cm H_2O
   5. Vital capacity of ≥8 to 10 mL/kg

Failure to Wean Off of Cardiopulmonary Support

A. Inadequate cardiac reserve
B. Volume overload/pulmonary edema
C. Pulmonary disease is present
D. Poor metabolic/nutritional status
E. Increased metabolic demand: fever or sepsis
F. Impaired neurologic function

Postoperative Complications Associated with Surgical Correction for Congenital Heart Disease

Diaphragmatic Paralysis

Etiology. Diaphragmatic paralysis occurs due to direct trauma during surgery (transection or traction) or cold exposure during external cooling for hypothermic cardiac arrest.

Diagnosis. Children have paradoxic breathing when spontaneously breathing and may fail to wean off of mechanical ventilation. An elevated hemidiaphragm is usually seen on chest radiograph after surgery.

Investigations. Paradoxic motion of the diaphragm off positive pressure ventilation during spontaneous ventilation can be diagnostic of diaphragmatic paralysis. Fluoroscopy or ultrasound can be performed to confirm the diagnosis.

Management and Prognosis. Unilateral diaphragmatic paresis will spontaneously recover; however, many patients require prolonged mechanical ventilation. Surgical plication of the paralyzed diaphragm will restrict its movement to paradoxic breathing and should be considered if there is failure to wean from mechanical ventilation after 2 weeks.

Chylothorax

Etiology. Chylothoraces can develop as a result of transection of the lymphatics/thoracic duct during surgical dissection, or the lymphatic duct can spontaneously rupture due to obstruction of flow into the systemic venous circulation. High central venous pressure associated with superior vena cava syndrome, right heart failure, constrictive pericarditis, and clot obstructing venous return to the right atrium can cause chylous pleural effusions.

Diagnosis. A chylothorax usually manifests as a pleural effusion that evolves when the child begins enteral feeding. Fluid obtained via thoracentesis may be turbid and "milky" (due to triglycerides in the fluid) when consuming a diet with long-chain fatty acids or remain serosanguinous if on hyperalimentation.

Investigations. Laboratory analysis of the fluid obtained via thoracentesis will show a high triglyceride level. Triglyceride levels of >110 mg/dL are pathognomonic for a chylothorax, whereas a level of <50 mg/dL indicates that chylous fluid is unlikely. If triglyceride levels are between 50 and 110 mg/dL, a lipoprotein electrophoresis can be performed to search for chylomicrons, which confirm the diagnosis (Staats). Chyle is rich in protein (>3 g/dL) and immunoglobulins and contains a large number of lymphocytes of T-cell origin.

Management and Prognosis. Long-chain fatty acids ingested in the gastrointestinal tract are absorbed by lymphatics and increase lymph flow. Medium-chain triglycerides bypass lymphatics and are directly absorbed into the enterohepatic circulation. Treatment involves chest tube drainage and a diet devoid of long-chain fatty acids. Enteral feedings that are high in protein and have medium-chain triglycerides (Portagen) are first attempted. If chylous drainage persists, oral feedings are withheld, and central venous hyperalimentation is instituted. Anatomic pathology should be evaluated after surgery to eliminate the possibility of a surgically correctable cause of persistent chylous effusions. If the child becomes malnourished and immunocompromised, consider surgical ligation of the thoracic duct, pleurodesis, or placement of a pleuroperitoneal shunt.

Cardiac Dysrhythmias

See Chapter 7.2, Arrhythmias in the Pediatric Intensive Care Unit.

Cardiac Tamponade

Etiology. Cardiac tamponade after cardiac surgery is caused by the presence of fluid collecting within the pericardial sac, which impedes adequate diastolic relaxation and cardiac filling and thus impairs myocardial function. Cardiac tamponade can occur if mediastinal drainage is not adequate or if brisk bleeding occurs related to poor coagulation status or leakage of blood around suture lines.

Diagnosis. The classic presentation of cardiac tamponade is pulsus paradoxus, high central venous pressure, and a narrow pulse pressure when this condition develops over time. After cardiac surgery, cardiac tamponade can manifest acutely and as hypotension, bradycardia, and cardiac arrest. When cardiac tamponade presents insidiously, it manifests as myocardial dysfunction with signs of low cardiac output, rising ventricular end-diastolic pressures, a widened mediastinum on chest radiograph, and muffled heart sounds on auscultation.

Management and Prognosis. If cardiac tamponade is suspected, mediastinal drains should be inspected and "stripped" to remove clots. Volume expansion and correction of coagulation abnormalities can help to maintain cardiac output while pericardiocentesis or open pericardiotomy is performed. Pericardial tamponade that develops slowly over time can be drained by pigtail catheter insertion under fluoroscopic or echocardiographic guidance.

Pulmonary Hypertension

See Chapter 6.6: Use of Nitric Oxide in Pulmonary Hypertension.

Postoperative Sequelae to Palliative and Corrective Repairs for Congenital Heart Disease

Pulmonary-to-Systemic Shunts

- Blalock-Taussig: subclavian-to-pulmonary artery shunt
- Modified Blalock-Taussig: synthetic shunt placed between subclavian artery and ipsilateral pulmonary artery
- Waterston: ascending aorta-to-right pulmonary shunt
- Potts: descending aorta-to-left pulmonary artery shunt

A. Occlusion of the shunt
1. Clinical presentation
a. Loss of shunt murmur on auscultation

      b. Acute deterioration in arterial saturation or persistent cyanosis

  2. Diagnosis

      a. Two-dimensional echocardiogram can be used to assess shunt flow and size, inadequate vessel size, or obstruction at the anastomotic site

      b. Chest radiograph shows limited pulmonary blood flow

  3. Management

      a. Assess patency of airway and ventilation

      b. Maintain adequate systemic pressure to encourage left-to-right shunting

      c. Maintain adequate preload and oxygen-carrying capacity (hematocrit of 40 to 45 g/dL) to maintain oxygen delivery

      d. Prostaglandins (E_1) can be used to maintain ductal patency if not surgically ligated during surgery and may augment pulmonary blood flow (0.1 μg/kg/min)

      e. Emergency surgical repair to replace the shunt is necessary if total shunt occlusion occurs and the majority of pulmonary blood flow is dependent on this shunt

B. Pulmonary edema

  1. Clinical presentation

      a. Rales and rhonchi on auscultation

      b. Excessive arterial saturation in a cyanotic heart disease patient on room air oxygen

      c. Pleural effusion on the side of the shunt

      d. Signs of congestive heart failure

  2. Diagnosis

      a. Two-dimensional echocardiogram with Doppler to assess shunt flow and left ventricular volume overload

      b. Chest radiograph shows increased pulmonary vascular markings on side of the shunt with pleural effusions and pulmonary edema

      c. Cardiac catheterization can be used to evaluate shunts in complicated heart lesions

  3. Management

      a. Positive pressure ventilation with PEEP can maintain airway patency

      b. Inotropes can be used to support the volume-overloaded ventricle

      c. Digoxin has minimal effects on vasomotor tone and can be useful in increasing myocardial contractility

      d. If no improvement, assess need to revise and place smaller shunt

Vena Cava-to-Pulmonary Artery Anastomoses

- Glenn: superior vena cava-to-right pulmonary artery shunt
- Bidirectional Glenn: superior and inferior vena cavae-to-pulmonary artery shunt

A. Superior vena cava syndrome

  1. Clinical presentation

      a. Facial edema, periorbital swelling, venous congestion of the upper body, and high central venous pressure

      b. Pleural effusions, ascites, and hepatomegaly can develop

2. Diagnosis
   a. Two-dimensional echocardiography can be used to isolate shunt obstruction and clot and assess right atrial outflow obstruction
   b. Chest radiograph shows decreased pulmonary vascular markings
3. Management
   a. Thrombolytics (urokinase, streptokinase, recombinant tissue-type plasminogen activator) can be used in an attempt to lyse a clot
   b. Persistent or elevated central venous pressure may indicate a need to revise the shunt or for palliative repair
B. Inadequate pulmonary blood flow
   1. Clinical presentation
      a. Persistent cyanosis or acute deterioration in arterial oxygen saturation
      b. Pulmonary blood flow is determined by the pressure gradient between the systemic vein and pulmonary artery and by the resistance to blood flow into the lung; therefore, conditions that increase pulmonary vascular resistance will impair pulmonary blood flow (e.g., pulmonary disease, pulmonary vascular disease)
   2. Diagnosis
      a. Two-dimensional echocardiography can help to assess shunt patency, right ventricular compliance, cardiac function, and pulmonary artery pressure
      b. Cardiac catheterization may be needed to isolate cause of limited pulmonary blood flow if shunt is inadequate, and shunt obstruction may be amenable to balloon angioplasty
      c. Chest radiograph demonstrates diminished pulmonary vascular markings
   3. Management
      a. Assess patency and adequacy of ventilation; minimize the use of high mean airway pressures on mechanical ventilation
      b. Obtain two-dimensional echocardiogram to assess shunt function and surgical repair for cause of decreased pulmonary blood flow
      c. Optimize preload and oxygen-carrying capacity (hematocrit of 40 to 45 g/dL)
      d. Augment cardiac output with agents that decrease pulmonary vascular resistance (e.g., dobutamine, amrinone); optimize preload before using systemic pulmonary vasodilators (e.g., nitroprusside, prostaglandins) to prevent systemic hypotension
      e. If hypoxemia does not resolve, consider surgical revision of Glenn shunt

Pulmonary Artery Banding

A. Separation of the band and failure of banding
   1. Clinical presentation
      a. Failure to restrict pulmonary blood flow in patients with large left-to-right shunts results in pulmonary edema and congestive heart failure
      b. A functional band will result in a slight decrease in arterial saturation due to a restriction in pulmonary blood flow in single ventricle without restriction to pulmonary blood flow; pulmonary artery bands that are

"too loose" will have arterial oxygen saturations remaining at >90% in room air
2. Diagnosis
   a. Two-dimensional echocardiography can be used to determine position and gradient across the band
   b. Chest radiograph is compatible with congestive heart failure and pulmonary edema
3. Management
   a. Assess the need for surgical revision of banding
   b. Support cardiac function with adequate preload and inotropic support until surgical correction
B. Migration of the band with obstruction to the right pulmonary artery
   1. Clinical presentation
      a. Banding that is too tight will result in diminished pulmonary blood flow and therefore a decrease in arterial saturation
      b. Tight banding may be manifested as hypercyanotic episodes
   2. Diagnosis
      a. Two-dimensional echocardiography with Doppler to determine gradient across the band and position on the right pulmonary artery
      b. Chest radiograph shows decreased pulmonary vascular markings to the right lung compared with the left lung
   3. Management
      a. Assess airway, breathing, and circulation
      b. Maintain adequate preload and cardiac output with inotropes if needed
      c. Consider surgical revision of banding

Septal Defect Closure (Atrial, Ventricular, and Atrioventricular Septal Defects)

A. Persistent atrial or septal communication
   1. Clinical presentation
      a. Small communications may be clinically insignificant
      b. Large communications present with persistent or new holosystolic murmur (ventricular septal defect) or presence of systolic ejection murmur with fixed splitting of the second heart sound heard at the left sternal border (atrial septal defect) if there is increased pulmonary blood flow from a residual left-to-right shunt
   2. Diagnosis
      a. Two-dimensional echocardiography with Doppler is used to assess repair, valvular competency, cardiac function, and the presence of residual septal defects
      b. Cardiac catheterization is used when two-dimensional echocardiography cannot be used to assess the contribution of a left-to-right shunt in complex congenital heart lesions
   3. Management
      a. A hemodynamically insignificant communication often does not require surgical correction

     b. Patients with residual defects should have bacterial endocarditis prophylaxis

B. Pulmonary hypertension (see Chapter 6, Respiratory)

C. Dysrhythmias (see Chapter 7.2, Arrhythmias in the Pediatric Intensive Care Unit)

D. Valvular insufficiency

  1. Clinical presentation

    a. Mitral insufficiency can occur after atrial septal defect repair manifested by a midsystolic click or pansystolic murmur radiating to the axilla.

    b. Tricuspid insufficiency can be seen after ventricular and atrioventricular septal defect repair and manifests as a plateau pansystolic murmur that can be differentiated from the holosystolic murmur of a residual ventricular septal defect

    c. Aortic insufficiency can occur after ventricular and atrioventricular septal defect repair (5% of patients) and manifests hemodynamically with a wide pulse pressure and diastolic decrescendo murmur

  2. Diagnosis

    a. Two-dimensional echocardiography and color Doppler echocardiography are useful in the assessment of valvular dysfunction

    b. Cardiac catheterization is reserved for complex heart lesions

  3. Management

    a. The degree of valvular dysfunction and hemodynamic effects will determine the need for medical treatment (e.g., digoxin) and possible surgical repair

    b. A mild degree of valvular insufficiency is common after surgical repair of ventricular and atrioventricular septal defect and is usually hemodynamically well tolerated

Coarctation of the Aorta

A. Hypertension

  1. Clinical presentation

    a. Postoperative rebound hypertension is seen more commonly in patients who have surgical repair while in adolescence

    b. Hypertension is rarely seen in infants after surgical resection of coarctation

  2. Diagnosis

    a. A significant pressure gradient is usually absent on blood pressure measurement of upper and lower extremities

    b. Pain relief, sedation, and anxiolysis should be controlled when evaluating the degree of hypertension and need for medical therapy

  3. Management

    a. Assess the need for appropriate analgesia and anxiolysis

    b. β-blockers (e.g., propranolol, esmolol) are most commonly used for treatment of hypertension; esmolol has the advantage of having a short half-life, allowing one to titrate the dose of β-blockade via infusion

    c. Smooth muscle relaxants (e.g., nitroprusside, hydralazine) as well as drugs that alter adrenergic metabolism (e.g., methyldopa) have been used to treat postoperative hypertension

d. In patients with hypertension before surgery, blood pressure after surgical repair should not be inadvertently lowered too rapidly or it will result in splanchnic hypoperfusion; mean arterial blood pressure should be maintained at 80 to 95 mm Hg in hypertensive patients

e. Uncontrolled hypertension after surgery increases the risk for separation of the repair at the suture lines, intracranial hemorrhage, and nonocclusive mesenteric arteritis (ischemic bowel disease)

B. Left subclavian artery compromise
 1. Clinical presentation
  a. Usually occurs after coarctation repair with subclavian artery flap in infancy
  b. Clinical examination of the left arm and monitoring of perfusion and pulses are important after surgical repair
 2. Diagnosis
  a. Knowledge of the surgical repair is important
  b. Clinical examination is used for diagnosis
 3. Management
  a. Avoid blood pressure monitoring and blood draws from the left arm
  b. Do not put warm soaks on the poorly perfused arm, as this will increase oxygen consumption in an already ischemic vascular bed
  c. Observe pulses and perfusion of the left arm, and if distal perfusion remains cool and pulseless and has marginal capillary filling, consider vascular repair to prevent the risk of limb loss

C. Postcoarctectomy syndrome (nonocclusive mesenteric arteritis)
 1. Clinical presentation
  a. Occurs 48 to 96 hours after surgery and is most likely to occur in older children with preoperative hypertension
  b. Infants usually develop splanchnic ischemia secondarily as a manifestation of organ system failure secondary to shock at the time of presentation
 2. Diagnosis
  a. Children develop symptoms resembling an acute abdomen (abdominal pain, ileus, distention) that are accompanied by bloody stools and a leukocytosis
  b. Abdominal radiograph shows an ileus pattern with air-fluid levels; other gastrointestinal studies (computed tomography scan, ultrasound) are negative for obstruction, abscess, or other acute intra-abdominal emergencies
 3. Management
  a. Control hypertension
  b. Maintain adequate volume/fluid status
  c. Keep the patient nothing by mouth (NPO) and place a nasogastric tube for low intermittent nasogastric suction
  d. Start H_2 blockers and/or carafate
  e. Start hyperalimentation if kept NPO for >48 hours
  f. Broad-spectrum antibiotics are usually instituted and continued until symptoms abate

      g. When abdominal examination improves and the patient is clinically stable for ≥48 hours, diet can be advanced slowly

D. Other postoperative complications associated with coarctectomy
1. Recurrent laryngeal nerve injury
2. Thoracic duct injury
3. Anastomotic stenosis
4. Unilateral vocal cord paralysis
5. Spinal cord ischemia

Tetralogy of Fallot

A. Residual right ventricular outflow obstruction
1. Clinical presentation
   a. Obstruction correlates with type of preoperative outflow obstruction: infundibular obstruction has better outcome than when pulmonary valve is also involved
   b. A good result is a pulmonary artery pressure of <20 mm Hg or a low right-to-left systolic pressure ratio
2. Diagnosis
   a. Two-dimensional echocardiography can be used to assess the extent of residual obstruction
   b. Cardiac catheterization may be required to assess site and degree of obstruction
3. Management
   a. A high right ventricular systolic pressure after surgical repair is indicative of a poor operative result
   b. Isolate sites of obstruction to assess need for surgical repair
B. Restrictive pulmonary blood flow
1. Clinical presentation
   a. Despite adequate surgical repair, patients have high pulmonary vascular resistance distal to the pulmonary valve
   b. Restrictive pulmonary blood flow can be secondary to hypoplastic pulmonary vascular bed, obstructive pulmonary vascular disease due to a large systemic-to-pulmonary artery shunt, or obstruction to pulmonary venous return
2. Diagnosis
   a. Two-dimensional echocardiography is used to assess pulmonary blood flow
   b. Cardiac catheterization is reserved for complicated heart lesions in which echocardiography cannot adequately evaluate the cause of restricted pulmonary blood flow
3. Management
   a. Maximize medical therapy to augment pulmonary blood flow
   b. Pulmonary vasodilators (prostaglandin E_1, amrinone) can be used to augment pulmonary blood flow after surgery
   c. Patients who do not improve with medical therapy after a few days and do not have a surgically correctable lesion have a guarded prognosis

C. Other complications
   1. Aneurysmal dilatation of the repair of right ventricular outflow tract
   2. Arrhythmias

Transposition of the Great Vessels: Atrial and Arterial Switch Operations

A. Sequelae after atrial and arterial switch operations
   1. Atrial switch operations (Mustard and Senning procedures) in which a baffle or patch is used to redirect venous blood from the right atrium to the left atrium to the pulmonary circulation; complications include residual atrial shunts (baffle leaks), superior vena cava obstruction, sinoatrial nodal injury (sick sinus syndrome), pulmonary venous obstruction (baffle obstruction), residual subpulmonic obstruction, tricuspid insufficiency, subpulmonic obstruction, and residual ventricular septal defect
   2. Arterial switch operation (Jatene procedure) involves switching the great vessels and reanastomosing the coronary arteries as a "button" to the new aortic root; complications include coronary ostial stenosis, myocardial infarction, and the potential for outflow gradients secondary to obstruction at suture lines
   3. All patients with transposition of the great arteries are at risk for pulmonary vascular disease and abnormalities in right and left ventricular function
B. Diagnosis
   1. Two-dimensional echocardiography with Doppler and ECG can be used to delineate the cause of most complications
   2. Cardiac catheterization can be used if echocardiography does not isolate the specific problem
C. Management
   1. Specific management for the above complications has been discussed previously
   2. Baffle leaks and baffle obstruction may require surgical repair; arterial switch is the preferred operation in infancy when right ventricular pressures are high or in older patients with an unrestrictive ventricular septal defect
      Long-term follow-up of patients with arterial switch operation is under way.

Fontan Procedure

A. Sequelae after the Fontan operation for tricuspid atresia and univentricular hearts with pulmonary outflow obstruction
   1. Systemic venous return is directed by a conduit (Glenn shunt baffle to the pulmonary circulation); the entire cardiac output returns to and perfuses the lung without an intervening pump and is dependent on the transpulmonary gradient (right atrial [RA] pressure being greater than pulmonary artery [PA] pressure) for pulmonary blood flow
   2. Conditions under which PA pressure is elevated (pulmonary vascular disease, pulmonary disease, high pulmonary venous pressure, left ventricular

dysfunction, tricuspid insufficiency, and residual right-side outflow obstruction) will decrease pulmonary blood flow

3. Sinus rhythm should be maintained since the "atrial" kick is important in maintaining cardiac output and tachyarrhythmias and heart block are poorly tolerated

4. Superior vena caval obstruction and persistently elevated RA pressures require further evaluation of the adequacy of surgical repair

B. Diagnosis

1. Monitoring of central venous (CV), PA , left atrial (LA) pressures is useful in the management of low cardiac output after surgery

a. With low CV, PA, and LA pressures, consider fluid replacement for hypovolemia

b. With high CV and PA pressures and low LA pressure (<10 mm Hg), consider pulmonary hypertension secondary to pulmonary vascular disease, pulmonary disease, or pulmonary venous obstruction

c. CV pressures that are excessively high in relation to PA pressures signify obstruction in caval-to-pulmonary artery anastomosis

d. High CV, PA, and LA pressures usually signify poor ventricular compliance and cardiac dysfunction

2. Two-dimensional echocardiography with Doppler is useful for evaluation of adequacy of surgical repair

3. Cardiac catheterization can be used to assess complex lesions and adequacy of the surgical repair

C. Management

1. When positive pressure ventilation is used, it should be optimized to maintain functional residual capacity of the lung to prevent atelectasis and alveolar hypoxia from causing an increase in pulmonary vascular resistance

2. Low cardiac state should be treated according to etiology of cardiac dysfunction

3. Medical antishock trousers (MAST) can be used to limit the amount of fluids given parenterally in the early postoperative recovery period (24 to 48 hours) and can help sustain high CVP (14 to 18 mm Hg) or CVP minus LA pressure gradient of <7 mm Hg

4. Persistently high CVPs after repair require assessment of the adequacy of the surgical repair

D. Other complications associated with Fontan repair

1. Systemic venous hypertension

a. Chylothoraces

b. Protein-losing enteropathy

c. Superior and inferior vena caval syndrome

d. Atrial dysrhythmias and heart block

e. Hepatic insufficiency

2. Hypoxemia after surgical repair

a. Persistent right-to-left shunts (atrial septal defect, venous connection to left atrium)

b. Pulmonary disease

c. Low cardiac output state

Truncus Arteriosus Repair

A. Sequelae after repair of truncus arteriosus
   1. The degree of preoperative common atrioventricular valvular incompetency and degree of pulmonary vascular disease will dictate the postoperative course
   2. Children with truncus arteriosus have an increased incidence of DiGeorge syndrome (21%) (Van Mierop), and associated anomalies may also affect outcome; risk factors associated with poor outcome include interrupted aortic arch, common truncal valve insufficiency, coronary anomalies, and repairing patients >100 days old (Nicholas)
B. Diagnosis
   1. Monitoring of PA, RA, and LA pressures can aid in the diagnosis and management of pulmonary hypertension, valvular insufficiency, and cardiac dysfunction
   2. Two-dimensional echocardiography with Doppler is useful during and after surgery in assessing the cause of cardiac dysfunction
   3. Cardiac catheterization is reserved for evaluating cardiac dysfunction that cannot be adequately evaluated with the use of echocardiography
C. Management
   1. Pulmonary hypertension is more common in infants repaired when >3 months old
   2. Cardiac failure is usually secondary to truncal valve insufficiency or due to right heart failure secondary to poor ventricular compliance and the inability to tolerate elevations in pulmonary vascular resistance
      a. Adequate preload and inotropic support is used to augment ventricular function (e.g., dopamine, dobutamine, amrinone)
      b. Atrioventricular pacing can be used to augment cardiac output
      c. Pulmonary vasodilators are often used to decrease right ventricular afterload (e.g., nitroprusside, nitroglycerin, prostaglandins, nitric oxide)
   3. Late complications include obstruction of the conduit and truncal valve incompetence that may require further surgical correction

Norwood Procedure for Hypoplastic Left Heart Syndrome

A. Sequelae after stage I repair for hypoplastic left heart syndrome (HLHS): construction of right ventricular-to-aortic conduit and placement of central shunt for pulmonary blood perfusion
   1. Clinical presentation
      a. Excessive pulmonary blood flow is the most common problem encountered in the early postoperative period; it manifests as high arterial oxygen saturation with low arterial pressures in the systemic circulation
      b. Patients with high pulmonary-to-systemic blood flow ratios develop pulmonary edema, have low systemic blood pressures, and therefore are at risk for coronary hypoperfusion (myocardial ischemia)
      c. After a stage I Norwood procedure for HLHS, <5% of patients have insufficient pulmonary blood flow (low pulmonary-to-systemic blood flow ratio)

2. Diagnosis
   a. Pulmonary and systemic perfusion can be assessed clinically by monitoring capillary perfusion, hemodynamics (CV and mean arterial pressures), and arterial oxygen saturation with the use of pulse oximetry
   b. Two-dimensional echocardiography with Doppler is useful in postoperatively assessing central shunt flow and myocardial function
3. Management
   a. Perioperative care is directed toward maintaining a pulmonary-to-systemic blood flow ratio close to 1 after a stage I Norwood procedure
   b. Pulmonary vascular resistance can be regulated by reducing FIO_2, ≤ 0.30 and by stabilizing alveolar $PaCO_2$ with inspired CO_2 to achieve a $PaCO_2$ of 40 mm Hg and a tidal volume of 15 to 20 mL/kg, limiting peak inspiratory pressure to 35 cm H_2O
   c. Inotropic support (dopamine 5 $\mu g/kg/min$) is instituted if central filling pressures are >15 mm Hg and signs of poor cardiac output are manifested
   d. Digoxin and diuretics are usually instituted within 24 to 48 hours after surgical repair
   e. Metabolic acidosis should be treated with sodium bicarbonate to optimize myocardial performance
   f. Inspired CO_2 can be used after extubation in patients with a pulmonary-to-systemic blood flow of >1
   g. Failure to wean can be related to poor myocardial performance, pulmonary pathology, or both; aortic arch obstruction and limited pulmonary blood flow secondary to a small atrial communication or shunt obstruction can appear late in the postoperative course
B. Sequelae to stage II repair (bidirectional Glenn procedure) for HLHS
   1. Clinical presentation
      a. Stage II repair consists of bidirectional Glenn shunt to unload the systemic right ventricle and provide pulmonary blood flow from the superior vena cava; inferior vena caval blood flows into the common atrium and mixes with the pulmonary venous blood to the right ventricle and then into the systemic circulation; central shunts are ligated
      b. Pulmonary vascular resistance (PVR) will determine pulmonary blood flow; if superior vena caval pressure rises secondary to pulmonary pathology (edema, atelectasis, or increased pulmonary venous pressure), pulmonary blood flow will be limited, causing progressive cyanosis and effusions to develop (e.g., pleural)
      c. Systemic hypotension can be related to hypovolemia (low superior vena caval pressure, low PVR) or poor myocardial function (high right ventricular end-diastolic pressure secondary to right ventricular dysfunction or AV valve incompetence)
   2. Diagnosis
      a. Hemodynamic monitoring of atrial pulmonary filling pressures is useful in assessing PVR during the early postoperative period
      b. Two-dimensional echocardiography can be used to assess repair, AV valve competency, and ventricular function
      c. Cardiac catheterization used to further evaluate residua after repair

3. Management
   a. Mechanical ventilatory support is aimed at optimizing alveolar ventilation to achieve a $Paco_2$ of 30 to 35 mm Hg at low intrathoracic pressure
   b. Volume status and oxygen-carrying capacity should be optimized
   c. Inotropic agents that are also pulmonary vasodilators (e.g., amrinone) have been useful in supporting patients with myocardial diastolic dysfunction and increased PVR
   d. Effusions should be drained when affecting ventricular filling and pulmonary compliance
C. Sequelae to complete Fontan (stage III)
   1. Inferior caval blood flow connected to the pulmonary circulation by a conduit or baffle; atrial communication closed or fenestrated
   2. Postoperative management parallels Fontan procedure for univentricular hearts

BIBLIOGRAPHY

Dajani AS, et al: Prevention of bacterial endocarditis. Recommendations by the American Heart Association. JAMA 264:2919–2922, 1990.
Garson A, Bricker JT, McNamara DG (eds): The Science and Practice of Pediatric Cardiology, Vol I, II, III. Malvern, Lea & Febiger, 1990.
Nichols DG, Cameron DE, Greeley WJ, et al (eds): Critical Heart Disease in Infants and Children, Vol. I. St. Louis, Mosby–Year Book, 1995.
Staats BA, et al: The lipoprotein profile of chylous and non-chylous effusions. Mayo Clin Proc 55:700, 1980.
Van Mierop LH, Kutsche LM: Cardiovascular anomalies in DiGeorge syndrome and importance of neural crest as a possible pathogenetic factor. Am J Cardiol 58:133–137, 1986.

7.5 Cardiovascular Pharmacology

HERSCHEL C. ROSENBERG, MD, FRCP(C)

Cardiac output can be increased by increasing either the heart rate or the stroke volume. Newborns have little cardiac reserve and thus rely principally on heart rate to modify cardiac output. In the older child, changes in cardiac output are achieved largely through changes in stroke volume. Stroke volume can be altered pharmacologically via two primary mechanisms: inotropic drugs and vasodilators (Fig. 7–11). *Inotropic drugs* increase contractility by stimulating the cardiac muscle to a higher inotropic state. Alternatively, cardiac output can be

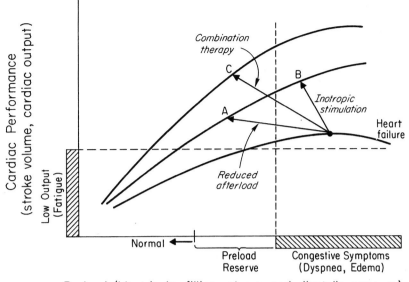

Preload (Ventricular filling volume, end-diastolic pressure)

Figure 7–11. Cardiac output can be increased through the use of inotropic agents to increase cardiac contractility, moving the heart to a steeper function curve. A similar effect can be achieved through the use of vasodilators to reduce the afterload on the heart and, in effect, shift to a new curve. (From Freidman WF, George BL: New concepts and drugs for congestive heart failure. Pediatr Clin North Am 31:1197, 1984.)

increased by using *vasodilators* to pharmacologically decrease the afterload against which the heart muscle must work.

Inotropic Drugs

DIGOXIN

Drug Properties

Digitalis glycosides have the longest history as inotropic agents and the most widespread acceptance in pediatrics. Digoxin is the most widely used of this class of drugs (Table 7–14). Digoxin acts by inhibiting membrane Na^+,K^+-ATPase, resulting in an increased concentration of sodium but also calcium anions. The increased calcium within the cell enhances contractility. Apart from its positive inotropic effect, digoxin also has major electrophysiologic effects. Although the drug has a direct effect on conduction tissue, the major physiologic effect of digoxin is vagotonic, acting to slow the sinoatrial node as well as slowing conduction and prolonging the refractoriness of the atrioventricular node.

Digoxin is extremely well absorbed orally, although it is usually used intravenously in the intensive care setting. Because the drug is tightly bound to muscle,

Table 7–14. DOSING GUIDE

Digoxin	
Digitalizing dose (divided into three IV doses over 24 hr)	
<37 weeks:	0.015 mg/kg
Term and older:	0.030 mg/kg (maximum, 1.0 mg)
Maintenance dose	
<37 weeks:	0.003 mg/kg/day (0.004 mg/kg PO)
Term and older:	0.007 mg/kgday
Isoproterenol	0.1–2.0 μg/kg/min
Norepinephrine	0.05–1.0 μg/kg/min
Epinephrine	0.05–1.0 μg/kg/min
Dopamine	2.0–20 μg/kg/min
Dobutamine	1.0–20 μg/kg/min
Amrinone	
Loading dose:	0.75–3.0 mg/kg
Maintenance dose:	3.0–10.0 μg/kg/min
Phenoxybenzamine	1 mg/kg as slow IV load
Captopril	0.5–6.0 mg/kg/day in three divided doses
Nitroglycerin	0.5–10.0 μg/kg/min
Nitroprusside	0.1–10 μg/kg/min

intramuscular use results in very erratic absorption and is contraindicated. Digoxin has a long half-life ($\approx$35 hours). In the premature infant, this can be considerably prolonged. Consequently, it is customary to administer a loading dose over 24 hours before commencing once- or twice-daily maintenance therapy (Table 7–14). The drug is primarily excreted by the kidneys. In the presence of renal impairment, it may be adequate to provide a loading dose alone. Digoxin has significant toxicity, particularly in the face of hypokalemia. *The drug is easily administered but difficult to remove.* As a consequence, except in the treatment of life-threatening arrhythmias, a conservative approach to its administration is appropriate.

Clinical Use

Digoxin has been partly supplanted in the intensive care setting by intravenous inotropes. Its greatest use remains in the newborn with critical left ventricular outflow tract obstruction. In these patients, digoxin may rapidly reverse severely *impaired myocardial function* and provide a "honeymoon period" during which definitive surgical correction can take place. It also has a role in the child with *inappropriate tachycardia* or the child who has improved on intravenous inotropes and now requires *long-term inotropic support.*

SYMPATHOMIMETIC AGENTS

Sympathomimetic agents have become the standard in the treatment of impaired myocardial function in the intensive care unit. They are distinguished by acting on cardiac and peripheral vascular adrenergic receptors. Three major classes of receptors have been identified (Fig. 7–12). All three classes interact with

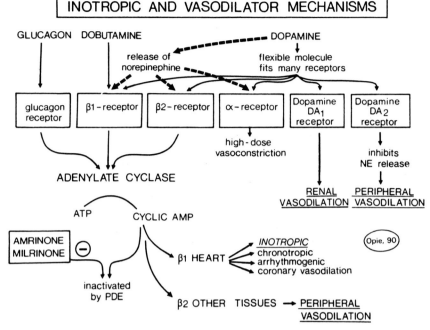

INOTROPIC AND VASODILATOR MECHANISMS

Figure 7–12. Sympathomimetic agents induce their dominant physiologic effects by acting on the three major classes of adrenergic receptors. In contrast, phosphodiesterase inhibitors (PDE) exercise their effects by preventing the breakdown of cyclic AMP. (From Marcus FL, Opie LH, Sonnenblick EH: Digitalis and other inotropes. *In* Opie LH (ed): Drugs for the Heart, 3rd ed. Philadelphia, WB Saunders, 1991, p. 141, copyright by Lionel H Opie.)

nucleoside regulatory proteins (G proteins), resulting in an increase in adenylate cyclase activity and a rise in cyclic AMP. *The drugs are effective in increasing cardiac output and blood pressure, but they do so at the cost of increased myocardial work.* In the patient with an injured myocardium, this should be carefully considered, particularly when higher doses are used.

ISOPROTERENOL

Drug Properties

Isoproterenol is a synthetic, pure β-adrenergic receptor agonist. In addition to its inotropic effect, it has a major chronotropic effect, accelerating the heart rate. It is also a systemic vasodilator. The drug has a variable effect on blood pressure, tending to leave systolic blood pressure unchanged while decreasing diastolic pressure. As a consequence, myocardial demand increases, but myocardial supply may actually decrease because of the lower diastolic perfusion pressure.

Clinical Use

For the reasons given, isoproterenol has largely been replaced by other inotropic agents. It may still have a role in the child with *pulmonary hypertension* because of its vasodilatory effects. In newborns, who appear to have a limited inotropic reserve, the drug may be more effective in increasing cardiac output because of its *dominant chronotropic effect*. Like all of the intravenous catecholamines, the drug has a short half-life and must be administered via continuous intravenous infusion.

NOREPINEPHRINE

Drug Properties

In contrast to isoproterenol, norepinephrine is predominantly an α-adrenergic receptor agonist. Although it is a positive inotrope, its dominant effect is vasoconstriction. *Norepinephrine is effective in increasing systemic blood pressure but often at the cost of impaired cardiac output because of the increased afterload on the heart.* As an endogenous catecholamine, the drug has an extremely short half-life and must be administered via continuous infusion. Because of the intense vasoconstriction induced by the drug, *extravasation can result in ischemic injury, and administration through a central line is mandatory.*

Clinical Use

The drug must be used with caution but can have a role in the patient with low systemic vascular resistance, as might occur with *bacterial sepsis* or *drug reaction*.

EPINEPHRINE

Drug Properties

Epinephrine is a balanced α,β-agonist with predominant β_1 (cardiac) effects. As a result, it has both inotropic and chronotropic (increased heart rate) properties.

Clinical Use

The drug has been largely supplanted by newer intravenous inotropes. It has a unique role in *anaphylaxis* and is frequently used in patients with *refractory cardiogenic shock*.

DOPAMINE

Drug Properties

Dopamine is an endogenous precursor of norepinephrine. At low doses, it has positive inotropic effects and *induces dilatation of selective vascular beds through specific dopaminergic receptors*. By increasing renal plasma flow, dopamine may encourage diuresis. At higher doses, the predominant effect is direct and indirect (through norepinephrine release) α-adrenergic stimulation, resulting in vasoconstriction (see Fig. 7–12). Again, blood pressure may be supported but at the cost of greatly increased myocardial work. At higher doses, dopamine also exerts a vasoconstrictor effect on the pulmonary vascular bed.

Clinical Use

Dopamine has become the *predominant intravenous inotrope in pediatric practice.* Although low doses of dopamine appear to be useful in the distressed neonate to maximize cardiac function, high doses should be used with caution because of the risk of pulmonary hypertension. Similar to norepinephrine, *extravasation may result in skin sloughing, and the drug should be administered as a continuous infusion through a central line.*

DOBUTAMINE

Drug Properties

Dobutamine is a synthetic sympathomimetic agent with effects similar to those of dopamine, to which it is structurally related. It has predominant β_1 effects, with weaker effects on β_2- and α-adrenergic receptors. Dobutamine has a more marked effect on decreasing pulmonary wedge pressure, although it lacks the selective renal vasodilatory effect of low-dose dopamine. The drug also has less tendency to accelerate the heart rate.

Clinical Use

Dobutamine is becoming increasingly popular in the pediatric intensive care unit. Cardiac output generally is increased more by dobutamine than by dopamine. In the neonate, dobutamine is less effective in supporting the blood pressure. The drug appears to be particularly useful in patients with *impaired myocardial function* and elevated pulmonary wedge pressure and systemic vascular resistance.

PHOSPHODIESTERASE INHIBITORS

Phosphodiesterase inhibitors are a newer class of inotropic drugs typified by amrinone. These drugs act by inhibiting cellular phosphodiesterase, increasing the intracellular concentration of cyclic AMP. The increased levels of cyclic AMP in turn enhance contractility (see Fig. 7–12). Although initially developed as oral inotropic agents, their chronic use has been associated with increased mortality, and they are now used primarily through the intravenous route in acute care settings. Although they clearly *exhibit positive inotropic effects in vitro, clinically their effects are dominated by vasodilation.*

AMRINONE

Drug Properties

Amrinone is a bipyridine derivative that was the first and remains the most widely used of the phosphodiesterase inhibitors. Although initially available orally, chronic oral use was associated with a high incidence of side effects, and the drug is now used exclusively intravenously in acute care settings. Short-term intravenous use appears to be safe, although there is a high incidence of thrombocytopenia with prolonged use at high doses. Although possessing a half-life of 2 to 4 hours, the drug is usually given as an initial intravenous bolus followed by a continuous infusion. Amrinone is primarily excreted by the kidneys. As stated, the drug clinically acts predominantly as a vasodilator, decreasing capillary wedge pressure and increasing cardiac output primarily by decreasing afterload.

Clinical Use

Amrinone is frequently used in concert with sympathomimetic agents in *refractory low output states* associated with elevated systemic vascular resistance. Amrinone also appears to be an effective (but not selective) *pulmonary vasodilator* and may be particularly useful in the patient with myocardial dysfunction associated with pulmonary hypertension. *Amrinone, in the newborn, has been associated with adverse outcomes.* There is evidence of a greatly prolonged half-life, particularly in sick newborns, which may account for the observed toxicity.

ENOXIMONE

Enoximone is a newer phosphodiesterase inhibitor. Experience in children is limited, but it may have fewer side effects than amrinone.

Vasodilators

Vasodilators have largely replaced inotropic agents as first-line therapy in the treatment of patients with chronic congestive heart failure. They also fill an expanding role in the acute management of low cardiac output. Through arterial dilation, these drugs decrease the afterload on the heart, improving cardiac function and cardiac output. Although in normal subjects vasodilators tend to decrease blood pressure, in the setting of the failing heart, the increase in cardiac output usually compensates for the decline in systemic vascular resistance, and blood pressure is largely unaffected. Most of these drugs also have a variable effect on the capacitance (venous) side of the vasculature, potentially ameliorating pulmonary venous hypertension and pulmonary edema.

NITROPRUSSIDE

Drug Properties

Nitroprusside is a direct-acting, balanced vasodilator with potent effects on both arteries and veins. The drug has a very short half-life that allows careful titration of response via continuous infusion. *In patients with elevated systemic vascular resistance and decreased circulating volume, however, there may be large swings in blood pressure*. Therapy with nitroprusside is limited by the accumulation of thiocyanate. Treatment beyond 2 to 3 days requires monitoring of thiocyanate levels to avoid cyanide poisoning. The drug is sensitive to light, and the infusion must be protected from light sources. Nitroprusside has an effect on the pulmonary vascular bed that is similar to its systemic effect and is an effective but nonspecific pulmonary vasodilator.

Clinical Use

Nitroprusside has its primary application in *hypertensive emergencies*. The drug can be used for short-term *afterload reduction* in patients with low cardiac output associated with an elevated systemic vascular resistance.

NITROGLYCERIN

Drug Properties

In contrast to nitroprusside, nitroglycerin has dominant effects on the systemic veins. It has a slightly longer half-life but still is best administered via continuous infusion. It does not share the potential toxicity of nitroprusside and has the added advantage of improving coronary blood flow. It also is a fairly effective pulmonary vasodilator.

Clinical Use

Given the effect of nitroglycerin on the capacitance vessels, it has particular use in patients with markedly elevated pulmonary venous wedge pressure. The drug may be better tolerated than nitroprusside in the patient with critically low cardiac output. Long-term therapy is limited by the development of tolerance.

PHENOXYBENZAMINE

Drug Properties

Phenoxybenzamine is a unique vasodilator. It induces an irreversible blockade of α-adrenergic receptors. The drug has a half-life of <24 hours, but its pharmacologic effect is determined by the rate at which new α-adrenergic receptors are generated.

Clinical Use

There has been a resurgence of interest in phenoxybenzamine with the increase in neonatal cardiac surgery. There is some evidence that α-blockade may be *protective to the newborn myocardium*. Use of the drug is largely limited to the neonate after cardiopulmonary bypass.

ANGIOTENSIN-CONVERTING ENZYME INHIBITORS

Drug Properties

Angiotensin-converting enzyme (ACE) inhibitors are mentioned last because, as oral agents, they have a limited role in the acute care setting. Although enalapril is available for intravenous use, experience in children is limited. These drugs induce vasodilation by blocking the vasoconstriction induced by activation of the renin-angiotensin system. In addition to decreasing afterload and improving cardiac output, ACE inhibitors have been demonstrated uniquely to prolong survival in adults with chronic congestive heart failure, probably by suppressing levels of norepinephrine and vasopressin. The various ACE inhibitors have similar efficacies and side effects, varying primarily in their pharmacokinetic properties, with captopril having the shortest half-life. This does, however, allow for more rapid titration of effect in the acutely ill child.

Clinical Use

ACE inhibitors have become the drugs of choice for *long-term afterload reduction*. Their role in the patient with chronic congestive heart failure is second only to that of diuretics. Like all vasodilators, *ACE inhibitors are relatively contraindicated in the presence of left ventricular outflow tract obstruction.*

8

Central Nervous System

8.1 Central Nervous System Monitoring

IDO YATSIV, MD

Several groups of pediatric patients with central nervous system (CNS) pathology present in a critically ill state requiring intensive monitoring and treatment aimed at the CNS.

These groups consist of patients with trauma (head or multiple, involving the CNS), CNS infections, encephalopathies (hypoxic-ischemic, metabolic, and toxic), and status epilepticus and patients who undergo elective brain surgery. Accurate continuous CNS monitoring is an essential aspect of the management of these children. Patients with CNS compromise often have increased intracranial pressure (ICP), abnormal brain electrical activity, and metabolic derangement. In addition to basic cardiopulmonary monitoring, these patients often require determination of ICP, electrophysiologic monitoring, and, in selected cases, measurement of cerebral oxygen metabolism.

Pathophysiology

INTRACRANIAL PRESSURE

Monro and Kellie proposed the fundamental model of compartmentalization of the skull. The model assumes that the skull is a cavity with a fixed volume. The different skull compartments are *neural tissue,* comprising 80 to 90% of the intracranial volume; *cerebrospinal fluid* (CSF), comprising 5 to 10%; and *vascular bed,* comprising 5 to 10%. The most characteristic response of neural tissue to any injury is *swelling*, leading in a closed cavity to increased ICP, unless a parallel reduction in volume occurs. This can occur through a decrease in CSF or in vascular volume or through therapy aimed at reducing brain edema.

179

Increased ICP can be harmful in two ways:

1. Herniation: The main open area in the skull is the foramen magnum. Thus, in an intact skull, the only possible motion of brain tissue is caudal, resulting in herniation either at the tentorial level or into the foramen magnum.
2. Inadequate cerebral perfusion: The CNS is dependent on continuous oxygen delivery and has a very limited tolerance to ischemia or hypoxia. Cerebral perfusion is determined by the *cerebral perfusion pressure* (CPP), which is related to the *mean arterial pressure* (MAP) and the ICP by the following relation: CPP = MAP – ICP. To keep adequate oxygen delivery, cerebral blood flow is maintained relatively constant along a broad range of CPPs, a mechanism known as *cerebral autoregulation.* It is controversial whether this autoregulatory mechanism remains intact in the injured CNS.

There are two main objectives in neurointensive care:

- Prevention of herniation
- Maintenance of adequate brain perfusion

Both goals require continuous monitoring of ICP. This requirement led to the development of several methods of ICP monitoring that are discussed in this chapter.

Electrophysiology

Focal and generalized seizures accompanying head trauma, certain encephalopathies, and other CNS pathology occur at a varying incidence. Accurate rapid diagnosis and prompt control of generalized seizures are essential to prevent additional damage to an already compromised CNS. Prolonged seizures result in severe physiologic derangements, including *hypoxemia,* metabolic and respiratory *acidosis, hypotension, hyperthermia, increased ICP,* and up to a fivefold *increase in oxygen consumption* that outweighs the increase in cerebral blood flow. These seizures are usually obvious in nonparalyzed patients. Some patients in the pediatric intensive care unit, however, are paralyzed with muscle relaxants and cannot demonstrate seizure activity. In such patients, monitoring of brain electrical activity is advisable. Continuous monitoring of brain electrical activity is also required in patients undergoing *barbiturate coma,* for either intractable seizures or uncontrollable increase in ICP. In these patients, a state of electrical *burst suppression* is desired. Bedside electroencephalography (EEG) and other electrophysiologic measurements are discussed.

Evaluation of Children with Altered Mental Status

The majority of children with brain pathology present with altered mental status, so we focus on the workup of that state. The following aspects must be examined:

- Patient history
- Physical examination
  - ☐ Degree of altered mental status
  - ☐ Respiratory pattern
  - ☐ Pupillary response
  - ☐ Extraocular movements
  - ☐ Motor examination
  - ☐ Glasgow Coma Scale score
- Ancillary tests
  - ☐ ICP monitoring
  - ☐ EEG and evoked response tests
  - ☐ Specific blood tests (glucose, electrolytes and anion gap, calcium, magnesium, arterial blood gases, toxicology screen)

HISTORY

History is often vague or absent in patients with altered consciousness. When available, special effort must be aimed at determining the sequence of events leading to the patient's present state, including exact mechanism and estimated velocity of impact for trauma cases, immediate neurologic response, seizure activity, and evaluation of transport records.

PHYSICAL EXAMINATION

Degrees of Mental Status

The commonly accepted classification of altered mental status is as follows:

1. Awake: The patient is alert, does not need any stimulation. Wakefulness does not mean the patient is necessarily coherent.
2. Lethargy: The patient seems to be asleep but can be aroused to an awake state when stimulated lightly, either verbally or with mild physical stimulus. When stimulation is stopped, the patient drifts back to his or her original state.
3. Stupor: The patient responds to potent stimuli by withdrawal or moaning. He or she never regains full consciousness.
4. Coma: The patient does not have purposeful responses to any kind of stimuli.

Respiratory Pattern
(Fig. 8–1)

1. Cheyne-Stokes respiration: In this pattern, there is an alternating rhythm between deep hyperventilation and apnea. This pattern is typical to bihemispheric involvement such as hypoxia, drug ingestion, or a metabolic abnormality.
2. Central neurogenic hyperventilation: The patient is hyperventilating contin-

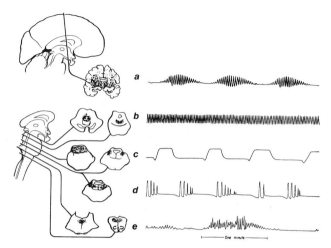

Figure 8–1. Abnormal respiratory patterns associated with pathological lesions (shaded areas) at various levels of the brain. *a,* Cheyne-Stokes respiration. *b,* Central neurogenic hyperventilation. *c,* Apneusis. *d,* Cluster breathing. *e,* Ataxic breathing. (From Plum F, Posner JB: The Diagnosis of Stupor and Coma, 3rd ed. Philadelphia, FA Davis, 1980.)

uously without a metabolic derangement, usually resulting in metabolic alkalosis. This pattern results from *midbrain lesion.*

3. Apneustic breathing: The patient breathes in a prolonged inspiratory phase followed by a short exhalation. This type of breathing is associated with involvement of the *pons.*

4. Cluster breathing: Clusters of breaths that follow each other in an irregular fashion. This is a characteristic pattern in *low pontine and high medullary lesions.*

5. Ataxic breathing: Irregularity of irregular breathing pattern distinctive to *medullary involvement.*

Pupillary Response
(Fig. 8–2)

In principle, bilateral cortical involvement does not affect pupillary size. An exception is the response to various drugs such as amphetamines or opiates, which can result in either mydriasis or miosis, respectively.

Lesions of the midbrain present with pupillary dilation, usually as a result of parasympathetic inhibition. Pontine damage results in constricted "pinpoint" pupils, and medullary involvement does not influence the pupils.

Extraocular Movements
(Fig. 8–3)

Conjugated eye movements in response to vestibular stimulus involve several brain stem structures, the midbrain, pons, and medulla; thus, a *positive vestibulo-*

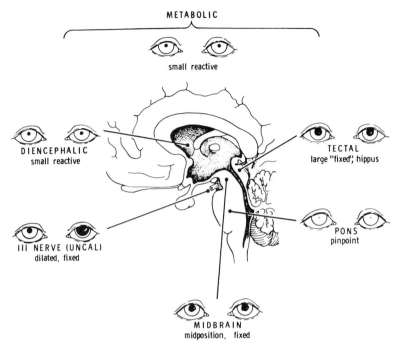

Figure 8–2. Pupils in comatose patients. (From Plum F, Posner JB: The Diagnosis of Stupor and Coma, 3rd ed. Philadelphia, FA Davis, 1980.)

ocular reflex represents an intact brain stem. Stimulation of the vestibular apparatus involves the eighth cranial nerve, whose nucleus is in the medulla. The information is processed by the paramedian pontine reticular formation, which is responsible for the coordination of lateral conjugated eye movements. The synchronized movement requires a link between the sixth and third nerve nuclei, a link achieved through the medial longitudinal fasciculus, running from the pons to the medulla. In practice, the vestibulo-ocular reflex is achieved by flushing an ear canal with 60 mL of ice-cold water. This results, in the intact brain stem, in inactivation of the vestibular apparatus in that side enabling the active opposite other side to cause both eyes to move *toward* the side of the injected ear.

Motor Examination
(Fig. 8–4)

The motor examination can contribute to the assessment of mental status through evaluation of the patient's motor response to painful stimuli or *posturing*. There are two postures that an unconscious patient can have: *decorticate* and *decerebrate*.

Decorticate posture occurs in patients with lesions *above the red nucleus* of the midbrain. In response to pain, they extend their feet and flex their arms. In

CONDITION: OCULAR REFLEXES IN UNCONSCIOUS PATIENTS

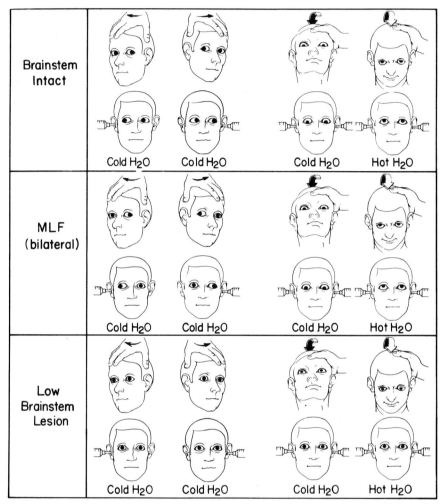

Figure 8–3. Ocular reflexes in unconscious patients. *Top rows,* Oculocephalic reflex. *Bottom rows,* Oculovestibular reflex. (From Plum F, Posner JB: The Diagnosis of Stupor and Coma, 3rd ed. Philadelphia, FA Davis, 1980.)

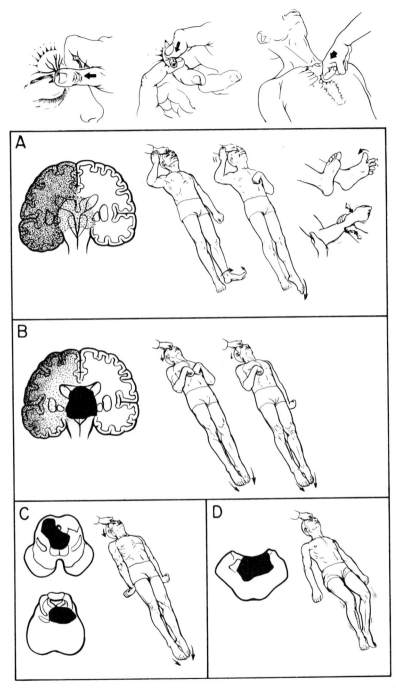

Figure 8–4. Motor responses to noxious stimuli in patients with acute cerebral dysfunction. *A,* Partial hemiplegia, as a result of massive unilateral cortical damage. *B,* Decorticate rigidity, a large lesion above the red nucleus. *C,* Decerebrate rigidity, a large lesion at or below the red nucleus. *D,* Flaccidity ("spinal shock"). (From Plum F, Posner JB: The Diagnosis of Stupor and Coma, 3rd ed. Philadelphia, FA Davis, 1980.)

decerebrate posturing, the lesion is in a site *between the red nucleus and the midmedulla,* and the patient *extends* all four extremities with internal rotation of the legs. *Brain-dead* patients do not posture.

Glasgow Coma Scale Score

It is possible to quantify and summarize the findings of the physical examination according to a scaling system. The most frequently applied scoring system is the Glasgow Coma Scale (GCS), which was developed by Teasdale and Jennet and based on data collected from head-injured adult patients (see Chapter 13). The GCS has been successfully applied in comparing patient populations, in making therapeutic decisions, and in predicting outcome both in adults and in children. A modification was made by ME James to adjust for infants and toddlers.

ICP Monitoring Devices

There are two groups of ICP monitoring devices: invasive and noninvasive (Table 8–1). Noninvasive devices use the open fontanelle as a "window" to assess ICP. These devices remain experimental, have not gained wide acceptance, and are not discussed in this chapter.

VENTRICULOSTOMY

Lundberg described the use of a fluid-filled catheter system in 1960. Measurement of pressure from the ventricles has been the gold standard in the determination of ICP. A ventriculostomy has two main advantages:

- It reflects most accurately an evenly distributed ICP, unlike measurements at other sites, which may reflect regional compartments.
- By establishing a connection to the ventricular system, it enables CSF drainage, which can be used therapeutically to decrease the CSF volume and reduce ICP.

Table 8–1. INTRACRANIAL PRESSURE MONITORING DEVICES FOR CENTRAL NERVOUS SYSTEM REGION MONITORED AND COMPLICATIONS

Device Type	Area Monitored	Infection Risk	Incidence
Ventriculostomy	Ventricles	+ + +	65–72%
Fiberoptic-tipped intraparenchymal catheter	Brain tissue, ventricles, or any other area	Rare	48–65%
Subdural bolt	Subdural space	+	5–24%
Subdural or epidural catheters	Subdural or epidural space	+	10–15%
External devices	Fontanelle	No infection	Rare

Placement of a ventriculostomy is not always an option because it requires patent ventricles and in many patients with head trauma, the patient's ventricles are compressed and cannot be penetrated by the time the patient reaches the trauma center. The main drawbacks of this method are the development of ventriculitis (6 to 21% in different reports) and intracranial hemorrhage (1 to 2%). Insertion of a ventriculostomy can be done by the bedside: a hole is drilled over the right frontal area anterior to the coronal suture 2 cm lateral to the midline. The catheter is inserted through the dura and arachnoid and is directed to the intersection of lines that pass through the pupil and the tragus of the ear, at a depth of 4 to 6 cm. The external portion of the catheter is tunneled beneath the skin to reduce the likelihood of infection.

Fiberoptic-Tipped Intraparenchymal Catheter

Advancement in electro-optics has enabled the development of very small pressure transducers. The fiberoptic catheters have a microtransducer based on a pressure-sensitive membrane at the tip of a catheter. These devices can measure pressure inside any tissue, including brain parenchyma, CSF, or blood. The transducing system is a closed one, resulting in a very low rate of infection. The devices have been shown to have a very close correlation to ventriculostomies and have a minimal drift with time. In contrast to other systems, calibration is done *only once*, before insertion. The only drawback of these catheters is the inability to drain CSF through them. As with other systems, subcutaneous tunneling of the proximal catheter is recommended, and some recommend antistaphylococcal prophylaxis.

SUBARACHNOID/SUBDURAL MONITORS

Subdural Bolt

When perforation of brain tissue is undesirable, pressure measurement can be obtained from the subarachnoid or subdural spaces. The most common monitor of these compartments is the subdural bolt. The bolt is a fluid-filled pressure monitor that is screwed through a burr hole after the dura and arachnoid have been cut, thus making a fluid column continuity from the CSF to an external transducer. The main advantage of the bolt is its superficial location, which prevents disruption of brain parenchyma.

The bolt has several limitations:

- Compared with other methods, pressures measured with the bolt do not always reflect intraventricular pressures and may result in a wide variability depending on the exact location of the device.
- The bolt tends to become occluded with brain tissue, especially in patients who have increased ICP. In these instances, the pressure wave becomes dampened, and the bolt might need to be flushed with a minimal volume.
- Despite the communication with CSF, it is not possible to drain sufficient fluid to reduce increased ICP.

■ To have a firmly secured bolt, the skull bones have to be well ossified, which limits its use to children who are older than 6 months.

Subdural/Epidural Catheter

The subdural or epidural spaces can also be monitored with a catheter. Direct visualization is recommended for safe placement of the catheter, usually requiring an operating room, although bedside placement has been reported. In acute cases, epidural catheters have poor correlation compared with intraventricular devices but have better correlation in a long-term setting.

ELECTROPHYSIOLOGIC MONITORING (ELECTROENCEPHALOGRAPHY AND EVOKED POTENTIALS)

Clinical monitoring of patients with CNS involvement is frequently limited by the need to sedate or paralyze them. The primary methods of monitoring the function of the CNS are the EEG and the various evoked-potential systems. Electrophysiologic monitoring can be used for diagnosis and assessment of response to therapy and could help in predicting viability and outcome.

Electroencephalography

Electroencephalography records spontaneous electrical activity at different points on the scalp, reflecting, mainly, superficial cortical activity. EEG tracings are examined manually for frequency, amplitude, and activity patterns. EEG can be used to identify seizure activity in patients receiving muscle relaxants or having focal activity that might be overlooked; it can also indicate the depth of coma. It is clear that EEGs that show either low-amplitude, slow (<4 Hz) patterns or are isoelectric indicate a poor prognosis. There are conflicting reports as to the predictive value of EEG in patients with tracings that are marginally abnormal. Recently, computer techniques have been developed that analyze continuous EEG tracings and evaluate trends over time. Initial studies point toward a better correlation between these methods and prognosis.

Sensory-Evoked Responses

Sensory-evoked potentials (SEP) are the brain electrical responses to various sensory stimulation. These responses are extremely small (1 to 2 μV) and cannot be differentiated from the electrical background. They are isolated through the use of computerized amplification: the electrical response to a series of $\leq$1000 stimuli is collected, thus erasing the background effect. Three forms of evoked potentials are used clinically:

Somatosensory-Evoked Potentials (SSEP). These potentials reflect the response to a weak electrical current placed on a peripheral nerve, usually in a limb.

Auditory Brainstem Responses (ABR). These responses reflect the response of the auditory tract: auditory nerve (wave I), cochlear nucleus (III), and the inferior colliculus in the midbrain (V). Waves II and IV do not always appear, and there is controversy regarding their origin.

Visually Evoked Potentials (VEP). These potentials represent a potential recorded over the occipital cortex that reflects the response to repeated light flashes directed to the eyes.

In contrast to EEG, SEP reflect deep CNS structures, such as the brain stem. They are much less influenced by drugs than is EEG and therefore have an important role in the investigation of patients who are sedated with barbiturates or other drugs. SEP and ABR have a role in evaluating coma level, in differentiating brain dysfunction (elevated ICP, ischemia or drug induced), and in prognostication. To improve the accuracy of grading systems, the three SEP forms were designed. These methods are used to assess statistically accumulated data and, combined, have better correlation to outcome than each form alone.

Table 8–2 summarizes the characteristics of the four electrophysiologic monitoring methods discussed.

Laboratory Studies

Every critically ill patient requires a thorough laboratory workup, with some tests repeated frequently. The CNS-injured patient requires special focus on the following aspects:

Table 8–2. USE OF ELECTROENCEPHALOGRAPHY AND SENSORY-EVOKED POTENTIAL MONITORING IN HEAD INJURY

	EEG	SSEP	ABR	VEP
CNS structures assessed	Cerebral cortex (surface)	Peripheral nerve, spinal cord, brain stem, sensory cortex	Brain stem	Retina, visual cortex
Use	Depth of coma Seizure detection Brain death	Cerebral ischemia, increased ICP, mass lesions	Brain stem injury, uncal herniation, deep coma	Increased ICP, optic nerve injury
Prognosis for death with severely abnormal tracing	Accurate	Accurate	Accurate	Moderately accurate
Prognosis for good outcome when responses are not severely abnormal	Inaccurate	Accurate	Accurate	Inaccurate
Problems	Scalp injuries Metabolic disorders Affected by drugs	Peripheral nerve and spinal cord injury	External auditory injuries	Ocular injuries

From Sloan TB: Electrophysiologic monitoring in head injury. New Horizons 3:431, 1995.
EEG, electroencephalography; SSEP, somatosensory-evoked potentials; ABR, auditory brain stem responses; VEP, visually evoked potentials; CNS, central nervous system; ICP, intracranial pressure.

Serum Sodium and Osmolarity. Serum Na$^+$ tends to have significant changes in these patients. CNS injury often results in either the syndrome of inappropriate secretion of antidiuretic hormone (SIADH) or in diabetes insipidus (DI). Both are serious complications that warrant rapid diagnosis and treatment, and both manifest in changes in serum and urine Na$^+$ and in urine output. In addition, mannitol, which is given to reduce increased ICP, produces changes in serum osmolarity and Na$^+$, making essential the frequent determination of serum electrolytes and osmolarity.

Blood Glucose. Patients with CNS injury often present with altered mental status, and low blood glucose can easily be missed. In animal experiments, high glucose levels have been shown to have adverse effects on outcome. It is therefore recommended that glucose be maintained in a normal physiologic range regardless of therapy.

Hemoglobin. The aim of brain resuscitation is the maintenance of adequate O$_2$ delivery. CNS-injured patients, especially multiple-trauma patients, often become anemic. It is recommended that a hemoglobin level of >100 gm/L be preserved. Polycythemia should be avoided as well because it increases blood viscosity, thus impeding perfusion.

Summary

Much controversy remains regarding the exact therapeutic maneuvers in children with CNS injury. There is no question, however, that these patients present an exceptionally complex array of physiologic and biochemical changes that warrant close and aggressive monitoring and treatment.

BIBLIOGRAPHY

Ghajar J, Hariri RJ, Narayan RK, et al: Survey of critical care management of comatose head-injured patients in the United States. Crit Care Med 23:560, 1995.

Greenberg RP, Newlon PG, Hyatt MS, et al: Prognostic implications of early multimodality evoked potentials in severely head-injured patients. J Neurosurg 55:227, 1981.

James ME: Neurologic evaluation and support in the child with an acute brain insult. Pediatr Ann 15:16–22, 1986.

Lundberg N: Continuous recording and control of ventricular fluid pressure in neurosurgical practice. Acta Psychiatr Neurol Scand 36(Suppl 149):1–193, 1960.

Monroe A: Observations on the Structure and Functions of the Nervous System. Edinburgh, 1783, footnote 1:5. Quoted by Kellie (1824).

Sloan TB: Electrophysiologic monitoring in head injury. New Horizons 3:431, 1995.

Sohmer H: Auditory nerve and brainstem responses (ABR): physiological basis and clinical uses. *In* Desmedt JE (ed): Neuromonitoring in Surgery. Elsevier Science Publishers B.V., 1989, pp. 23–47.

Teasdale G, Jennet B: Assessment of coma and impaired consciousness. Lancet 2:81, 1974.

Temkin NR, Dikman SS, Wilensky AJ, et al: A randomized, double-blind study of phenytoin for the prevention of post-traumatic seizures. N Engl J Med 323:497, 1990.

8.2 **Status Epilepticus**

NARENDRA C. SINGH, BSc, MB, BS, FRCPC, FAAP

Status epilepticus is a life-threatening emergency characterized by an epileptic seizure lasting longer than 30 minutes or repeated seizures for 30 minutes without the patient regaining consciousness. Status epilepticus may manifest clinically in different forms (Fig. 8–5). Because convulsive tonic-clonic seizures are life threatening and can result in significant long-term sequelae, this chapter focuses primarily on the assessment and management of tonic-clonic seizures.

Pathophysiology

A multitude of events can precipitate a derangement between neuronal excitation and inhibition, resulting in uncontrolled neuronal discharge. This discharge initiates a chain of events that result in obvious clinical signs but also subclinical and dangerous events that result in neuronal damage. The five major factors that influence the degree of neuronal damage are *duration, hypoxia, hypoglycemia, etiology*, and *age* (Fig. 8–6).

Differential Diagnosis

The etiology of status epilepticus is unknown in 50% of cases. Of the remaining 50%, the majority are as a result of a chronic seizure disorder, a febrile event, an infectious process (e.g., encephalitis, meningitis), or an acute metabolic event (e.g., hypoglycemia) (Table 8–3).

Figure 8–5. Clinical classification of status epilepticus.

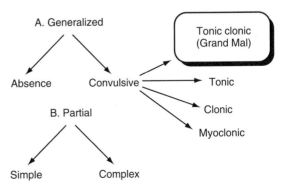

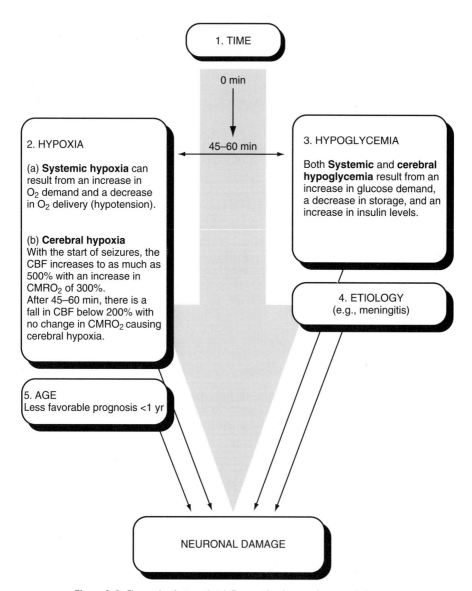

Figure 8–6. Five major factors that influence the degree of neuronal damage.

Table 8–3. ETIOLOGY OF STATUS EPILEPTICUS

Etiology	%
Idiopathic	
Febrile	25
Afebrile	25
Chronic encephalopathy	17
Infectious	12
Trauma	2
Other	7

Management

The goals of management (Fig. 8–7) are to (1) prevent secondary injury (e.g., hypoxia, acidosis, hypotension, hypoglycemia), (2) provide anticonvulsant treatment to stop the seizure and prevent recurrence, and (3) determine the etiology.

PREVENT SECONDARY INJURY (ABCD)

Airway
Assess patency of the airway. The patient may require suctioning and the chin-lift or jaw-thrust maneuver to open the airway.
Administer 100% O_2 by mask.
Position the patient on his or her side, especially if vomiting, to prevent aspiration.

Breathing
Assess the adequacy of ventilation. Most patients in early status epilepticus will continue to ventilate adequately; however, if ventilation is inadequate, then bag-and-mask ventilate. Consider using cricoid pressure to limit gaseous distention of the stomach, which may result in vomiting and aspiration.
If unable to bag-and-mask ventilate adequately, then consider intubation (see below).

Circulation
Assess hemodynamic function (e.g., heart rate, blood pressure, peripheral perfusion).
Establish peripheral venous access.
Draw blood for initial investigations (see Etiology).

Dextrose
Check the blood sugar with a Chemstrip.
Administer dextrose (1–2 mL/kg of 25% dextrose) if glucose level is low.

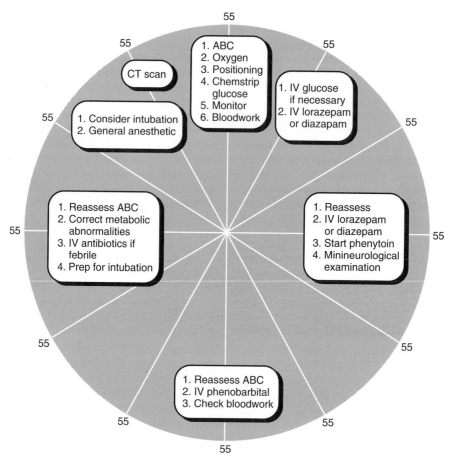

Figure 8–7. Time clock for the management of status epilepticus.

Disability

Rule out focal signs (e.g., unequal pupils) that would suggest trauma or a focal lesion.

DRUG THERAPY

All drugs should be administered intravenously when possible since intramuscular and rectal routes are slow and unreliable (Table 8–4). Preparation should be made to ventilate at any time since respiratory depression may result from anticonvulsant therapy and prolonged seizures. It is therefore necessary to *recheck the ABCs* before and after readministration of any drug or administration of another drug.

1. *Lorazepam* (0.05 to 0.1 mg/kg). This is the drug of choice for initial cessation of seizure activity. The advantage over diazepam is that it is

Table 8–4. DRUGS USED IN THE MANAGEMENT OF STATUS EPILEPTICUS

Drug	Dose	Onset	Duration	Comments
Lorazepam	0.05–0.1 mg/kg (maximum, 4 mg)	2–8 min	3–24 hr	Sedating, respiratory depression, laryngospasm, hypotension
Diazepam	0.1–0.3 mg/kg (maximum, 10 mg)	1–2 min	20–30 min	
Midazolam	0.1–0.3 mg/kg (maximum, 5–10 mg)	1–5 min	<2 hr	
Phenytoin	20 mg/kg *slowly* (1 mg/kg/min)	15–30 min	>24 hr	Hypotension, conduction defects, less sedating
Phenobarbital	20 mg/kg	20–30 min	>24 hr	Sedating, respiratory depression, synergistic with benzodiazepines

    longer acting and therefore the patient is less likely to require polyphar-macy, with resultant respiratory depression.

2. Repeat lorazepam in 10 minutes if no response.
3. *Alternative:* If vascular access is not obtained within 5 to 10 minutes, then rectal lorazepam (0.01 mg/kg) can be administered. Intramuscular *midazolam* has also been demonstrated to be effective in stopping seizures.
4. *Phenytoin* (20 mg/kg IV slowly [1 mg/kg/min]). This is the second-line drug, and it is advantageous over phenobarbital in that respiratory depres-sion occurs less frequently, especially after use of a benzodiazepine, and the effects are less sedative. The disadvantage is that it has to be given slowly (1 mg/kg/min) because bradycardia and hypotension may occur. This may be started 10 minutes after the first dose of lorazepam if the seizure does not resolve. It may also be started with the second dose of lorazepam because the onset of action is relatively slow.
5. *Phenobarbital* (20 mg/kg). This is the third-line drug of choice; however, it may cause respiratory depression, especially after the administration of a benzodiazepine.
6. *Paraldehyde* can also be used in some patients instead of barbiturate coma. Because of its foul smell and difficulty in administration, *it is not used routinely.* Before administration, it must be diluted to a 5% solution (5 mL of 100% paraldehyde diluted to a total of 100 mL with 5% dextrose in water or normal saline). A loading dose of 100 to 150 mg/kg should be given over 15 to 20 minutes. A continuous infusion should be started at 20 mg/kg/hr and may be increased gradually in refractory seizures to a maximum of 200 mg/kg/hr. The drug is incompatible with most plastics and should therefore be administered with a *glass syringe.* Potential side effects include pulmonary edema and hemorrhage as well as hepatic, renal, and cardiac toxicity.

Intubation and General Anesthetic

    If the above drugs fail to stop the seizure and laboratory evaluations fail to demonstrate a treatable cause (e.g., hyponatremia), then the patient should be intubated and ventilated to prevent significant cerebral hypoxia.

Intubation: The following drugs should be used: (1) *atropine* (0.01 mg/kg; minimum, 0.1 mg), (2) *sodium pentothal* (2 to 5 mg/kg), and (3) *succinylcholine* (1 to 2 mg/kg). Sodium pentothal will temporarily stop the seizure. Avoid using a long-acting muscle relaxant because the only indicator of cerebral activity is motor activity, which may be masked by paralysis. (For general anesthetic management, see Intensive Care Unit Management.)

Antibiotics/Antiviral

If the patient is febrile and the seizure is prolonged, meningitis or encephalitis cannot be ruled out. A blood culture should be drawn and a meningitis-treatment dose of a third-generation cephalosporin (cefotaxime [50 mg/kg/dose] or ceftriaxone [50 mg/kg/dose]) should be administered.

ETIOLOGY

History and *physical* may aid in establishing the etiology (e.g., meningitis, encephalitis, trauma, drugs).

Laboratory evaluation should include complete blood count, blood sugar, electrolytes, calcium, magnesium, and phosphate. Other tests may be done if the history suggests a specific etiology (e.g., toxicology screen). Blood cultures should be done in febrile patients.

Lumbar puncture should be done if meningitis or encephalitis is suspected. Delay the lumbar puncture in the presence of raised intracranial pressure, coagulopathy, cardiorespiratory compression, or local infection at the site.

Computed tomography scan should be considered in the presence of raised intracranial pressure, history of trauma, focal seizure activity, or focal deficit. It should also be considered in refractory seizures.

Intensive Care Unit Management

If the seizure is refractory, then a general anesthetic is necessary to abate the seizure and prevent long-term sequelae. After intubation and mechanical ventilation, adequate monitoring should be in place to evaluate the effectiveness of therapy and iatrogenic complications.

Monitoring

Electroencephalography is necessary to titrate the dose of phenobarbital.

Because pentobarbital may have cardiac side effects, arterial and central venous line placement as well as hemodynamic monitoring are necessary.

Pentobarbital (Barbiturate Coma)

Loading dose: 5 mg/kg IV is administered slowly every 5 minutes until burst suppression is observed on electroencephalography or a total of 20 mg/kg is administered.

Maintenance: 1 to 5 mg/kg/hr is administered to maintain burst suppression or a pentobarbital level is reached of 25 to 50 µg/mL.

Duration: This may be maintained for 24 to 48 hours and then withdrawn in the presence of electroencephalographic monitoring.

If the cardiac output and blood pressure are impaired, an inotrope such as dopamine may be started.

Prognosis

Neurologic sequelae occur five times as often in infants less than 1 year of age than in children more than 3 years old. The sequelae can include chronic seizure disorder, mental retardation, focal deficits, and behavioral disorders.

BIBLIOGRAPHY

Barnett TM, Wasserman GS: Seizures and status epilepticus. *In* Reisdorff EJ, Roberts MR, Wiegenstein (eds): Pediatric Emergency Medicine. Philadelphia, WB Saunders, 1992, pp. 1008–1014.

Johnston MV: Neuroexcitatory syndromes. *In* Holbrook PR (ed): Textbook of Pediatric Critical Care. Philadelphia, WB Saunders, 1993, pp. 218–229.

Mayhue FE: Intramuscular midazolam for status epilepticus in the emergency department. Ann Emerg Med 17:643, 1988.

8.3 **Meningitis and Encephalitis**

CATHERINE A. FARRELL, MD, FRCPC

Meningitis and encephalitis are the most common forms of acute infection of the central nervous system (CNS) encountered in childhood. The term *meningitis* refers to an inflammatory process principally confined to the meninges. The term *encephalitis* implies that the cerebral matter is involved in the inflammatory or infectious process. In some situations, both the meninges and the cerebrum are affected; this may be referred to as *meningoencephalitis.*

The incidence of bacterial meningitis varies according to age, being relatively more frequent in the newborn (1 to 10 in 10,000) and infant less than 1 year old (75 in 100,000) than in children in the second year of life (25 in 100,000) and older (2 in 100,000 by age 5). The overall incidence of encephalitis for all ages is estimated to be 7.4 in 100,000.

Pathophysiology

The development of meningitis is the consequence of colonization and proliferation of the meningeal pathogen in mucosal tissue of the nasopharynx, invasion of and diffusion through the intravascular space, and invasion of the subarachnoid space via the choroid plexus, with inflammation of the meninges. Passage across the blood-brain barrier often occurs, so there meningoencephalitis may occur. Meningitis may result from the contiguous spread of organisms in an adjacent space, for example, as the result of a penetrating wound or skull fracture, sinusitis, or a ruptured abscess.

Several factors may lead to cerebral edema and increased intracranial pressure in meningitis, including disturbances of cerebral autoregulation, dysfunction of the blood-brain barrier, and a vasculitic process with vasospasm, thrombosis, and resulting ischemia. The cerebral edema may be both *vasogenic* (related to fluid flux across a disturbed blood-brain barrier) and *cytotoxic* (due to the direct effects of bacteria and inflammatory mediators stimulated by their presence).

The pathophysiology of encephalitis includes two different mechanisms of transmission of the infecting agent. The first involves the hematogenous spread after penetration into the lymphatic system of a virus acquired through the respiratory tract, the gastrointestinal tract, or after an insect bite. The multiplication of the virus in the lymphatic system is followed by dissemination through the bloodstream to the CNS. Certain viruses (e.g., herpes simplex and rabies) spread through peripheral nerves to eventually reach the CNS and undergo replication locally. In some cases (e.g., varicella), the encephalitis is postinfectious and entails an immune response provoked by the infecting organism, which causes inflammation in various regions of the CNS.

Etiology

BACTERIAL MENINGITIS

Newborns (≤1 Month Old)

Group B β-hemolytic *Streptococcus*
Gram-negative bacilli (e.g., *Escherichia coli, Klebsiella* sp., *Pseudomonas aeruginosa*)
Listeria monocytogenes

Infants (<3 Months Old)

Group B β-hemolytic *Streptococcus*
Gram-negative bacilli (e.g., *E. coli, Klebsiella* sp.)
L. monocytogenes
Haemophilus influenzae, Streptococcus pneumoniae, Neisseria meningitidis (all three are relatively uncommon)

Infants and Children (>3 Months Old)

Bacterial meningitis: *H. influenzae*
S. pneumoniae
N. meningitidis

Other Meningitis-Causing Agents

Mycobacterium tuberculinum (TB)
Fungi: *Cryptococcus, Candida*
Viral (aseptic) meningitis: Enteroviruses (coxsackievirus, echoviruses)

ENCEPHALITIS

Herpes simplex, herpes zoster, Epstein-Barr virus, cytomegalovirus
Arthropod-borne viruses (e.g., St. Louis encephalitis, Western equine encephalitis)
Measles, mumps, varicella; enteroviruses, adenovirus
Rabies
Mycoplasma pneumoniae

Differential Diagnosis

The clinical presentations of meningitis and encephalitis may mirror each other, as well as those of a number of acute CNS disorders. Meningitis and encephalitis should be considered as possible diagnoses in any infant or child presenting with an altered level of consciousness or coma, particularly when signs of infection are present, such as fever or leukocytosis. Other causes of altered level of consciousness that should be considered are trauma, intoxication, tumor, intracranial hemorrhage, and thrombosis.

Clinical Evaluation

BACTERIAL MENINGITIS

Features that may be present in the history of a patient with bacterial meningitis include fever, lethargy or irritability, decreased appetite, vomiting, headache, photophobia, altered level of consciousness, and seizures.

Physical examination should include assessment of the following:

Airway. Consider whether the child's neurologic status is so compromised that he or she is unable to protect his or her airway.

Breathing. In the newborn and young infant, apnea episodes or irregular breathing may be present. With deepening coma, abnormal breathing patterns such as Cheyne-Stokes respiration may develop.

Circulation. The child may show signs of dehydration from vomiting or decreased fluid intake or may show signs of hemodynamic compromise related to sepsis.

Vital Signs. Fever (or hypothermia in the newborn and young infant) and tachycardia are often present. Both hypotension and hypertension are signs of impending crisis and require immediate action.

Ears, Nose, and Throat. An underlying otitis media or sinusitis may be present.

Neurologic Examination. The alteration of the level of consciousness may range from somnolence to deep coma (Glasgow Coma Scale may be useful to quantify trends) and may be associated with signs of raised intracranial pressure (ICP) (e.g., bulging fontanelle, pupillary changes, papilledema). Neck stiffness is the result of meningeal inflammation and irritation and may be elicited on direct examination or through use of the Kernig and Brudzinski tests. *Meningeal signs may be absent even in confirmed bacterial meningitis* in children younger than 2 years old. Focal neurologic signs such as hemiparesis or focal seizures may suggest an abscess or areas of ischemia. Cranial nerve involvement is infrequent, with the sixth, third, and fourth cranial nerves being those most often affected.

Skin. A petechial or purpuric rash, although most often associated with meningococcal disease, may occur in *Haemophilus* and even pneumococcal meningitis. Persistent or worsening jaundice may be a subtle sign of infection in the newborn.

VIRAL MENINGITIS

The signs and symptoms of viral meningitis may be confined to fever, headache, or neck stiffness alone or may include all of the signs and symptoms attributed to bacterial meningitis.

ENCEPHALITIS

The most frequent presenting symptom of encephalitis is an altered level of consciousness varying from somnolence to coma. Headache, vomiting, and behavioral changes may be present. Other elements to be sought in the history include recent travel, exposure to animals or insects, or contact with infected persons.

The characteristic rash of certain viral infections may be observed.

A key element in the physical examination is the neurologic examination. Herpes encephalitis frequently presents with seizures (often focal) that are difficult to control; focal neurologic deficits may be present. A temporal lobe focus is a classic finding on electroencephalography (EEG). Varicella CNS infection typically leads to cerebellar involvement with ataxia.

Investigations

SUSPECTED MENINGITIS

Lumbar puncture should be performed to obtain cerebrospinal fluid (CSF) for culture and analysis. Confirmation of the diagnosis of bacterial meningitis depends on the isolation of a bacterial pathogen on culture or its appearance on direct microscopic examination.

Analyses to be performed include the following:

- Complete blood cell count and differential
- Biochemistry: Glucose, protein, lactate (optional)
- Gram-stain and culture (bacterial and viral) (see Table 8–5 for comparison of CSF analyses according to pathogen)

Contraindications to performing a lumbar puncture include the following:

- Hemodynamic or respiratory compromise
- Raised ICP
- Local infection at puncture site
- Coagulopathy or thrombocytopenia

When in doubt, perform a blood culture and start antibiotic therapy. CSF can subsequently be obtained, once the patient has been stabilized, and sent for identification of bacterial antigens by *latex agglutination* or counterimmunophoresis (blood and urine may also be sent).

Other laboratory investigations include the following:

- Complete blood cell count and differential; coagulation profile if platelet count is low or there is a suspicion of disseminated intravascular coagulation
- Electrolytes
- Peripheral blood cultures
- Radiology: Chest radiography in an intubated patient
- Computed tomography scan in the presence of a focal neurologic deficit or suspected raised ICP

SUSPECTED ENCEPHALITIS

Lumbar puncture is also recommended, although it may often be negative. In herpes encephalitis, *polymerase chain reaction* analysis of the CSF may lead to a

Table 8–5. TYPICAL CEREBROSPINAL FLUID FINDINGS

Parameter	Bacterial Meningitis	Viral Meningitis	TB Meningitis	Herpes Encephalitis
White blood cell count ($\times 10^6$/L)	>500	>10	>500	
Differential	>90% neutrophils	Lymphocytes, monocytes	Lymphocytes	Lymphocytes
Protein (gm/L)	1.0–2.0	>0.5	>1.0	<1.0
Glucose (% of serum glucose)	<50%	Normal	<50%	Normal
Gram stain	Bacteria present	Negative	Negative (Ziehl-positive)	Negative

more rapid identification of the virus. Viral serology and viral cultures (CSF, nasopharyngeal secretions, urine, stool) should be performed. With the exception of a positive specific IgM response, their value lies in the retrospective confirmation of the diagnosis.

In addition, imaging studies such as computed tomography (CT) scan or magnetic resonance imaging (MRI) may be of use, for example, to document lesions in the temporal or fronto-orbital regions in herpes encephalitis.

Definitive identification may require a brain biopsy to obtain tissue for direct examination.

Management

The goals of management include the following:

- Identification and eradication of the causal pathogen
- Prevention, recognition, and treatment of raised ICP
- Maintaining hemodynamic stability and organ function in the context of sepsis
- Prevention and treatment of potential complications (e.g., seizures, syndrome of inappropriate secretion of antidiuretic hormone [SIADH], hypoxic-ischemic injury, subdural effusion)
- Identification and prophylactic treatment of contacts to prevent disease spread, where applicable

Criteria for intensive case unit admission include the following:

- Hemodynamic instability
- Raised ICP
- Status epilepticus
- Coma (Glasgow Coma Scale score of <9)

SUPPORTIVE CARE

Airway and Breathing

Indications for intubation include the following:

- Inability to protect airway (e.g., Glasgow Coma Scale score of <8)
- Status epilepticus
- Raised ICP

Maintain arterial oxygen tension (Pao_2) at >100 mm Hg.

Hyperventilation to carbon dioxide tension (Pco_2) should be 30 to 35 mm Hg in the case of raised ICP.

Hemodynamic

Monitor as outlined in "Surveillance and Monitoring." The goal is the maintenance of normovolemia and adequate cerebral perfusion pressure.

If the patient is *hemodynamically unstable* and there are signs of decreased perfusion or hypotension:

- Give a fluid bolus of normal saline or Ringer's lactate (20 mL/kg) and repeat as necessary.
- If there is no response to fluid bolus, suspect septic shock (especially in meningococcal or group B *Streptococcus* meningitis), and begin vasopressor and inotropic support (see Chapter 9.1).

If the patient is hemodynamically stable:

- Give IV fluids (5% dextrose in 0.2%, 0.45%, or 0.9% sodium chloride [NaCl] depending on the patient's sodium requirement) at daily maintenance (1500 mL/m²/day).
- Fluid restriction is not initially indicated as patients often are initially dehydrated, and on-going fluid restriction may increase the risk of cerebral ischemia from low cerebral perfusion pressure.
- Fluid restriction is indicated only in the presence of the SIADH (see under "Metabolic").

Neurologic

Close surveillance of the neurologic examination is essential. In both meningitis and encephalitis, potential emergencies include raised ICP and seizures.

Raised ICP. Intubation, hyperventilation, sedation, and neuromuscular paralysis are recommended. *Mannitol* should be used with caution, in doses of 0.25 to 1.0 gm/kg. Barbiturate coma is rarely indicated and is a criterion for invasive measurement of ICP and consideration of use of continuous EEG monitoring.

Seizures. Seizures occur in 20% to 30% of patients before admission for bacterial meningitis and are a frequent mode of presentation of encephalitis.

Treatment. To stop seizures, administer lorazepam (0.05 to 0.1 mg/kg IV) or diazepam (0.1 to 0.3 mg/kg IV). Subsequently, phenytoin (20 mg/kg IV loading dose, followed by maintenance dose of 5 mg/kg/day) for patients at risk of recurrent seizures or presenting in status epilepticus (see Chapter 8.2).

Venous thrombosis. Sagittal sinus thrombosis may present with signs of paralysis or cortical blindness. Cavernous sinus thrombosis produces chemosis, proptosis, and an ophthalmoplegia. Treatment is supportive, with anticoagulation being indicated rarely, in severe cases.

Dexamethasone therapy. The medical literature provides conflicting evidence on the benefits of early dexamethasone therapy to reduce the consequences of the inflammatory process involved in meningitis due to *H. influenzae* and *S. pneumoniae*, with the specific goal being the reduction of eighth nerve damage and hearing loss.

Current recommendations are to consider use of dexamethasone in children older than 2 to 3 months with bacterial meningitis at a dosage of 0.6 mg/kg/day IV q6h for 4 days, starting, if possible, before the first dose of antibiotic is given.

There is no indication for the use of corticosteroids in viral meningitis. The same applies to encephalitis, although some authors favor the use of corticosteroids in herpes encephalitis with multiple foci of inflammation and cerebral infarction documented on computed tomography scan.

Metabolic

Electrolyte disturbances may occur in both meningitis and encephalitis.
SIADH. Diagnosis is based on the following criteria:

- Hyponatremia (Na <130 mmol/L)
- Urinary sodium >60 mmol/L; urine specific gravity >1.020 despite hyponatremia
- Serum osmolarity <275 mOsm/L; urine osmolarity >300 mOsm/L
- Absence of hypovolemia, raised blood urea nitrogen, renal or adrenal dysfunction

Treatment. Restrict fluid to as little as 60% of maintenance requirements (or lower if necessary).
Diabetes insipidus. Diabetes insipidus is extremely rare in bacterial meningitis or in encephalitis, with the exception of bacterial meningitis occurring in the neonatal period.
Treatment. Administer intravenous fluids to provide for insensible losses (5% dextrose in water/NaCl 0.45% with 30 mmol/L KCl at 300 to 400 mL/m^2) and hourly replacement of urinary losses with a hypotonic solution (NaCl 0.2% to 0.45% or 2.5% dextrose in water, with 3 to 4 mmol/L of potassium chloride [KCl]).

EMPIRIC ANTIBIOTIC THERAPY IN BACTERIAL MENINGITIS

Age <1 month. Ampicillin (75 to 150 mg/kg/day IV q8h if <7 days old; 100 to 200 mg/kg/day IV q6h if >7 days old) **and** cefotaxime (100 mg/kg/day IV q12h if <7 days, 100 to 150 mg/kg/day q8h IV if >7 days old); **or** ampicillin (same doses) **and** gentamicin (5 mg/kg/day q12h IV if <7 days old, 5 to 7.5 mg/kg/day q8h IV if >7 days old)
Age 1 to 3 months. Ampicillin (200 to 300 mg/kg/day IV q6h) **and** cefotaxime (200 mg/kg/day IV q6h or q8h)
Age >3 months. Cefotaxime (200 mg/kg/day IV q6h or q8h, maximum 12 gm/day) **or** ceftriaxone (80 to 100 mg/kg/day IV q12h, maximum 4 gm/day) **or** ampicillin (200 to 300 mg/kg/day IV q6h, maximum 12 gm/day) **and** chloramphenicol (100 mg/kg/day IV q6h, maximum 4 gm/day)

EMPIRIC ANTIVIRAL THERAPY IN ENCEPHALITIS

In any unstable or deteriorating patient, especially in the presence of EEG or CT scan findings suggestive of herpes encephalitis, empiric therapy should be begun:
Age <1 year. Acyclovir 30 mg/kg/day IV q8h
Age >1 year. Acyclovir 750 mg/m^2/day IV q8h

SURVEILLANCE AND MONITORING

All patients admitted to the intensive care unit with meningitis or encephalitis initially require continuous cardiorespiratory monitoring and frequent (at least every hour) vital signs assessment, including Glasgow Coma Scale score and determination of pupil size and response. Intake and output should be accurately measured and recorded. Any intubated patient, those in respiratory distress, and those with uncertain airway or breathing control status should have continuous monitoring of O_2 saturation. Hemodynamically unstable patients may benefit from invasive monitoring via an indwelling arterial catheter as well as a central venous line for central venous pressure measurement. It is rarely necessary to place a Swan-Ganz (pulmonary artery) catheter for thermodilution cardiac output measurement.

Laboratory investigations include daily complete blood count, coagulation profile if abnormality is suspected, electrolytes every 8 to 24 hours, serum and urine osmolarity if there is a suspicion of SIADH, daily blood urea nitrogen and creatinine, and arterial or capillary blood gases every 6 hours in intubated patients or in presence of problems of respiratory drive.

Complications

Complications include seizures, brain abscess, subdural fluid collection, hearing loss (5 to 33% of patients with meningitis), and other pathologies (e.g., reactive arthritis, osteomyelitis, pericarditis, pneumonia).

Prognosis

The mortality rate for bacterial meningitis is approximately 5%. Morbidity varies according to series and may approach 25%. The most common sequela is hearing loss, which may be temporary or permanent. Brain stem auditory-evoked potentials or an audiogram should be performed before discharge in all patients. Prognosis in meningitis is related to the pathogen (e.g., hearing loss is more common with pneumococcal meningitis than with other childhood pathogens), age (e.g., higher mortality and morbidity are associated with neonatal meningitis), and severity of illness.

The prognosis in most cases of viral meningitis is excellent; a full recovery ensues within several days. Neurologic sequelae may occur in the very young infant after viral meningitis.

The prognosis of encephalitis varies according to the pathogen. Among the arbovirus (arthropod-borne) encephalitides, St. Louis encephalitis has the mildest clinical course and carries the best prognosis, and Eastern equine encephalitis has the worst prognosis. Untreated herpes encephalitis has a mortality rate of 70%, and neurologic complications occur almost universally in survivors. Early treatment with acyclovir greatly reduces mortality, but neurologic sequelae of varying degrees occur in >50% of patients.

Prevention/Prophylaxis

Prophylaxis with rifampin is indicated for close contacts of patients with bacterial meningitis due to *H. influenzae* or *N. meningitidis*. For *H. influenzae*, administer rifampin (20 mg/kg [maximum of 600 mg] PO once daily for 4 days) to all household members if there is a child younger than 4 years old in the household. For *N. meningitidis*, administer rifampin (20 mg/kg/day [maximum 600 mg] PO b.i.d. for 2 days).

BIBLIOGRAPHY

Kennedy C: Acute viral encephalitis in childhood. Br Med J 310:139, 1995.
Prober C: The role of steroids in the management of children with bacterial meningitis. Pediatrics 95:29, 1995.
Quagliarello V, Scheld WM: Bacterial meningitis: pathogenesis, pathophysiology, and progress. N Engl J Med 327:84, 1992.
Report of the Committee on Infectious Diseases of the American Academy of Pediatrics: Red Book, 23rd ed. Elk Grove Village, Illinois, American Academy of Pediatrics, 1994.
Wald ER, Kaplan SL, Mason EO, et al: Dexamethasone therapy for children with bacterial meningitis. Pediatrics 95:21, 1995.
Walsh-Kelly C. Nelson DB, Smith DS, et al: Clinical predictors of bacterial versus aseptic meningitis in childhood. Ann Emerg Med 21:910, 1992.

8.4 Severe Traumatic Brain Injury in Children

PATRICK M. KOCHANEK, MD
P. DAVID ADELSON, MD
ROBERT S. B. CLARK, MD
DONALD W. MARION, MD

Trauma is the leading cause of death in the United States in persons younger than 18 years old, and head injury is a key contributor to outcome in >50% of these victims. This chapter focuses on the management issues in infants and children with severe traumatic brain injury because this is the group of patients in whom highly specialized assessment, monitoring, and management in the pediatric intensive care unit (ICU) are essential to optimal outcome. The designation of *severe traumatic brain injury* is generally applied to patients with an initial presenting Glasgow Coma Scale (GCS) score of ≤8.

Pathophysiology

The pathobiology and pathophysiology of severe traumatic brain injury are complex and varied. The clinical picture in the acute setting depends importantly on the etiology of the insult, age of the patient, and presence of secondary insults.

PATHOLOGY

Contusion, hematoma, ischemic injury, and axonal injury are the four key pathologic entities associated with severe traumatic brain injury (Fig. 8–8). *Contusions* represent localized traumatic, necrotic, and hemorrhagic lesions. They are observed in about 42% of adults with fatal head injury. The incidence of contusion in children with severe traumatic brain injury is less well defined. *Hematomas* can be subdural, epidural, or parenchymal. There is a 30% incidence of hematoma in adults and in infants and children younger than 4 years old. In contrast, the incidence of hematoma is only 17% in children between the ages of 5 and 15. *Ischemic neuronal necrosis* and/or *infarction* are common and key findings in cases of severe traumatic brain injury. They are seen in about 90% of fatal cases. The traumatically injured brain is particularly susceptible to hypoxic-ischemic insults. Moderate levels of hypoxia, which produce no pathologic effects in the normal brain, can induce permanent damage in the traumatically injured brain. *Axonal injury* is an important and unique finding of traumatic brain injury and can be local or diffuse. Stretching or transection of axons by shearing forces is caused by a rotational acceleration-deceleration type of injury.

ETIOLOGY

Motor vehicle accidents account for the majority of cases in children older than 4 years old. In contrast, falls and assaults account for 48% of the cases in infants and children younger than 4 years old.

PHYSIOLOGY

Cerebral Blood Flow and Metabolism

In most cases of severe traumatic brain injury, a characteristic pattern of changes occurs in cerebral blood flow (CBF) and metabolism (Fig. 8–9). During the first few hours after trauma, CBF is reduced and arteriojugular venous difference in oxygen content is increased, suggesting hypoperfusion or ischemia. Early

Figure 8–8. Pathology of severe traumatic brain injury.

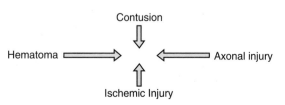

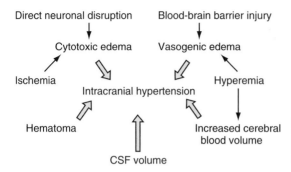

Figure 8–9. Pathophysiologic disturbances observed in severe traumatic brain injury and associated with intracranial hypertension.

post-traumatic cerebral ischemia is an important therapeutic target. During the more delayed phases (by 24 hours after trauma), a much more complex situation generally develops. In some regions of the brain, severe injury is accompanied by sustained hypoperfusion or infarction. In other regions, flow begins to increase despite no increase in cerebral metabolic rate for oxygen, and a state of relative hyperemia may occur (i.e., uncoupling of flow and metabolism). The contribution of glucose utilization to cerebral metabolic rate, however, is still under investigation, and the exact nature of the relationship between CBF and metabolism in these regions requires further study. Nevertheless, increases in CBF and cerebral blood volume in some brain regions between 48 and 72 hours after trauma contribute to intracranial hypertension. Pain, agitation, and seizures can also contribute to increases in cerebral metabolic rate and coupled increases in both cerebral blood volume and intracranial pressure (ICP). These are important areas for therapeutic manipulation.

Cerebral Edema

Blood-brain barrier injury and the development of cerebral edema important pathophysiologic disturbances associated with severe traumatic brain injury. They contribute to the development of coma, brain swelling, and intracranial hypertension. Peak edema generally occurs between 24 and 48 hours after injury. The intact blood-brain barrier is highly impermeable to polar molecules and charged species, including Na^+. Thus, osmotic rather than oncotic gradients are the key determinant of fluid flux across the intact blood-brain barrier. Unlike the systemic circulation, Na^+ gradients rather than albumin gradients govern fluid flux. Edema is another important therapeutic target. Unfortunately, most therapeutic efforts reduce water content only in noninjured brain regions.

Intracranial Hypertension

Post-traumatic intracranial hypertension has classically been defined as an ICP of >20 mm Hg for >5 minutes. It is observed in $>72\%$ of patients with severe traumatic brain injury and is inversely related to outcome. It is another key focus for therapy. As previously discussed, the origins of post-traumatic intracranial hypertension can be vascular or nonvascular. Specific causes include increases in cerebral blood volume and cerebrospinal fluid (CSF) volume, cytotoxic and vasogenic edema, and hematoma.

Children Versus Adults

Diffuse brain swelling is an entity that is observed twice as often in children younger than 16 years old than in adults. Although the exact pathophysiologic basis of this entity is still in question, a vascular origin, particularly hyperemia, is suggested. It may be quite important in children since a heterogeneous injury pattern with both ischemia and hyperemia can be seen, and the lower blood pressure limit of CBF autoregulation is less in children than in adults. Thus, even moderate increases in ICP may adversely affect regional cerebral perfusion. In addition, the diffuse swelling process may result from the development of edema and contribute to herniation.

Differential Diagnosis

The differential diagnosis of severe traumatic brain injury is generally straightforward. Nevertheless, the acquisition of information pertaining to the exact mechanism of injury can be important in making initial triage decisions. There are two clinical situations that are relatively unique to pediatrics in which issues surrounding the differential diagnosis of severe traumatic brain injury are important. First, the clinician must maintain a high index of suspicion of *nonaccidental trauma* when evaluating children younger than 1 year old who present with signs or symptoms of acute neurologic deterioration of any kind, particularly seizures or altered mental status. Second, an intracranial hemorrhage resulting from mild or moderate traumatic brain injury, with a resultant severe insult, should suggest the possibility of an *underlying coagulopathy* in the infant or child and merits laboratory assessment.

CLINICAL EVALUATION

Glasgow Coma Scale or a modified GCS (available for children) should be included in the initial evaluation (Table 8–6). The *airway* should be secured in children with a GCS score of 8 or less. In most cases, this can be accomplished through a rapid-sequence approach with preoxygenation (100% O_2), fentanyl (1 to 2 μg/kg IV), diazepam or midazolam (0.1 to 0.3 mg/kg IV), and vecuronium (0.2 to 0.3 mg/kg IV). Ideally, face-mask ventilation should be avoided *(always assume a full stomach)*, but if ventilation or oxygenation is inadequate or there is evidence of impending herniation, the patient must be ventilated. Apply gentle pressure to the cricoid to minimize the risk of aspiration. Direct laryngoscopy with a designated person assigned to *stabilize the cervical spine* (without traction) is the technique of choice. After intubation, mild hyperventilation is indicated (Fig. 8–10). However, if in the initial evaluation signs and/or symptoms of a focal lesion with intracranial hypertension and/or impending *herniation* are present (e.g., unilateral pupillary dilation, hypertension/bradycardia, developing hemiparesis),

Table 8–6. COMPONENTS OF THE INITIAL NEUROLOGIC ASSESSMENT FOR SEVERE TRAUMATIC BRAIN INJURY

Minineurologic Examination	Glasgow Coma Scale Score Modified for Children*	
Evaluate	*Motor*	
Level of consciousness	Obeys commands/spontaneous movement	6
Extremity movement	Localizes pain	5
Response to pain	Withdraws to pain	4
Deep tendon reflexes	Flexion to pain	3
Plantar response	Extensor to pain	2
Brain stem reflexes (pupils, extraocular movements, corneal, gag, cough)	No response	1
	Verbal	
	Oriented/appropriate for age	5
	Disoriented/cries but consolable	4
	Inappropriate/cries but inconsolable	3
	Incomprehensible/restless, lethargic	2
	No response	1
	Eyes	
	Open spontaneously	4
	Open to voice	3
	Open to pain	2
	No response	1

Modified from Luerssen TG: Acute traumatic cerebral injuries. *In* Cheek WR ed: Pediatric Neurosurgery, 3rd ed. Philadelphia, WB Saunders, 1994, p. 274.
*At present, this is not uniformly accepted as the definitive grading system for children. This scale is not supported by the extensive prognosis literature that the original Glasgow Coma Scale has in adults.

immediate intervention is essential and should include a cerebral protective intubation with thiopental (5 to 7 mg/kg IV), lidocaine (1 mg/kg IV), and vecuronium (0.2 to 0.3 mg/kg IV). In addition, mannitol (0.5 gm/kg IV) should be administered, and hyperventilation should be instituted. Additional thiopental, mannitol, and hyperventilation should be titrated as the patient is being taken for emergency computed tomography (CT) scan. During intubation and subsequent management, rigorous attention must be given to *maintenance of adequate blood pressure,* and all treatments must be appropriately titrated. In light of the complex nature of the clinical presentation of patients with multiple trauma (ranging from cardiopulmonary arrest to hemodynamic stability), *intubation drugs must be tailored to the clinical situation.* Specific recommendations are outlined in Table 8–7. Once the airway, breathing, and circulation have been addressed in the trauma stabilization, completion of a *minineurologic examination* is appropriate, as is a *more complete trauma evaluation.* Intubation and stabilization should be followed by *emergency CT scan.* In most cases, evaluation and treatment can proceed as outlined (see Fig. 8–10).

Investigations

Additional monitoring investigations are critical to decision making in the management of these highly complex patients.

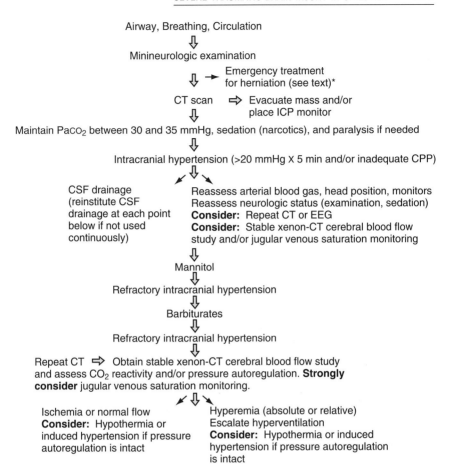

Airway, Breathing, Circulation
⇩
Minineurologic examination
⇩ → Emergency treatment
for herniation (see text)*
CT scan ⇨ Evacuate mass and/or
⇩ place ICP monitor
Maintain PaCO$_2$ between 30 and 35 mmHg, sedation (narcotics), and paralysis if needed
⇩
Intracranial hypertension (>20 mmHg X 5 min and/or inadequate CPP)
⇩

CSF drainage | Reassess arterial blood gas, head position, monitors
(reinstitute CSF | Reassess neurologic status (examination, sedation)
drainage at each point | **Consider:** Repeat CT or EEG
below if not used | **Consider:** Stable xenon-CT cerebral blood flow
continuously) | study and/or jugular venous saturation monitoring

⇩
Mannitol
⇩
Refractory intracranial hypertension
⇩
Barbiturates
⇩
Refractory intracranial hypertension
⇩
Repeat CT ⇨ Obtain stable xenon-CT cerebral blood flow study
and assess CO$_2$ reactivity and/or pressure autoregulation. **Strongly
consider** jugular venous saturation monitoring.
⇩

Ischemia or normal flow | Hyperemia (absolute or relative)
Consider: Hypothermia or | Escalate hyperventilation
induced hypertension if pressure | **Consider:** Hypothermia or induced
autoregulation is intact | hypertension if pressure autoregulation
 | is intact

* Mannitol, thiopental, and hyperventilation as needed en route to emergency CT scan for signs
of impending herniation.

Figure 8–10. Generalized management tree for severe traumatic brain injury and intracranial hypertension
in the pediatric intensive care unit. This is a general schematic protocol. Management frequently must
be tailored to each individual case.

COMPUTED TOMOGRAPHY

The use of CT scanning has revolutionized patient management in neurointensive care. However, one cannot rely on this parameter alone in clinical decision making. Data from the National Institutes of Health Traumatic Coma Data Bank (reported by Levin et al) reveal that there was a 10 to 15% incidence of significant intracranial hypertension, even in patients in whom the initial CT was normal.

INTRACRANIAL PRESSURE MONITORING

Unless contraindicated, ICP monitoring is recommended in patients with severe traumatic brain injury (GCS score of 8 or less and no eye opening).

Table 8–7. DRUGS FOR INTUBATION OF THE CHILD
WITH SEVERE TRAUMATIC BRAIN INJURY

Situation	Drug*
Cardiopulmonary arrest	Resuscitation drugs
Hemodynamically unstable	Fentanyl (2–4 µg/kg)
	Lidocaine (1 mg/kg)
	Vecuronium (0.3 mg/kg)
Hemodynamically stable	Fentanyl (2–4 µg/kg)
	Lidocaine (1 mg/kg)
	Diazepam or midazolam (0.1–0.3 mg/kg)
	Vecuronium (0.3 mg/kg)
Evidence of intracranial hypertension	Fentanyl (2–4 µg/kg)
(and hemodynamically stable)	Lidocaine (1 mg/kg)
	Thiopental (4–5 mg/kg)†
	Vecuronium (0.3 mg/kg)

*Drugs should be administered intravenously.
†Use with caution; see text for details.

Intracranial hypertension is seen in 50 to 70% of these patients, and more than half of patients who die due to head injury have uncontrolled ICP. Hydraulic-linked systems and catheter-tip sensor systems have been used for the measurement of ICP. The hydraulic-linked systems include the ventricular catheter, which is the gold standard for measurement of ICP. Currently, the subarachnoid screw and bolt are much less commonly used and may underestimate ICP when it is >30 mm Hg. Catheter-tip fiberoptic (Camino, NeuroCare, San Diego, CA) or micro-transducer (Codman, Johnson & Johnson, Raynhem, MA) devices are theoretically limited in that there is no means of in vivo zero calibration; however, they have minimal zero drift in clinical use. They are also limited because they cannot be used to treat intracranial hypertension by CSF drainage. They can be placed in subdural, intraventricular, or intraparenchymal sites.

MEASUREMENT OF CEREBRAL BLOOD FLOW

Several methods are available for the measurement of CBF after severe traumatic brain injury. Although these techniques are not standards of care, as our understanding increases of the complex pathophysiology of traumatic brain injury, it is becoming increasingly important to have this information to make rational patient care decisions. Stable xenon CT uses nonradioactive (stable) xenon (Xe) gas as the tracer and combines the inhalation of this gas with CT scanning and appropriate software to derive regional CBF from a wash-in or wash-out scan and a baseline CT scan. This technique, although not a method of on-line monitoring, provides excellent correlation of CBF and anatomy and can be particularly useful in patient management. It is the method of choice in this setting. Measurement of CBF with the ^{133}Xe method and blood velocity in the middle cerebral artery through the use of transcranial Doppler also have been used in several centers and are supplemental or alternative techniques. Some method of measuring or monitoring CBF is strongly encouraged. Although clinical decisions cannot be based solely on this single piece of information, knowledge of regional CBF can help guide therapy.

JUGULAR VENOUS SATURATION

This is a technique that was used by Obrist and coworkers in the late 1970s and early 1980s that was abandoned but is regaining popularity. Selecting a threshold of <50% saturation, Sheinberg and coworkers reported that the number of desaturations is associated with outcome. Only a portion of these desaturations, however, occurred in a situation in which there was not already an obvious need for intervention (i.e., arterial hypoxemia, hypotension), and there were many false-positives. In light of the heterogeneity of post-traumatic CBF, jugular venous saturation is similar to ICP in that if the value obtained is in a clinically unacceptable range, intervention is warranted, but values in the normal range do not preclude the existence of significant pathology. Although this monitoring technique is not a standard of care, its use has become more widespread and is encouraged. A protocol for responding to jugular venous saturation is given by Sheinberg and coworkers, along with illustrative examples of silent desaturations to 40% with excessive ventilation.

Management

The treatment of severe traumatic brain injury is based on the understanding of the components of the intracranial space: brain, blood, and CSF. Treatment modalities are used to attempt to alter the contribution of each of these components to intracranial hypertension (Table 8–8). A general schematic for management is given (see Fig. 8–10). Management issues addressed in this chapter relate specifically to those relevant to the management of the patient in the ICU. Communication between the neurosurgical and critical care teams is essential to provide optimal care to these complex patients.

HEAD POSITION

Head position has been an area of great controversy during the past 5 to 10 years. In general, the *30° head-elevated position* reduces ICP without deleterious effects on cerebral perfusion pressure (CPP) and is preferred. Head elevation and midline position improve jugular venous and possibly CSF drainage and decrease the contributions of these components to intracranial hypertension.

DRAINAGE OF CEREBROSPINAL FLUID

This technique effectively produces immediate reductions in ICP with minimal risk (other than insertion of the catheter) by directly reducing the CSF volume. However, despite widespread use, the effect of CSF drainage on ICP, CPP, CBF, and cerebral metabolic rate has received rather limited study. Recent studies suggest that the effect of CSF drainage on these parameters is similar to that

Table 8–8. INTERVENTIONS FOR SEVERE TRAUMATIC BRAIN INJURY
WITH SPECIFIC RECOMMENDATIONS AND/OR DOSES

Intervention	Standard Use or Dose
Head position	Head elevated 30° and in midline
Blood pressure	Rigorously avoid hypotension*
Cerebrospinal fluid drainage	Continuous or intermittent
Ventilation	$PaCO_2$ maintained at 30–35 mm Hg*
Mannitol	0.25–0.50 gm/kg IV q6h as needed
Barbiturates	Pentobarbital or thiopental: Load with ~30 mg/kg over a total of ~3 hours with intermittent doses of 3–5 mg/kg or a continuous infusion. Titrate to burst suppression on electroencephalogram unless intracranial pressure is adequately controlled with lower doses than needed to achieve burst suppression. Maintain on a continuous infusion of 1–2 mg/kg/hr. Carefully tailor to individual patient. Continuously monitor electroencephalogram. Larger or smaller doses may be required. Carefully avoid or treat hypotension or reduction in cardiac output.
Temperature	Aggressively treat fever and avoid iatrogenic hyperthermia. Avoid active rewarming if the child is hemodynamically stable and core temperature is ≥34°C.*

*See Fig. 8–10 and text for additional recommendations.

observed with mannitol administration. *Drainage of CSF is currently the first-line treatment of intracranial hypertension in the ICU.* CSF can be drained continuously or intermittently.

VENTILATION

The direct relationship between CBF and $PaCO_2$ in the normal brain and the resultant vasoconstrictor effect of hyperventilation on the cerebral arteriolar system is often used in the management of patients with severe traumatic brain injury. However, recent studies have reexamined the long-standing "blind" and prophylactic application of hyperventilation in the management of severe traumatic brain injury. Studies in experimental models have demonstrated that the effect of sustained hyperventilation on CSF pH and arteriolar diameter are short lived (i.e., vessel caliber returns to baseline within <20 hours). Chronic hyperventilation produces a loss of metabolic (bicarbonate) buffer in the CSF, putting the cerebral circulation at greater risk due to hypersensitivity of the vasculature to changes in CO_2. A randomized comparison of mild versus moderate hyperventilation in adults after severe traumatic brain injury revealed that prophylactic hyperventilation was not beneficial and may have actually been associated with a worse outcome ($PaCO_2$ = 32 versus 26 mm Hg). These findings parallel the findings of other recent reports demonstrating (1) hypoperfusion early after severe traumatic brain injury, (2) widened arteriojugular venous oxygen content difference early after trauma, and (3) jugular desaturation accompanying profound hypocarbia. It is important to recognize, however, that although the prophylactic application of hyperventilation may be detrimental, hypercarbia and even normocarbia are not advocated. *Mild hyperventilation* ($PaCO_2$ = 30 to 35 mm Hg) *is recommended.* Finally, the application of more profound levels of hypocarbia than a CO_2 of 30 to 35 mm Hg may be necessary in the management of severe traumatic brain injury in children, specifically due to the frequent contribution of hyperemia to the delayed rise in ICP that they exhibit. Except in the setting of impending herniation, it is recommended that the application and titration of this intervention to treat intracranial hypertension be guided by measurement of CBF and/or jugular venous saturation.

MANNITOL

Mannitol can attenuate intracranial hypertension through two separate mechanisms. Through an immediate reduction in blood viscosity, mannitol produces an immediate but transient reduction in cerebral blood volume without a change in CBF. This results in an immediate reduction in ICP that is transient. This mechanism (viscosity autoregulation) appears to operate only when pressure autoregulation of CBF is intact. When it is not intact, the decrease in viscosity will be accompanied by an increase in CBF and no change in vessel caliber, cerebral blood volume, or ICP. If a bolus of mannitol is given too rapidly and produces transient systemic hypertension in a patient with severe traumatic brain injury and defective pressure autoregulation, cerebral blood volume and ICP may actually increase. More prolonged decreases in ICP after mannitol administration are related to a dehydrating effect of mannitol via an osmotic effect. This effect probably operates only where there is an intact blood-brain barrier. *Mannitol should be administered every 6 hours as needed* at a dose of 0.25 or 0.50 gm/kg body weight. Additional doses can be administered for refractory intracranial hypertension (see Table 8–8 and Fig. 8–10). Mannitol administration is generally contraindicated when plasma osmolality is >330 mmol/L.

BARBITURATES

Barbiturates reduce ICP via a reduction in cerebral metabolic rate and a resultant secondary decrease in CBF and blood volume. They also have neuroprotectant effects. Although a randomized trial of barbiturate therapy in the treatment of severe traumatic brain injury in adults did not report a beneficial effect on outcome, these drugs can be effective when applied in the specific setting of *refractory intracranial hypertension* (see Table 8–8 and Fig. 8–10 for dosing recommendations). If either frequent dosing or barbiturate infusion is used, it is recommended that monitoring of the electroencephalogram be used to assess the cerebral metabolic response to treatment. The end point of barbiturate therapy is burst suppression. When barbiturates are used, it is essential that hypotension is avoided, and patients should be carefully monitored for reduction in blood pressure or cardiac output or inadequate systemic perfusion.

TEMPERATURE MANIPULATION

Two randomized trials of moderate hypothermia (body temperature of 32°C for 24 or 48 hours) have shown beneficial effects in adults after severe traumatic brain injury. Seizure incidence and ICP were reduced in the hypothermic groups. Meta-analysis of the two studies suggested a significant beneficial effect of hypothermia on neurologic outcome. A multicenter trial is under way of therapeutic hypothermia in severe traumatic brain injury in adults. Current recommendations include the use of hypothermia for the management of refractory intracranial hypertension (in selected cases). Careful attention should also be paid to *the prevention and aggressive treatment of fever or iatrogenic hyperthermia* after head injury. Active rewarming of hemodynamically stable patients with mild or moderate hypothermia ($>34°C$) should be avoided.

NUTRITION

The provision of adequate calories and protein substrate is essential during the catabolic response to critical illness, and the beneficial effects of early feeding (either enteral or parenteral) in the critically ill or injured patient are well described. If possible, jejunal feeding is associated with reduced morbidity and is recommended within 36 hours of admission. Often, a combination of parenteral alimentation and enteral feedings is used. Hyperglycemia should be avoided. Frequent monitoring of blood glucose and calorimetry are useful in this setting.

INDUCED HYPERTENSION

Whether pressure autoregulation of CBF is intact or defective, hypotension or an inadequate CPP should be rigorously avoided. If pressure autoregulation is impaired, CBF is directly related to CPP, and hypotension directly reduces flow. If pressure autoregulation is intact, as CPP is reduced, reflex cerebral vasodilatation occurs (which increases cerebral blood volume and ICP). This latter phenomenon occurs as CPP is reduced even within the autoregulatory range. An optimal CPP threshold of approximately 65 to 70 mm Hg is generally suggested for adults.

In selected cases of patients with refractory intracranial hypertension, induced arterial hypertension (CPP increased to between 100 and 140 mm Hg via infusion of phenylephrine) will reduce ICP. However, hypertension reduces ICP only when pressure autoregulation of CBF is intact because it is a hypertension-mediated reduction in vessel caliber that produces the reduction in cerebral blood volume (to maintain a constant CBF) and resultant reduction in ICP. It is also unclear what the short-term and long-term effects of the applied hypertension are on the development of cerebral edema. Greater hydrostatic pressure could exacerbate edema formation. The optimal management of blood pressure requires extensive monitoring of the involved factors and an in-depth understanding of the mechanisms at work. Induced hypertension is recommended only as a last resort in patients with intact pressure autoregulation and with careful monitoring of CBF and ICP. This situation is even more complex in the management of infants and children because a universal threshold value of CPP is not applicable; it is reasonable to assume that this value is directly related to age. Management *must* be tailored to and carefully titrated in each patient.

MISCELLANEOUS

Sedation and paralysis should be used as needed in the setting of intracranial hypertension once ICP monitoring has been established. *Narcotics and benzodiazepines* along with a nondepolarizing muscle relaxant are generally recommended. *Careful monitoring* of the level of sedation and muscle relaxation is warranted. Intermittent doses of thiopental and/or lidocaine are often needed to blunt excessive rises in ICP secondary to routine patient care maneuvers such as suctioning.

The maintenance of an adequate CPP is essential in the effective management of patients with severe traumatic brain injury, which is often accompanied by other extracranial injuries that produce shock or hypotension. *Volume expansion* is critical in this setting. However, judicious use of fluids is recommended to avoid iatrogenic exacerbation of edema. The use of *pressors* or *inotropes* may be necessary to optimize CPP in this setting. Dopamine, phenylephrine, or norepinephrine is most frequently recommended. Hypo-osmotic solutions should be avoided, and careful attention should be paid to the serum sodium concentration. If hyponatremia develops, it can usually be attributed to either syndrome of inappropriate secretion of antidiuretic hormone or cerebral salt wasting. Care should be taken to determine the correct cause of hyponatremia because the management of antidiuretic hormone excess involves fluid restriction, whereas that of cerebral salt wasting involves the administration of isotonic or hypertonic saline.

Corticosteroids ameliorate spinal cord injury in large part through the inhibition of lipid peroxidation. However, no beneficial effect of corticosteroids has been demonstrated in traumatic brain injury, and they are not recommended for clinical use.

Prognosis

Brain injury is the most important determinant of outcome in motor vehicle trauma. Approximately 20% of head injury cases result in severe traumatic brain injury. Although the mortality rate for children presenting with a GCS score of ≤8 is lower than that observed in adults (~60%), it is still approximately 33% overall. Within the pediatric population, outcome is particularly poor in the subgroup of infants and children younger than 4 years old (~60% mortality). Duration of coma, level of sustained intracranial hypertension, and presence of ischemic CBF are directly related to poor outcome. Morbidity in survivors includes disturbances in motor function, memory, cognition, and behavior. Plasticity of synaptic pathways in children does afford an added chance for good recovery.

BIBLIOGRAPHY

Bouma GJ, Muizelaar P, Bandoh K, Marmarou A: Blood pressure and intracranial pressure-volume dynamics in severe head injury: relationship with cerebral blood flow. J Neurosurg 77:15, 1992.

Clifton GL, Allen S, Barrodale P, et al: A phase II study of moderate hypothermia in severe brain injury. J Neurotrauma 10:263, 1993.

Fortune JB, Feustel PJ, Graca L, et al: Comparison of mannitol versus ventriculostomy drainage on cerebral blood flow after traumatic brain injury. J Neurotrauma 80:109, 1994.

Jane JA, Anderson DK, Torner JC, Young W (eds): Central nervous system trauma status report 1991. J Neurotrauma 9:S1, 1992.

Kochanek PM, Clark RSB, Adelson PD, Marion DW: Severe traumatic brain injury in children: pathobiology, management, and controversies. *In* Current Concepts in Critical Care Medicine. Anaheim, CA, Society of Critical Care Medicine, 1995, pp. 153–170.

Levin HS, Aldrich EF, Saydjari C, et al: Severe head injury in children: experience of the Traumatic Coma Data Bank. Neurosurg 31:435, 1992.

Marion DW, Obrist WD, Carlier PM, Penrod LE, Darby JM: The use of moderate therapeutic hypothermia for patients with severe head injuries: a preliminary report. J Neurosurg 79:354, 1993.

Muizelaar JP, Marmarou A, Ward JD, et al: Adverse effects of prolonged hyperventilation in patients with severe head injury: a randomized clinical trial. J Neurosurg 75:731, 1991.

Obrist WD, Langfitt TW, Jaggi JL, Cruz J, Gennarelli TA: Cerebral blood flow and metabolism in comatose patients with acute head injury. J Neurosurg 61:241, 1984.

Rosner MJ, Daughton S: Cerebral perfusion pressure management in head injury. J Trauma 8:933, 1990.

Sheinberg M, Kanter MJ, Robertson CS, et al: Continuous monitoring of jugular venous oxygen saturation in head-injured patients. J Neurosurg 76:212, 1992.

Ward JD, Becker DP, Miller JD, et al: Failure of prophylactic barbiturate coma in the treatment of severe head injury. J Neurosurg 62:383, 1985.

8.5 **Brain Death**

B. LOUISE PARKER, MD

TIMOTHY C. FREWEN, MD, FRCPC

Brain death is a relatively new concept in Western society in which the diagnosis of death is determined to be legally present when the *clinically assessable functions of the brain are irreversibly damaged.* Traditionally, the diagnosis of death was based on the lack of breathing effort, usually followed by the absence of a palpable heartbeat or pulse. Because these functions are preserved in patients in the modern intensive care unit (ICU), an alternative method of declaring death was necessary to establish the futility of further treatment directed solely at preserving cardiorespiratory function and to initiate the potential for organ donation in consenting patients and families.

Pathophysiology

The end effect of any brain insult that results in irreversible brain injury is severe neuronal injury and death, often occurring in the presence of a nonperfused cortex and brain stem. This diffuse neuronal injury can occur after severe diffuse metabolic derangement or as a result of raised intracranial pressure, catastrophic intracranial hemorrhage, trauma, or, commonly, hypoxic-ischemic insult (Table 8–9). No specific pathologic characterization of brain death has been described; however, extreme brain liquefaction necrosis has been correlated in the past with some patients meeting brain death criteria.

Table 8–9. ETIOLOGIES OF COMA LEADING TO BRAIN DEATH

Hypoxic ischemic encephalopathy
    After cardiorespiratory arrest
    Near–sudden infant death syndrome
    Near-drowning
    Perinatal asphyxia
Metabolic/endocrine derangement
Trauma
Vascular events
Infectious

Brain Death Criteria

The process of declaring brain death requires the clinician first to define, usually by history, a probable cause of brain injury and then to complete a careful yet simple series of bedside examinations to determine the cessation of brain stem neurologic function.

DIAGNOSIS

History

Determination of the cause of coma must be made to ensure that reversible conditions (toxic/metabolic disorders, sedative-hypnotic drugs, paralytic agents, hypothermia, hypotension) are absent (Table 8–10).

Clinical Examination

The following features of the neurologic examination must be present in the absence of significant systemic hypotension or hypothermia (rectal temperature of >34.2°C). Coma and apnea must coexist. There should be no evidence of consciousness, spontaneous movement, or vocalization.

Table 8–10. DIFFERENTIAL DIAGNOSIS OF BRAIN DEATH

Deep coma (from any cause, e.g., hypothermia, general anesthesia)
Drug intoxication
    Barbiturates
    Sedatives/hypnotics
    Neuromuscular blocking drugs
Shock
Peripheral neuromuscular junction disorder
    Peripheral nerve
    Muscle dysfunction
"Locked-in" syndrome

The absence of brain stem function must be demonstrated by the following:

- Midposition of fully dilated pupils that do not react to light
- Absence of spontaneous eye movements (including oculovestibular testing)
- Absence of corneal, gag, cough, suck, and rooting reflexes
- Absence of spontaneous or induced movements (although spinal cord reflexes in direct response to painful stimuli *may* exist in the presence of brain death)

Apnea Test. To perform the apnea test, the patient should first receive assisted ventilation with 100% oxygen for at least 10 minutes before testing to ensure an arterial carbon dioxide tension ($Paco_2$) of 35 to 45 mm Hg at the beginning of the test and, if possible, sufficient hyperoxia to prevent a dangerous fall in arterial oxygen tension (Pao_2) during apnea. A further safeguard against hypoxia during apnea is achieved by providing a minimum of 6 L/min flow of oxygen down the endotracheal tube through an insufflating catheter connected to an oxygen source.

A *positive apnea test* indicating the absence of brain stem–mediated respiratory function is considered present when the arterial $Paco_2$ is >60 mm Hg in the absence of systemic hypoxemia.

The *recommended observation period* between clinical neurologic examinations to verify the presence of brain death varies with the age of the patient and the choice of ancillary tests. The American Academy of Pediatrics guidelines suggest that infants *younger than 7 days* cannot be declared brain dead (Table 8–11). The declaration of brain death in infants between *7 days* and *2 months old* requires two examinations and two isoelectric electroencephalograms (EEGs) that are performed ≥48 hours apart. The declaration in infants between *2 months* and *1 year old* requires two examinations and two isoelectric EEGs that are performed ≥24 hours apart or one examination and one isoelectric EEG *plus* an absent cerebral blood flow study. Children older than *1 year* require an observation time of 12 hours *unless* the coma is due to hypoxic-ischemic encephalopathy, then the recommended observation time is 24 hours.

Ancillary Tests

Angiography. The absence of intracranial blood flow determined with the use of four-vessel cerebral angiography has been the gold standard in the past to diagnose brain death but is impractical for most ICU patients. In general, this test is not required to diagnose brain death unless the clinical criteria cannot be applied.

Electroencephalogram. Although EEGs are an American Academy of Pediatrics requirement in the very young, they are not routinely used to assist in the diagnosis of brain death. British and Canadian recommendations do not require the use of an EEG in the diagnosis of brain death in infants and children (Table 8–12).

Radioisotope Scanning. This can be used as a bedside test in the ICU and correlates well with four-vessel angiography. In the cases in which clinical criteria cannot be safely tested, this is a useful ancillary test. If radionucleotide blood flow testing or cerebral angiography or both are used to declare brain death, there must be no evidence of cerebral blood flow or perfusion or both. Cases have been

Table 8–11. AMERICAN ACADEMY OF PEDIATRICS GUIDELINES FOR THE DETERMINATION OF BRAIN DEATH IN CHILDREN

History: Determine the cause of coma to eliminate remedial or reversible conditions
Physical examination criteria
  Coma and apnea
  Absence of brain stem function
    Midposition or fully dilated pupils
    Absence of spontaneous oculocephalic (doll's eye) and caloric-induced eye movements
    Absence of movement of bulbar musculature and corneal, gag, cough, sucking, and rooting reflexes
    Absence of respiratory effort with standardized testing for apnea
  Patient must not be hypothermic or hypotensive
  Flaccid tone and absence of spontaneous or induced movements excluding activity mediated at spinal cord level
  Examination should remain consistent for brain death through the predetermined period of observation
Observation period according to age
  Age 7 days to 2 months: Two examinations and EEGs 48 hours apart
  Age 2 months to 1 year: Two examinations and EEGs 24 hours apart and/or one examination and an initial EEG showing electrocerebral silence combined with a radionuclide angiogram showing no cerebral blood flow
  Age of >1 year: Two examinations 12 to 24 hours apart; EEG and isotope angiography are optional

Data from Task Force on Brain Death in Children: Guidelines for the determination of brain death in children. Pediatrics 80:298, 1987.
EEG, electroencephalogram.

reported of clinical brain death with continued blood flow as determined with radioisotope scanning.

Other Ancillary Tests. Other ancillary tests to declare brain death have been recommended (e.g., evoked potentials, Doppler ultrasonography). However, each of these ancillary tests has unique technical limitations and none is sufficiently

Table 8–12. CANADIAN MEDICAL ASSOCIATION CRITERIA FOR THE CLINICAL DIAGNOSIS OF BRAIN DEATH

1. An etiology has been established that is capable of causing brain death and potentially reversible conditions have been excluded.
2. The patient is in deep coma and shows no response within the cranial nerve distribution to stimulation of any part of the movements; "decorticate" or decerebrate posturing arising from the brain are present.
3. Brain stem reflexes are absent.
4. The patient is apneic when taken off the respirator for an appropriate time.
5. The conditions listed above persist when the patient is reassessed after a suitable interval.

Data from Canadian Medical Association: CMA Position Statement: guidelines for the diagnosis of brain death. Can Med Assoc J 136:200A, 1987.

standardized or widely studied to be recommended in the declaration of brain death.

Maintenance of Organ Perfusion

Brain death is usually the starting point for organ transplantation. If the process of organ donation is contemplated, it is important that the solid organs of the dead patient continue to be adequately perfused after brain death declaration. In such cases, inotropic support, antibiotics, metabolic needs, and other methods of ensuring organ survival will be necessary until donation occurs.

BIBLIOGRAPHY

Ashwal S, Schneider S: Brain death in children: part I. Pediatr Neurol. 3:5, 1987.
Ashwal S, Schneider S: Brain death in children: part II. Pediatr Neurol. 3:69, 1987.
Ashwal S, Schneider S: Brain death in the newborn. Pediatrics 84:429, 1989.
Canadian Medical Association: CMA Position Statement: guidelines for the diagnosis of brain death. Can Med Assoc J 136:200A, 1987.
Parker BL, Frewen TC, Levin SD, et al: Paediatric brain death: current practice in a Canadian paediatric critical care unit. Can Med Assoc J 153:909, 1995.
Singh NC, Reid RH, Loft JA, et al: Usefulness of (Tc[99m]) HM-PAO scan in supporting clinical brain death in children: uncoupling flow and function. Clin Intens Care 5:71, 1994.
Task Force on Brain Death in Children: Guidelines for the determination of brain death in children. Pediatrics 80:298, 1987.
Volpe JJ: Brain death determination in the newborn. Pediatrics 80:293, 1987.

9

General Critical Care

9.1 Septic Shock

JOSEPH A. CARCILLO, MD

Septic shock is a pediatric emergency characterized by cardiovascular dysfunction that requires immediate resuscitative efforts to prevent progressive end-organ damage and death. Septic shock may be present when a child with a clinical suspicion of infection, an abnormal temperature, and tachycardia develops at least one of the following *manifestations of decreased organ perfusion:* altered mental status, oliguria, delayed capillary refill, bounding peripheral pulses, or increased lactate level. These signs occur before hypotension. Decreased blood pressure is a late sign of septic shock. Early recognition of signs of decreased perfusion before the onset of hypotension, appropriate therapeutic response, and removal of the nidus of infection are the keys to survival in children with septic shock.

Pathophysiology

Systemic infection with bacteria, virus, or fungus has been associated with cytokine and nitric oxide production and multiorgan system dysfunction in children.

Cardiovascular collapse can occur as a result of a myriad of combinations of pathophysiologic response to systemic infection. The initiating infection activates a number of inflammatory cascades resulting in cellular and microvascular alterations. One such cascade includes the stimulation of inducible nitric oxide synthase increasing the production of nitric oxide which, in turn, causes vasodilation, increased capillary leak, and ultimately cardiovascular collapse.

Children may have decreased oral intake and increased loss of fluids (vomiting or diarrhea) during systemic illness. Sepsis can cause a *diffuse capillary leak syndrome* that further exacerbates hypovolemia. Severe *hypovolemia* can lead to shock and death. In the presence of intravenous volume loading in children with septic shock, the cardiovascular system demonstrates combinations of cardiac and vascular failure. Children can have *cardiac dysfunction* that requires inotropic support; *vascular dysfunction* that requires vasopressor support; or a combination of cardiac and vascular dysfunction, or failure, that requires both inotropic and vascular support. Other organ dysfunctions associated with septic shock include *noncardiogenic pulmonary edema,* or the adult respiratory distress syndrome (ARDS); renal failure; and disseminated intravascular coagulation (DIC). Each of these may improve with treatment of the shock state.

Differential Diagnosis

The *inflammatory triad* of fever, tachycardia, and peripheral vasodilatation is commonly seen in children with benign viral or bacterial infections that respond to management with antipyretics or antibiotics or both. Signs of hypoperfusion suggest the possibility of early septic shock.

Inflammatory triad + signs of hypoperfusion = early septic shock

The diagnosis of septic shock should be considered when the child with the inflammatory triad develops altered mental status, which manifests as irritability, decreased interaction with parents, sleepiness, or stupor. Children with septic shock and coma can awake with a normal mental status after volume resuscitation. Signs of decreased perfusion include bounding pulses and brisk capillary refill as a manifestation of early vascular failure or diminished pulses and decreased capillary refill as a manifestation of hypovolemia or cardiac failure. In children with invasive monitoring, the presence of a *low diastolic blood pressure and a wide pulse pressure* suggests early warm shock. Low mean arterial blood pressure occurs in the late stage of septic shock. Similarly, decreased urine output from an unobstructed catheterized child with the inflammatory triad suggests septic shock as a leading diagnosis.

Clinical Evaluation

The key to clinical evaluation is to recognize warm septic shock. *Warm septic shock is often missed during clinical examination.*

Warm Septic Shock	**Cold Septic Shock**
Fever	Fever or hypothermia
Tachycardia	Tachycardia
Bounding pulses	Poor pulses
Altered mental status	Altered mental status
Wide pulse pressure (decreased diastolic blood pressure)	Narrow pulse pressure
Diminished perfusion	Diminished perfusion
Decreased urine output	Decreased urine output
Decreased or brisk capillary refill	Decreased capillary refill
Warm extremities	Mottled extremities

This state frequently responds to volume alone or minimal vasoactive support if the nidus of infection can be eradicated. Cold septic shock can occur in children if warm septic shock is not recognized and treated during its early stage. These patients will always require sophisticated cardiovascular support.

Laboratory Investigations

The diagnosis of septic shock is attained through clinical examination. Initial resuscitation is given according to clinical examination. Laboratory tests should not delay the institution of therapy.

Management

The goal of management is to prevent end-organ damage by correcting hypovolemia and supporting cardiac and vascular dysfunction.

IMMEDIATE RESUSCITATION

Airway

Children with sepsis rarely have difficulty with airway patency unless it is associated with end-stage shock and severe depression of mental status. The airway patency should be ensured.

Breathing

As many as 80% of children with septic shock will require intubation and intermittent mandatory ventilation for respiratory distress or central line placement. Ventilation decreases the work of breathing and allows the dysfunctional heart to work more efficiently.

Intubate and ventilate on the basis of clinical evidence of respiratory distress or failure. Blood gas determinations are not required, and the decision to ventilate a patient with severe septic shock is not based on confirmatory laboratory data.

Intubation and positive pressure ventilation can induce hypotension in the hypovolemic patient. Volume load the child and consider intubation with *ketamine* (2 mg/kg) or a combination of *fentanyl* (2 μg/kg) and a nondepolarizing neuromuscular blockade agent, such as *vecuronium* (0.2 mg/kg). Use the Sellick maneuver if the child has eaten within 8 hours of presentation.

Circulation

Volume Resuscitation

Volume resuscitation is required by virtually all children with septic shock. Isotonic solutions, including normal saline, lactated Ringer's solution, and 5%

albumin, can be used with discretion. Saline is least expensive and does not require normal liver function to metabolize lactate.

Push 20-mL/kg volumes of saline and assess perfusion until the child has an improved mental status, warm extremities with strong pulses, a capillary refill time of <2 seconds, a brisk urine output response, and a return to a normal diastolic and mean arterial blood pressures.

Listen to the lung fields, and feel the liver edge with each volume bolus. The appearance of rales or an advancing liver edge before restoration of normal perfusion suggests that further fluid resuscitation will not be helpful and underlines the need for vasoactive support.

On average, children with septic shock will show some response with 40 to 60 mL/kg volumes of saline; however, some will require <20 mL/kg, while others may require as much as 200 mL/kg.

Vasoactive Support

Vasoactive support should be directed at improving perfusion and blood pressure.

Titrate the vasoactive agents to attain normal perfusion (capillary refill of <2 seconds, 2+ pulses, normal mental status, and >1 mL/kg/hr urine output) and blood pressure (normal diastolic and mean arterial blood pressures for age).

Children may require inotropic support or vasopressor support or a combination of both.

Inotropic agents will improve perfusion and blood pressure in children with cardiac failure.

Vasopressors will improve diastolic blood pressure and perfusion in children with vascular failure and good cardiac function. However, in children with vascular failure and *marginal* cardiac output, vasopressors will improve diastolic blood pressure but impair perfusion.

Add inotropic support to patients who show decreased perfusion when vasopressor support is used for a low diastolic blood pressure.

Dopamine is a good initial drug to use because it has inotropic qualities in low concentrations (5 to 8 μg/kg/min) and vasopressor qualities in high concentrations (10 to 20 μg/kg/min).

Some children will require more potent agents. *Epinephrine* is a good first choice because it has inotropic qualities in low concentrations (0.01 to 0.05 μg/kg/min) and vasopressor qualities at higher concentrations (>0.1 μg/kg/min). *Norepinephrine* may be useful due to the strong vasoconstriction property in patients with persistently low diastolic pressure. Low diastolic pressure may further contribute to the deterioration in cardiac function.

Use high-dose dopamine, norepinephrine, or phenylephrine to attain a normal systemic vascular resistance for age. In some children, this may result in a decrease in cardiac output and oxygen delivery to a level that diminishes oxygen consumption. These children will require the addition of an inotropic agent to attain a normal systemic vascular resistance and an oxygen delivery that allows optimal oxygen consumption.

Use dobutamine, low-dose dopamine, or low-dose epinephrine to attain a normal cardiac index (>3.5 L/min/m²) in patients with cardiac failure. Add an

Table 9–1. EFFECT OF VASOACTIVE AGENTS ON PERFUSION

	Inotropic Support	Vasopressor Support	Combination
Cardiac dysfunction (low CO)	Improves MAP and perfusion	With or without effect on MAP, decreases perfusion	
Vascular dysfunction (high CO, low SVR)		Improves diastolic blood pressure and perfusion	
Combined dysfunction (with or without high CO, low SVR)		Improves diastolic blood pressure, decreases perfusion	Improves diastolic blood pressure and perfusion

MAP, mean arterial pressure; CO, cardiac output; SVR, systemic vascular resistance.

afterload-reducing agent if the cardiac index is still <3.5 and systemic vascular resistance index is >1200 (Tables 9–1 and 9–2).

Steroids

For shock in children with purpura fulminans or a history of chronic steroid use, give 50 mg/kg *hydrocortisone* IV, followed by continuous infusion at 50 to 60 mg/kg/day.

ANTIBIOTICS

Antibiotics should be administered according to the setting of infection and age of the child.

The use of antibiotics should not delay administration of fluid or vasoactive support in the immediate resuscitative stage (Table 9–3).

MONITORING

An *arterial line* should be placed for continuous monitoring of systolic and diastolic blood pressures and for titration of therapy. Give inotropes to increase the steepness of the upstroke (to increase contractility), vasopressors to summate

Table 9–2. CARDIOVASCULAR GOALS OF IMMEDIATE RESUSCITATION (FIRST HOUR)

Normal Diastolic Blood Pressure for Age		Normal Perfusion
Infant (6 mo)	>53 mm Hg	Normal mental status
Toddler (2 yr)	>53 mm Hg	Capillary refill <2 sec
School-age child (7 yr)	>57 mm Hg	2 + distal pulses
Adolescent (15 yr)	>66 mm Hg	Urine output >1 mL/kg/hr

Table 9–3. ANTIBIOTIC THERAPY IN SEPTIC SHOCK

Empirical therapy	
Outpatient sepsis	
>2 mo	Third-generation cephalosporin
<2 mo	Ampicillin and gentamicin
	or
	Ampicillin and cephalosporin
Nosocomial sepsis	Staphylococcal and Gram-negative coverage; consult hospital susceptibility data
Nosocomial sepsis after 7 days on antibiotic with or without low absolute neutrophil count	Rule out candidemia
Herpes or varicella sepsis	Acyclovir

a reflection wave (to increase systemic vascular resistance), and volume to maintain the same systolic pressure during positive pressure inhalation and exhalation (to increase preload).

A *central line* should be placed in patients requiring large fluid volumes to titrate the volume status.

A *Swan-Ganz catheter* should be placed in children who do not attain normal perfusion and blood pressure or acid-base status with volume resuscitation and minimal vasoactive support.

A *Foley catheter* should be placed for close monitoring of urine output and fluid balance.

Measure cardiac output, arterial and mixed venous oxygen saturation, pulmonary artery pressure, central venous pressure, pulmonary capillary wedge pressure, arterial or venous base deficit, and/or lactate (Table 9–4). Calculate systemic

Table 9–4. CARDIOVASCULAR AND OXYGEN UTILIZATION VARIABLES

	Normal Values
$SVRI = \dfrac{MAP - CVP}{CI} \times 80$ $PVRI = \dfrac{MPAP - PAOP}{CI} \times 80$ $Cao_2 = 1.36 \times hemoglobin \times \%O_2\ sat + (0.003 \times Pao_2)$ $AVDo_2 = Cao_2 - Cmvo_2$ $Do_2 = Cao_2 \times CI \times 10$ $\dot{V}o_2 = AVDo_2 \times CI \times 10$ $O_2\ ext = \dot{V}o_2/Do_2$	CI: 3.5–5.0 L/min/m^2 SVRI: 800–1400 dyne-sec/cm^5/m^2 PVRI: 70–230 dyne-sec/cm^5/m^2 Cao$_2$: 15–20 vol% AVDo$_2$: 3–5 vol% Do$_2$: 550–650 mL/min/m^2 $\dot{V}$o$_2$: 130–190 mL/min/m^2 Sao$_2$: >90% Svo$_2$: 70–75%

SVRI, systemic vascular resistance index; MAP, mean arterial pressure; CVP, central venous pressure; PVRI, pulmonary vascular resistance index; MPAP, mean pulmonary artery pressure; PAOP, pulmonary artery occlusion pressure; Cao$_2$, arterial oxygen content; Pao$_2$, partial pressure arterial oxygen; AVDo$_2$, arteriovenous oxygen content difference; Cmvo$_2$, mixed venous oxygen content; Do$_2$, oxygen delivery; CI, cardiac index; $\dot{V}$o$_2$, oxygen consumption; O$_2$, oxygen extraction.

vascular resistance, pulmonary vascular resistance, oxygen delivery, oxygen consumption, and oxygen extraction.

Manipulate arterial oxygen content and vasoactive agents to attain normal perfusion pressure (mean arterial blood pressure minus central venous pressure) for age and an oxygen delivery that allows maximum oxygen consumption (critical point of oxygen delivery) and no base deficit. Accomplish this without inducing tachycardia (Fig. 9–1).

Oxygen delivery may be increased with infusions of packed red blood cells, an increase in cardiac output, or an increase in arterial oxygen saturation.

Children with an oxygen consumption of <120 mL/min/m^2 should be evaluated for cyanide toxicity if they are receiving nitroprusside.

Various combinations of inotropes, vasopressors, and even vasodilators may be used to attain these goals (Table 9–5).

Children who do not respond to vasopressors or inotropes despite adequate intravascular volume (pulmonary capillary wedge pressure of >12 cm H_2O) can

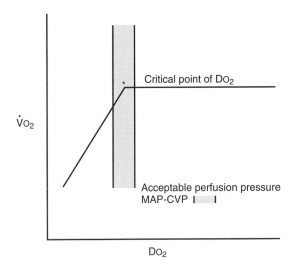

Normal MAP-CVP for age:

Infant (6 mo)	>56 mmHg
Toddler (2 yr)	>59 mmHg
School age (7 yr)	>65 mmHg
Adolescent (15 yr)	>75 mmHg

Figure 9–1. Cardiovascular goals in patients with intravascular monitoring. Oxygen delivery should be maintained at a level that ensures maximum oxygen consumption without increasing heart rate. Perfusion pressure (mean arterial pressure minus central venous pressure [MAP − CVP]) should be maintained in a normal range to ensure organ perfusion.

Table 9–5. PHARMACOTHERAPEUTIC AGENTS COMMONLY USED
TO MODERATE CARDIAC INDEX, SYSTEMIC VASCULAR
RESISTANCE INDEX, MEAN ARTERIAL PRESSURE,
OXYGEN CONSUMPTION, AND OXYGEN DELIVERY

Agent	Comments/Dose
Dopamine	Excellent first-line choice, 0–3 μg/kg/min dopaminergic agonist, 3–10 μg/kg/min β-agonist, >10 μg/kg/min α-agonist
Epinephrine	Excellent choice in patients who are unresponsive to dopaminergic agonist; at 0.01–0.05 μg/kg/min β-agonist, >0.05 μg/kg/min increasing α-agonist effect
Dobutamine	Excellent β-agonist with minimal tachycardia; may widen pulse pressure at concentration >10 μg/kg/min
Isoproterenol	Excellent β_1- and β_2-agonist; helpful during pulmonary hypertension; may increase pulmonary shunting; use 0.01–1 μg/kg/min
Norepinephrine	Excellent α-agonist with β-agonist activity that is frequently inapparent; use 0.05–1 μg/kg/min
Phenylephrine	Partial α-agonist; excellent combination agent with β-agonists
Norepinephrine and phentolamine	This combination allows β-agonist activity to be manifested through α-blockade; begin phentolamine at 1 μg/kg/min and advance according to outcome variable
Nitroglycerin	Excellent vasodilator; 1–3 μg/kg/min pulmonary vasodilator, >3 μg/kg/min systemic vasodilator
Nitroprusside	Premiere afterload reducing agent; frequently requires simultaneous administration of volume bolus; long-term use may be associated with cyanide toxicity

Higher concentrations of all agents may be used according to measured variables.

be given a trial of stress steroids or maintenance thyroxine. Effects should be noted in a matter of hours (Fig. 9–2).

NUTRITION

Surprisingly little work has been done on nutrition in children with septic shock.

- Shock is a contraindication, at present, to enteral feedings.
- The proper timing of introduction of central total parenteral nutrition is not known and is discretional.
- Hypoglycemia or hyperglycemia can occur during septic shock. Dextrose solutions should be adjusted according to need.
- Hypocalcemia should be monitored through measurement of ionized calcium. Treat hypocalcemia; this will improve cardiovascular function.

Complications

ADULT RESPIRATORY DISTRESS SYNDROME

Adult respiratory distress syndrome is defined as hypoxia and pulmonary edema in the presence of a pulmonary capillary wedge pressure of <16 cm H_2O.

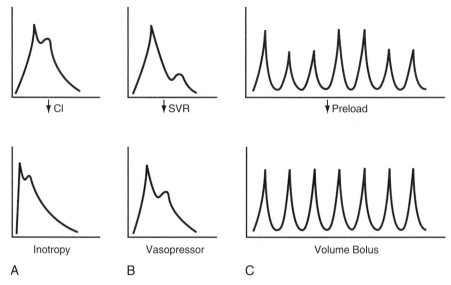

Figure 9–2. Use of arterial wave patterns to monitor therapies during septic shock. *A,* The upstroke is decreased due to a decreased dP/dt consistent with decreased contractility. The addition of inotropic support results in an increased dP/dt and a steeper upstroke. CI, cardiac index. *B,* The reflection wave separates from the arterial wave due to decreased systemic vascular resistance (SVR). The addition of a vasopressor results in increased vascular tone and summation of the arterial and reflection waves. *C,* Decreased preload is demonstrated by respiratory variation in the arterial systolic blood pressure. Volume loading and a normal preload result in the loss of variation in systolic blood pressure during changes in respiratory cycle.

Treat the reduction in functional residual capacity with positive end-expiratory pressure.

Treat decreased cardiac output from positive end-expiratory pressure–induced diminished venous return to the heart with volume boluses or increased vasoactive support or both.

RENAL FAILURE

Approximately 10% of children with septic shock will develop anuria and renal failure despite volume resuscitation and vasoactive support. These children have a high risk of mortality if not supported with hemo- or peritoneal filtration and/or dialysis.

Use diuretics liberally if urine output is <1 mL/kg/hr in the presence of a central venous pressure or pulmonary capillary wedge pressure of >8 cm H_2O. If urine output is <1 mL/kg/hr and central venous pressure or pulmonary capillary wedge pressure is <8 cm H_2O, then give volume boluses until pulmonary capillary wedge pressure is >8 cm H_2O; then, repeat the use of diuretics.

Augment cardiac output (cardiac index of >4 L/min/m²) and mean arterial pressure (mean arterial blood pressure minus central venous pressure normal for age) to obtain a normal renal blood flow and perfusion pressure. This is particularly important if there is increased abdominal pressure from ascites or other causes, as this can result in increased renal venous pressure and decreased perfusion.

Hemofiltration or dialysis or both should be initiated if the child has anuria or urine output of <0.5 mL/kg/hr despite central venous pressure or pulmonary capillary wedge pressure of >8 cm H_2O after 6 hours of resuscitation.

DISSEMINATED INTRAVASCULAR COAGULATION

Replace blood factors to maintain normal prothrombin and partial thromboplastin times, fibrinogen levels, and platelet count.

Cryoprecipitate has high concentrations of fibrinogen and von Willebrand factor and should be included in the management of disseminated intravascular coagulation.

Give antithrombin III infusion to children with low levels of antithrombin III or purpura fulminans.

Heparin may be used if considered necessary.

PROGNOSIS

The most recent multicenter trials of monoclonal antibody therapy in children with septic shock showed no difference in survival rates between treated and placebo groups; both groups had an 80% survival rate. Optimism is warranted in children undergoing therapy for septic shock.

BIBLIOGRAPHY

Carcillo JA: Management of pediatric septic shock. In Holbrook PR (ed): Textbook of Pediatric Critical Care. Philadelphia, WB Saunders, 1993, pp. 114–142.
Natanson C: NIH Conference: selected treatment strategies for septic shock based on proposed mechanisms of pathogenesis. Ann Intern Med 120:771, 1994.

9.2 **Near-Drowning**

JAMES S. HUTCHISON, MD, FRCPC, FAAP

Near-drowning occurs when a submersion victim is resuscitated and survives for at least 24 hours. Hypothermia is defined as an initial core temperature of <35°C recorded in the emergency department.

Epidemiology

Drowning is the third most common cause of death in children 1 to 14 years of age in Canada. Like other accidental causes of death and disability, drowning and near-drowning are more common in males. The peak incidences occur during the *toddler* years in both males and females and during *adolescence* and *early adulthood* in males. The majority of submersion accidents occur in pools, usually private pools (Table 9–6).

Pathophysiology

The pathophysiologic response to submersion has been divided into three stages (Figs. 9–3 to 9–5). In *stage one*, aspiration of a small volume of liquid triggers laryngospasm. In *stage two*, swallowing of liquid occurs. In *stage three*, hypoxic/ischemic central nervous system damage occurs. Pulmonary aspiration of immersion fluid or gastric contents or both occurs in 85% to 90% of victims. Irreversible central nervous system damage occurs after a period of 4 to 7 minutes of submersion. If pulmonary aspiration occurs, both fresh water and saltwater lead to washout of pulmonary surfactant, damage to alveolar basement membranes, and alveolitis. The combination of hypoxic/ischemic injury to the pulmonary microcirculation and pulmonary aspiration leads to "capillary leak" *pulmonary edema* and *adult respiratory distress syndrome*. Multiorgan system dysfunction can occur secondary to hypoxia/ischemia. Electrolyte changes and hemolysis induced by fluid and electrolyte shifts across the alveolar-capillary membrane are unlikely to be clinically important.

Hypothermia is common and in anecdotal cases has been associated with a better outcome due to cerebral protection. Likely, an "ideal" situation is needed

Table 9–6. RELATIVE CONTRIBUTION OF VARIOUS DROWNING MEDIA TO DROWNING ACCIDENTS

Medium	Percent of Drowning Accidents (%)
Saltwater	1–2
Fresh water	98
Swimming pools	
Private	50
Public	3
Lakes, rivers, streams, storm drains	20
Bathtubs	15
Buckets of water	4
Fish tanks or ponds	4
Toilets	1
Washing machines	1

From Orlowski P: Drowning, near drowning and ice-water submersions. Pediatr Clin North Am 34:75, 1987.

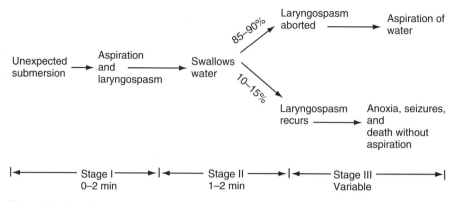

Figure 9–3. Stage 1. Aspiration of a small volume of liquid triggers laryngospasm. (From Orlowski JP: Drowning, near drowning and ice-water submersions. Pediatr Clin North Am 34:75, 1987.)

to promote rapid cooling and a rapid decrease in the cerebral metabolic rate, that is, icy water (<5°C), pulmonary aspiration, and young age.

Differential Diagnosis

Trauma may accompany the submersion event, particularly in adolescents where boats or other water vehicles or diving is involved. A diagnosis of nonaccidental submersion should be considered in infants and young children. Children with seizure disorders have a higher incidence of submersion accidents. Hypothermia is relatively common in submersion victims, even in warm climates.

Management

Management can be divided into three stages: on-scene and transport, emergency department, and intensive care unit.

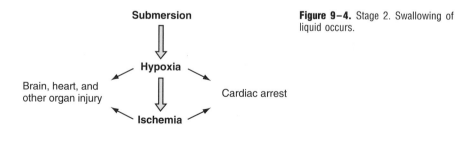

Figure 9–4. Stage 2. Swallowing of liquid occurs.

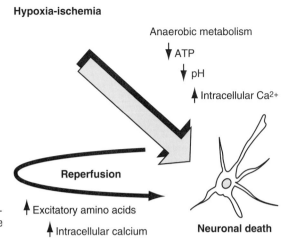

Hypoxia-ischemia

Anaerobic metabolism

↓ ATP

↓ pH

↑ Intracellular Ca^{2+}

Reperfusion

Figure 9–5. Stage 3. Hypoxic-ischemic central nervous system damage occurs.

↑ Excitatory amino acids

↑ Intracellular calcium

Neuronal death

ON-SCENE MANAGEMENT AND TRANSPORT

The *ABCs* must be addressed. Attention must be given to cervical-spine precautions for victims of boating and diving accidents.

Airway and Breathing

Place the victim in the left lateral decubitus position. Perform a chin-lift or jaw-thrust maneuver if the victim is not protecting their airway (i.e., does not have a cough or gag). Administer 100% oxygen immediately.

Apnea

The most important principle is the initiation of resuscitation *as soon as possible*. Mouth-to-mouth resuscitation and chest compressions are started and maintained if necessary during transport to a hospital. Cricoid pressure should be maintained during cardiopulmonary resuscitation to prevent aspiration of gastric contents. The administration of 100% oxygen, early placement of nasogastric tube, and suctioning of gastric contents are ideal.

EMERGENCY DEPARTMENT MANAGEMENT

Airway and Breathing

Provide a patent airway with a chin-lift or jaw-thrust maneuver. Suction the mouth and pharynx with a large-bore, rigid suction device. Cervical-spine precautions should be maintained in cases of suspected trauma.

Provide 100% oxygen. If the patient is apneic, comatose, or in severe respiratory failure, provide bag-to-mask ventilation with 100% oxygen. Then, gently *intubate* orally with the appropriate-size *cuffed endotracheal tube.* The cuffed tube may be necessary to prevent aspiration of gastric contents and to prevent loss of pressure during positive pressure ventilation. Because the patient is at risk of developing pulmonary edema, he or she may eventually require high peak-inspiratory and positive end-expiratory pressures on the ventilator for maintenance of adequate oxygenation and alveolar ventilation.

Circulation

Assess the patient's pulse, blood pressure, and peripheral perfusion. Begin or continue chest compressions if the patient is without a pulse. Start two intravenous or intraosseous lines and connect the patient to a cardiac monitor. The initial intravenous resuscitation fluid should be normal saline or Ringer's lactate solution. Most patients will be hypovolemic because of capillary leak and cold-induced diuresis. Intravascular volume status should be carefully assessed, and shock should be treated with 20 mL/kg IV or intraosseous (IO) crystalloid or colloid, repeated as necessary. Hyperglycemia has been associated with a poor neurologic outcome; therefore, glucose should be withheld from intravenous fluids until serum glucose is documented to be normal. The 1992 Pediatric Advanced Life Support guidelines should be followed for appropriate management of cardiac arrest.[2]

Disability

Assess the reactivity of pupils and Glasgow Coma Scale score.

Hypothermia

The hypothermic victim should be rewarmed, and resuscitation should be maintained until core temperature is >35°C (Table 9–7). Wet clothing should be removed, and the patient should be dried and insulated to prevent conductive and

Table 9–7. REWARMING TECHNIQUES

Temperature	Method	Technique
≥32°C	Passive external (truncal only)	Forced air or plumbed heating blanket, thermal pads, warm packs, and warm cloth blankets
<32°C	Active internal	Warm humidified air (set ventilator humidifier at 40–45°C)
		Warm intravenous fluids*
		Warm peritoneal lavage: 10–20 mL/kg repeat lavages with K+-free crystalloid dialysate*
		Extracorporeal venovenous or venoarterial bypass

*Use an in-line countercurrent heat exchanger or other device that ensures warming of the fluid to 40–45°C at high flow rates. Place the device as close as possible to the patient.

evaporative heat loss. If the patient has a core temperature of ≥32°C, passive warming techniques should be used. Active core rewarming techniques should be used if the patient has a core temperature of <32°C, cardiovascular instability, or attempts at external rewarming have failed. The brain-dead patient is poikilothermic and difficult to rewarm. *Ventricular fibrillation is common* and refractory to treatment in the hypothermic patient, and aggressive rewarming is needed. Defibrillation should be attempted no more than three times (at 2 J/kg, 4 J/kg, and 4 J/kg) before rewarming to ≥30°C. At that temperature, along with continued aggressive rewarming, attempts at defibrillation and administration of medications should be done. *Epinephrine* (0.1 mg/kg) and *lidocaine* (1 mg/kg ×2) followed by *bretylium* (5 mg/kg and 10 mg/kg IV or IO) should be administered. *Medications should be administered less frequently than usual* because metabolism is slowed. Bretylium may be more effective than lidocaine in refractory cases. Consider extracorporeal rewarming in the hypothermic patient with ventricular fibrillation.

Tubes

Place a nasogastric tube and Foley catheter to decompress the stomach and bladder, respectively.

Laboratory Tests

Arterial blood gases, complete blood count, electrolytes, glucose, calcium, urea, creatinine, liver function tests, prothrombin time, partial thromboplastin time, fibrinogen, fibrin degradation products, and lactate should be measured. Fluid, electrolyte, and acid-base imbalances are common.

Radiologic Investigations

Chest, anteroposterior, and lateral cervical-spine radiographs should be taken in patients with suspected trauma. Computed tomography scan of the head is not helpful initially unless cranial trauma is suspected.

Clinical Evaluation

Reassess intermittently the ABCs.

History

Document the events surrounding the submersion and rescue, including the estimated length of submersion and resuscitation, who was involved, when and where the submersion and resuscitation occurred, water temperature, and occurrence of trauma.

Document past medical history, including allergies and medications.

Physical Examination

Perform a full examination, including a search for signs of trauma.

INTENSIVE CARE UNIT MANAGEMENT

Patient management is supportive, with the goal being prevention of secondary injury to the brain and other organs as a result of hypoxia, ischemia, or metabolic imbalance.

Neurointensive Care

In the comatose child, the head should be kept in the midline, and the head of the bed should be elevated 15 degrees (Table 9–8). Stimuli should be kept to a minimum, and intravenous sedatives and analgesics should be administered and titrated to the response of the patient. Once adequate perfusion has been established, fluid is restricted to 50% to 60% of maintenance. *Ventilate to a carbon dioxide partial pressue (PCO_2) of 30 to 35 mm Hg.* Aggressive therapies, including intracranial pressure monitoring, aggressive prolonged hyperventilation, barbiturate coma, and induced hypothermia, have not been shown to improve outcome, although randomized, controlled trials of their efficacy have not been done.

Respiratory Care

Pulse oximetry and end-tidal carbon dioxide should be monitored continuously. Arterial blood gases should be monitored intermittently. Chest radiographs are done as needed. Positive pressure ventilation with optimum positive end-expiratory pressure and inhaled bronchodilators are administered as needed to prevent hypoxia and hypoventilation. Intermittent tracheal suctioning is used to prevent obstruction of the endotracheal tube.

Cardiovascular Care

If myocardial hypoxic/ischemic injury is suspected, invasive hemodynamic monitoring should be done, including continuous arterial and central venous

Table 9–8. GUIDELINES FOR NEUROINTENSIVE CARE

Therapy	Comments/Drugs
Nursing	Head in midline, head of bed elevated 15°, minimal handling
Sedation	Midazolam 0.1–0.2 mg/kg/hr IV loading dose, then 0.5–5 μg/kg/min IV infusion or lorazepam 0.05–0.1 mg/kg IV q6h
Analgesia	Morphine 0.1 mg/kg IV bolus followed by 10–80 μg/kg/min IV infusion or fentanyl 0.5–10 μg/kg/min IV
Fluids	50–60% maintenance IV
Mechanical ventilation	Avoid hypoventilation, PCO_2 30–35 mm Hg

pressure monitoring. Intravenous fluid boluses, diuretics, and inotropes such as *dopamine* and *dobutamine* may be necessary to maintain optimum blood pressure and oxygen delivery to the tissues.

Other Care

Renal and hepatic dysfunctions and disseminated intravascular coagulation may occur. Metabolic and hematologic balances are maintained. *Antibiotics are not used routinely;* however, they are indicated for victims of immersion in contaminated liquid and the choice of antibiotic should be based on Gram-stain. Steroids have not been shown to be effective in the management of cerebral edema and the pulmonary manifestations associated with near-drowning.

Prognosis

The ultimate outcome relates to the *length of submersion* and *hypoxic/ischemic injury to the brain.* Immediate attempts at resuscitation by the rescuers or bystanders improve the prognosis. Children with a prolonged submersion (>25 min) or prolonged resuscitation (>25 min) have a poor prognosis for neurologic recovery. Other indicators of unfavorable prognosis are apnea and coma on presentation to the emergency department and initial arterial pH <7.1. The mechanism of death from near-drowning is almost invariably cerebral edema, herniation, and brain death. Deaths from pulmonary causes are rare.

Hypothermia has been associated with a *worse* prognosis when the submersion occurs in water that is not icy. The degree of hypothermia correlates with the length of submersion. In the hospital, aggressive resuscitation of the nonhypothermic near-drowning victim arriving with an absence of vital signs results in eventual death or survival in a persistent vegetative state. Withdrawal of life support should be considered in these patients after successful resuscitation if they remain comatose after a 24-hour period of mechanical ventilation.

Severe neurologic impairment occurs in 5% to 12% of survivors of a near-drowning. One third of "normal" survivors have minimal cerebral dysfunction based on psychometric testing. The neurodevelopmental handicaps experienced by children after near-drowning represent a large burden to families and society.

BIBLIOGRAPHY
Levin DL, Morriss FC, Toro LO, et al: Drowning and near-drowning. Pediatr Clin North Am 40:321, 1993.
Pediatric Advanced Life Support, Part VI, 268:2268, 1992.

9.3 Hepatic Failure

ANNIK DE JAEGER, DGHV, CK
JACQUES LACROIX, FRCPC, FAAP

Hepatic failure is present when one or many of the main liver functions are so impaired that it becomes life threatening. The failure is considered *severe* when the level of the clotting factors produced by the liver is <50% and there is encephalopathy. By definition, hepatic failure is *fulminant* if failure develops within 2 weeks after the onset of symptoms. There is no consensus regarding the interval from onset of jaundice to encephalopathy, although it is generally accepted that patients with a shorter interval have a different evolution and a better prognosis (more severe cerebral edema and less severe ascites).

Pathophysiology

The liver synthesizes a great amount of important substances (e.g., glucose, proteins, and clotting factors), metabolizes many others (e.g., ammonia and all drugs and compounds metabolized by the cytochrome P-450 system), and excretes many metabolites (e.g., bilirubin). If the insult is sufficiently severe, the liver will be unable to carry out its metabolic work; this can cause *hypoglycemia, hyperammonemia, hyperbilirubinemia,* and *a low concentration of clotting factors.* Liver cell necrosis is manifested by an increased level of liver enzymes (alanine transaminase [ALT] and aspartate transaminase [AST]).

The pathophysiology of *hepatic encephalopathy* is not completely understood: it appears to be caused by the accumulation of substances usually metabolized in the liver, e.g., ammonia, short-chain fatty acids, benzodiazepine-like substances, enkephalins, octopamine, mercaptans (producing the typical fetor hepaticus), γ-aminobutyric acid, and many others.

Table 9–9 gives the most frequent *etiologies.* In infants, most cases are caused by an infectious process or an inborn error of metabolism (e.g., tyrosinemia, galactosemia, and fructosemia). In older children, autoimmune diseases, toxic liver disease (e.g., due to acetaminophen, *Amanita phalloides,* and halothane), or idiosyncratic hypersensitivity (e.g., valproate) should also be considered. Wilson's disease should be excluded in all children older than 5 years. In adolescents, drug toxicity (e.g., methylendioxymethamphetamine ["ecstasy"]) and suicide attempts should be considered.

Differential Diagnosis

The differential diagnosis of hepatic failure includes all causes of coma and liver disease. However, many diseases can insult the liver and brain without

Table 9–9. ETIOLOGY

Etiology	Proportion of Cases at Bicêtre, France	Age	
		≤3 mon	>3 mon
Infectious disease	62%		
Hepatitis A		−	+ +
Hepatitis B		+ +	+ + +
Hepatitis C		±	+ + +
Other infections		+	±
Intoxication	19%	+	+ +
Metabolic diseases	9.5%	+	±
Autoimmune diseases	3%	±	+
Other (vascular disease, cancer)	6.5%	±	±

+ + +, Common; + +, less common; +, rare; −, never.
Adapted from Devictor D, Paradis K, Gauthier M: Insuffisance hépatique grave. *In* Lacroix J, Gauthier M, Beaufils F (eds): Urgences et Soins Intensifs Pédiatriques, 1st ed. Montréal/Paris, Presses de l'Université de Montréal and Doin éditeurs, 1994, pp. 271–291.

causing true hepatic failure. The most common are (1) metabolic (e.g., Reye syndrome, congenital urea cycle disease), (2) infectious (e.g., adenovirus, toxic shock syndrome), (3) toxic (e.g., aspirin, phenytoin), and (4) hemorrhagic (e.g., syndrome of hemorrhagic shock with encephalopathy).

Clinical Evaluation

The symptoms and signs most frequently reported are weakness, weight loss, fetor hepaticus, vomiting, jaundice (which is almost always present, with the exception of acetaminophen poisoning or Reye-like syndrome), hepatomegaly, signs of coagulopathy (e.g., bleeding, purpura), altered state of consciousness, convulsion, and asterixis (flapping movements of the fingers and hands on dorsiflexion of the wrist with the arm fixed in extension). An ophthalmologic examination with a slit lamp (to detect a Kayser-Fleischer corneal ring) is indicated for all children older than 10 years, unless the hepatic failure is clearly related to cause other than Wilson's disease.

The symptomatology of hepatic encephalopathy is related to metabolic abnormalities and cerebral edema. The severity of hepatic encephalopathy is estimated with the use of *staging*. Early symptoms can be very subtle, such as deterioration in handwriting, increasing combativeness, or altered mood (*grade I*). *Grade II* is characterized by inappropriate behavior or drowsiness. *Grade III* is defined by stupor (the patient is responsive to painful stimuli and can be aroused but falls asleep at once when the stimulus is withdrawn). Flaccid coma indicates *grade IV* (decorticate or decerebrate posturing is possible). Grades III and IV are frequently associated with *cerebral edema.* Some physicians consider intracranial pressure monitoring to be mandatory under these circumstances; however, a lethal intracranial bleed can occur, and the coagulopathy should be controlled before any intracran-

Table 9–10. CLINICAL MONITORING

A and B, Airway and breathing: Respiratory rate, pulse oximeter
C, Circulation: Hourly vital signs (heart rate, blood pressure), hourly fluid balance (ingesta and excreta), with or without urinary catheter, with or without arterial line, with or without central venous pressure
D, Others: Neurologic signs each hour (Glasgow Coma Scale score, pupils, oculomotor reflex, with or without intracranial pressure), weight daily

ial device is inserted. The risk of intracranial bleeding is lower with the use of extradural transducers.

A patient with acute or subacute hepatic failure should be closely monitored. Table 9–10 lists clinical data that should be evaluated.

Laboratory Investigations

The laboratory test results characteristic of hepatic failure are hyperammonemia, high bilirubin level, and low levels of clotting factors, which demonstrates hepatic dysfunction; increased level of transaminases (ALT and AST), which suggests liver cell necrosis; and increased level of alkaline phosphatase or γ-glutamyltranspeptidase, which suggests bile duct injury.

Table 9–11 lists analyses that can be useful in finding the cause of the hepatic failure and tests that should be done repeatedly for monitoring.

Management

NONSPECIFIC TREATMENT MODALITIES

The goals of management are to treat primary hepatic injury and to prevent secondary injury. An extensive etiologic search is necessary to determine whether

Table 9–11. LABORATORY INVESTIGATION AND MONITORING

Investigation: Coombs, viral serology (hepatitis A, B, C, and D; herpes; echovirus; adenovirus; Epstein-Barr virus; cytomegalovirus), viral cultures (throat, stool, and urine), toxicologic screening, with or without enzymatic function (galactosidase, fructosemia, and so on), serous α_1-antitrypsin, with or without ceruloplasmin, with or without copper (serum and urine), with or without amino acids (blood and urine), serous autoantibodies (anti-DNA, antimitochondrial, and so on), with or without hepatic biopsy.
Monitoring: Hemoglobin and hematocrit, platelets, coagulogram, factor V, glycemia, ALT, AST, bilirubin, alkaline phosphatase, γ-glutamyl transferase, ammonia, blood urea nitrogen and creatinine, blood gases, electrolytes, ionized calcium, magnesium, phosphorus, with or without others (albumin, α-fetoprotein, abdominal echography, EEG, and so on)

specific treatment is indicated. *Primary injuries*, which are immediately related to liver failure, include coma, hypoglycemia, and coagulopathy. *Secondary injuries* are pulmonary edema, cerebral edema, shock, renal insufficiency, infections, pancreatitis, and death.

Airway and Breathing

Hypoxia is common and usually caused by pulmonary edema. All patients should be monitored with the use of continuous pulse oximetry. *Oxygen* may be the only treatment needed. Some patients benefit from *continuous positive airway pressure* or *positive end-expiratory pressure*, but these modalities increase hepatic vein pressure and, theoretically, can increase liver cell ischemia; therefore, they should be used cautiously, and low pressure is recommended. *Mechanical ventilation* should be used when hypercapnia or hypoxia develops. Early *intubation* and mechanical ventilation are recommended for patients in grade III or IV to supply adequate oxygenation and prevent aspiration. If *hypocapnia* is indicated to treat intracranial hypertension, the alveolar carbon dioxide tension ($Paco_2$) should be maintained between 25 and 35 mm Hg with pH <7.50.

Circulation: Fluids, Electrolytes, and Coagulation

A *urinary bladder catheter, arterial line,* and *central venous pressure* monitoring should be used in patients in grade III or IV and should be considered in grade II patients. The goal is to keep the patient normovolemic (central venous pressure of 2 to 6 mm Hg) with normal electrolyte levels.

1. *Fluid* and *sodium balance* should be very closely monitored. There always is some renal dysfunction with hyponatremia and fluid retention; therefore, initial fluid restriction should be two thirds of maintenance volume and should not contain sodium. Total sodium intake should not exceed losses (<2 mEq/kg/day). Developing renal failure can sometimes be reversed with a continuous infusion of *dopamine* (2 to 4 μg/kg/min). Furthermore, dopamine could increase splanchnic and hepatic blood flow.
2. *Spironolactone* (1 to 3 mg/kg/day PO) could be useful if diuretics are needed or there is a trend to hypokalemia. Diuretics should be used with close monitoring of diuresis and central venous pressure because a precipitous drop in intravascular volume may result in irreversible renal failure.
3. Supplementation with *potassium* (>2 mmol/kg/day) is frequently needed because secondary hyperaldosteronism associated with hepatic failure results in significant kaliuresis.

Hypovolemic shock can occur through hemorrhage or dehydration; *blood products, plasma volume expanders, saline,* and vasoactive drugs, such as *dopamine* and *norepinephrine,* should be given as needed to reestablish the hemodynamic status.

Hemorrhage could be caused by coagulopathy or upper gastrointestinal bleeding. Coagulopathy is caused by low clotting factor production by the liver (factors II, V, VII, IX, and X), low platelet counts, and, sometimes, disseminated intravascular coagulation (DIC); active bleeding should be treated with *fresh frozen plasma or platelets* (2 units/10 kg) or both. However, fresh frozen plasma is a salt/water/ nitrogen load that can contribute to the development of coma and cerebral edema.

Dextrose and Drugs

Hypoglycemia occurs in approximately 40% of cases of severe acute hepatic failure. It can be severe, prolonged, and undetected in comatose patients. The patient's blood sugar should be checked frequently (at least every 2 hours) with the use of Chemstrip or other method. A constant intake of sugar must be provided through a continuous infusion of 5% or 10% *dextrose*. A bolus of 25% dextrose (2 mL/kg) and adjustment of the continuous infusion may be needed.

Lactulose (0.5 gm/kg PO q2h initially and 0.25 gm/kg q6 to 48h after the appearance of loose stools) and/or *neomycin* (25 mg/kg PO q6h; maximum, 4 gm/ day) is frequently given to prevent and/or to treat hepatic encephalopathy. These drugs decrease the amount of ammonia absorbed by the colon. Some data suggest that their effect is additive. However, their usefulness is debated. Furthermore, the effect of lactulose should be closely monitored and adequately dose-titrated to achieve two to four semisolid bowel movements a day because severe lactulose diarrhea can result in excessive loss of free water and hyponatremia. Lactulose is contraindicated if galactosemia is suspected. It is probably better to avoid neomycin if renal function is altered. Some use *metronidazole* instead of neomycin because of the ototoxicity and nephrotoxicity of neomycin.

Convulsions can be caused by hypoglycemia, hyponatremia, intracranial bleeding, or hepatic encephalopathy. Sugar, sodium, or neurosurgical intervention could be necessary. *Phenytoin* is suggested. If the convulsion is attributable to the encephalopathy, the prognosis is so poor that a liver transplantation should be considered and discussed with the patient.

The etiology of the *upper gastrointestinal bleed* could be portal hypertension, gastroduodenal stress ulcer(s), or severe gastritis. Blood in the small bowel can worsen hepatic encephalopathy; therefore, a *gastric tube* should be inserted in all patients to detect early upper gastrointestinal bleeding and to wash out all blood pouring into the stomach. The prevention of upper gastrointestinal bleeding is important. *Sucralfate* (1 gm PO q6h) is the first-line drug. *Ranitidine* (2 to 6 mg/ kg/day by continuous infusion) could also be given, but some believe that H_2- blockers should be avoided because they could be hepatotoxic. However, 30% of deaths related to hepatic failure are caused by upper gastrointestinal bleeding; therefore, most recommend maintaining gastric pH >4.5 through the use of both sucralfate and ranitidine. *Antacids* and *omeprazole* are other options. Surgical intervention should be considered if the upper gastrointestinal bleeding is life threatening.

Vitamin K (0.2 mg/kg/day PO or IV; maximum, 10 mg/day) is frequently given, even though the liver is usually unable to use it to synthesize vitamin K–dependent clotting factors (factors II, VII, IX, and X).

Prophylaxis with antibiotics is the subject of controversy; it usually is not recommended. Fever, leukocytosis, worsening of the encephalopathy, or the ap- pearance of an hepatorenal syndrome should raise suspicion of infection. Lungs, blood (due to central catheters), and urinary tract (due to urinary catheter) are the most common sites, and cultures, for both bacteria and fungus, should be obtained frequently from these sites. Appropriate antibiotics should be prescribed early, before laboratory confirmation, taking into account the incidence and type and etiology of nosocomial infections in each medical center.

Flumazenil (0.2 to 0.5 mg/m^2/dose IV; maximum, 1 mg/dose), an antagonist of benzodiazepines, could awake some patients from a coma; however, its usefulness is not established.

Drugs altering consciousness (e.g., benzodiazepines, barbiturates, narcotics) and *drugs metabolized and/or excreted by the liver* (e.g., phenytoin, benzodiazepines, ranitidine, cyclosporin) should be avoided. If used, doses should be adjusted, taking into account the effect of the hepatic failure on their pharmacodynamics.

Other Nonspecific Treatment Modalities

The patient should be *isolated* if an infection is suspected.

Death is attributed to *cerebral edema* in >40% of cases of hepatic failure; the rate of cerebral edema in patients in grade III or IV is 50% to 85%. Clinical signs of cerebral edema appear when intracranial pressure is >30 mm Hg. However, the onset of these signs can be quite subtle, especially when sedatives and muscle-paralyzing agents are used. Moreover, it should be noted that the risk of death is high once the symptomatology of high intracranial pressure is clinically obvious. Therefore, it is clear that *intracranial pressure monitoring* could be useful, but the rate of severe complications is so high that its usefulness remains debated. *Head elevation* to 20° to 30° is suggested for all patients in grade III or IV encephalopathy. If an intracranial pressure–monitoring device is available, significant intracranial hypertension (>30 mm Hg) should be treated vigorously with *hyperventilation* (Paco$_2$ = 25 to 35 mm Hg) and *mannitol* infusion (0.25 to 0.5 gm/kg/dose IV over 20 minutes). Caution is needed when mannitol is used in the presence of renal failure. *Paralyzing agents* (e.g., *pancuronium* [0.1 mg/kg/dose IV q2 to 6h or by continuous infusion]) can be useful in severe cases. Despite the hepatic failure, some advocate the use of *barbiturates* (e.g., *thiopental* [2 to 5 mg/kg/hr]) in very severe cases; *hypothermia* is another option, despite its increased infection risk.

Nutrition is important. A specific diet is mandatory: intravenous or enteral intake should be low in protein (≤0.5 gm/kg/day) and sodium (≤2 mmol/kg/day) but high in sugar and potassium. A costly branched chain-enriched solution has been proposed, but its effectiveness has not been established.

Renal replacement therapy (dialysis or hemofiltration) is useful in the presence of renal failure to prevent fluid overload; it should be considered in the presence of persistent acidosis, hyperkalemia, or severe azotemia.

SPECIFIC TREATMENT MODALITIES

Some causes of hepatic failure warrant a specific treatment.

Acetaminophen intoxication. *N*-Acetylcysteine should be given as soon as possible. It has been suggested that *N*-acetylcysteine could be useful even after liver failure has appeared, but this remains debated in the literature.

Fructosemia or *galactosemia.* Do not give any fructose or lactose.

Wilson disease. Give D-penicillamine (1 to 2 gm/day PO q6 to 12h).

Autoimmune hepatitis. Administer steroids (e.g., *methylprednisolone* [2 mg/kg/day IV or PO]) with or without *azathioprine* (2 mg/kg/day IV or PO). Some data suggest that steroids are detrimental in cases of fulminant hepatic failure; therefore, steroids should only be given if the autoimmune process is well documented.

RESCUE THERAPY

Presently, there is no liver support system (e.g., charcoal hemoperfusion, plasmapheresis) that clearly improves the outcome of hepatic failure, and none are recommended for its clinical management. Liver *transplantation* is the only life-saving procedure in very severe cases; it must be considered in the presence of the following risk factors: fulminant hepatic failure without improvement despite full medical treatment, hepatic encephalopathy grade II or III, persistent gastrointestinal bleeding, persistent acidosis, progressive renal failure, level of factor V of ≤20% to 25% or prothrombin time of >50 seconds; or electroencephalogram type II (slow or abolished electroencephalographic activity) or worse. However, grade IV coma is a contraindication because the rate of mortality and severe neurologic sequelae is very high in survivors. Sepsis is another contraindication, whereas hepatorenal syndrome is not because renal function will resolve if the liver graft is successful.

Prognosis

Death is usually caused by cerebral edema, hemorrhage, nosocomial infections, renal insufficiency, or primary metabolic problems. Grade IV coma, increase in serum bilirubin associated with decrease in ALT and AST levels, lactic acidosis, level of factor V of <25%, prolonged prothrombin time unresponsive to vitamin K, and hepatorenal syndrome are decisive markers of a poor outcome. The death rate is >80% for patients in grade IV coma, and >40% of children in fulminant hepatic failure will die; liver transplantation must be considered in these cases. On the other hand, an increasing level of α-feto-protein suggests liver cell regeneration. A decreasing level of bilirubin and transaminases, a shortening of prothrombin and partial thromboplastin times, and an increasing albuminemia herald good prognosis.

BIBLIOGRAPHY

Caraceni P, Van Thiel DH: Acute liver failure. Lancet 345:163, 1995.

Harrison PM, Wendon JA, Gimson AES, et al: Improvement by acetylcysteine of hemodynamics and oxygen transport in fulminant hepatic failure. N Engl J Med 324:1852, 1991.

Keays R, Harrison PM, Wendon JA, et al: Intravenous acetylcysteine in paracetamol-induced fulminant hepatic failure: a prospective controlled trial. Br Med J 303:1026, 1991.

Mohan P, Kersner B: Hepatic failure. *In* Holbrook PR (ed): Textbook of Pediatric Critical Care. Philadelphia, WB Saunders, 1993, pp. 621–637.

Russell GJ, Fitzgerald JF, Clark JH: Fulminant hepatic failure. J Pediatr 111:313, 1987.

9.4 **Renal Failure**

R. MORRISON HURLEY, MD, MSc, FRCPC

Renal failure is the inability of the kidneys to maintain the homeostasis of body fluids and to clear wastes. If the deterioration in renal function is sudden, often with oliguria (urine output of <200 mL/m²/24 hr or <0.8 mL/kg/hr), it is called *acute renal failure* (ARF); if there is a slower progression of decrease in renal function, it is called *chronic renal failure* (CRF). Most renal failure in pediatric intensive care unit patients is acute; however, one should be able to distinguish ARF from CRF and to identify an acute renal injury in a child with preexisting chronic renal disease.

Pathophysiology of Acute Renal Failure

The basic defect is usually an acute reduction in glomerular filtration. This may be from a primary glomerular insult or a disease or secondary to pathologic processes occurring proximal (e.g., decreased intravascular volume, renal perfusion) or distal (e.g., obstruction) to the glomerulus.

Differential Diagnosis of Acute Renal Failure

Prerenal. The most common causes of ARF in pediatric renal critical care are prerenal; two major reasons are (1) decreased plasma volume and decreased effective intravascular volume (Table 9–12) and (2) ARF secondary to perinatal insults (newborns) associated with hypoperfusion and hypoxia (Table 9–13). Advances in critical care have contributed to the survival of neonates with very complex medical problems, and these neonates often develop ARF secondary to their underlying disorders or treatment interventions.

Intrarenal. If prerenal causes persist, there may be progression to intrinsic renal failure, acute tubular necrosis (ATN), or renal cortical or medullary necrosis. The effect of drugs and other toxins are particularly important in hospitalized children; these include aminoglycosides, cyclosporine, and antineoplastic agents. ATN from drugs and endogenous toxin is more common in those with decreased renal perfusion or chronic renal disease. Often, the cause of ARF is multifactorial as critically ill children may have sustained renal insults from multiple sources. Intrinsic acquired renal disease, e.g., hemolytic uremic syndrome, acute postinfectious glomerulonephritis, and interstitial nephritis, make up the majority of cases of non-ATN intrarenal ARF. Hemolytic uremic syndrome is one of the few causes of intrarenal failure in which anuria occurs. Although oliguria is the hallmark of the clinical diagnosis of ARF, some patients have a sudden deterioration in renal function without oliguria. In newborns, nonoliguric ARF is often associated with

Table 9–12. ACUTE RENAL FAILURE IN PEDIATRIC CRITICAL
CARE UNIT: CHILDREN AND ADOLESCENTS

Prerenal	*Intrarenal Continued*
Volume depletion/hemorrhage	Interstitial nephritis
Sepsis/burns	Drugs
Hypoalbuminemia	Antibiotics
Drugs	Furosemide
Nonsteroidals	Allopurinol
Angiotensin-converting enzyme	Systemic infections
inhibitors	Acute and subacute endocarditis
Hypotension/shock	Viral hepatitis
Congestive heart failure	Epstein-Barr
Hepatorenal syndrome	*Postrenal*
Intrarenal	Obstructive uropathy
Acute tubular necrosis	Bilateral
Hemolytic uremic syndrome	Posterior urethral valve
Acute glomerulonephritis	Neurogenic bladder
Nephrotoxins	Postoperative
Drugs	Unilateral (solitary kidney)
Antibiotics (aminoglycosides,	Ureteropelvic junction obstruction
amphotericin B)	
Cyclosporine	
Antineoplastic agents	
Contrast agents	
Endogenous (myoglobin, uric acid/	
phosphates)	

nephrotoxins, hypoxia/asphyxia, respiratory distress, and congenital renal anomalies. Interstitial nephritis associated with an immunologic reaction to systemic infections or drug hypersensitivity occurs occasionally.

Postrenal. Postrenal causes of ARF are rarely seen in the critical care unit. Other than in children with solitary kidneys or with chronic renal insufficiency, obstruction must be bilateral to cause decreased urine volume. If completely obstructed, anuria is the rule.

Clinical Evaluation and Laboratory Investigations

Prerenal and Intrarenal. The differentiation between these two conditions is the most frequent problem in evaluation. In addition to determination of whether the child has a reason to be in a state of renal hypoperfusion, the renal indices, especially the fractional excretion of sodium, can be very helpful (Table 9–14).

Postrenal. The most useful examination is a *renal ultrasound* to determine the number, size, and echogenicity of the kidneys and dilatation of the urinary tract. The ultrasound may be helpful in the differentiation of underlying chronic renal disease.

Table 9–13. ACUTE RENAL FAILURE IN PEDIATRIC
CRITICAL CARE UNIT: NEWBORNS

Prerenal	*Postrenal*
Hypoxia	Obstructive uropathy
Hypotension / shock	Bilateral
Congestive heart failure	Posterior urethral valve
Extracorporeal membrane oxygenation	Neurogenic bladder
Major vessel occlusion	Postoperative
Drugs	Unilateral (solitary kidney)
Indomethacin	Ureteropelvic junction obstruction
Tolazoline	
Hemorrhage	
Sepsis	
Postoperative	
Hydrops	
Intrarenal	
Acute tubular necrosis	
Nephrotoxins (see Table 9–12)	
Drugs	
Antibiotics (aminoglycosides,	
amphotericin B)	
Cyclosporine	
Antineoplastic agents	
Contrast agents	
Endogenous (myoglobin, uric acid /	
phosphates)	

Management

Management consists of prevention, supportive care, and dialysis.

PREVENTION

The best prevention is the recognition of the factors, especially volume depletion, that predispose the child to ARF. The use of diuretics prophylactically, although intuitively attractive, has produced conflicting results. Continuous infusion of furosemide has been shown to provide a more controlled and predictable urine output in postoperative pediatric cardiac patients. There are suggestions from uncontrolled studies that oliguric renal failure may be converted to nonoliguric renal failure. This may simplify supportive management. Although the effect on the course of renal failure is not clear, the recommendations are (1) to *ensure euvolemia* with fluid challenges (normal saline [10 to 20 mL/kg over 30 minutes]), (2) to *correct other factors that contribute to hypoperfusion* where possible (e.g., hypoxia, acidosis, hypoalbuminemia, congestive heart failure), (3) when the above have failed, to try a trial of *intravenous furosemide* (1 to 5 mg/kg/dose) or *furosemide infusion* (0.1 mg/kg/hr); *mannitol* (0.5 mg/kg/bolus) has been used in this situation, but there is a serious risk of volume expansion and congestive heart

Table 9–14. INDICES OF ACUTE RENAL FAILURE

	Prerenal		Renal	
	Neonates	*Older Children*	*Neonates*	*Older Children*
UNa (mEq/L)	≤20	<10	>50	>50
FeNa (%)	≤2.5	≤1	>3	>2
UOsm (mOsm/L)	≥350	≥500	≤300	≤300
U/POsm	≥1.2	≥1.5	0.8–1.2	0.8–1.2
Blood urea nitrogen/ creatinine	>10	>20	Progressive increases in both	
Response to volume	Increased urine output		No effect	

failure, and (4) to *maintain increased urine flow* and alkalinization of the urine, which may help prevent ARF in children with myoglobinuria or hyperuricosuria.

SUPPORTIVE CARE

The essence of supportive care is to prevent or treat the predictable results of renal failure.

Fluid Balance and Sodium

Restore and *maintain euvolemia.* If the child is volume deplete, give fluid boluses; if the child is volume overloaded, restrict fluids and give furosemide by bolus or infusion if necessary. If the child does not respond, he or she may have established ATN rather than merely renal hypoperfusion. For most children with ARF, daily maintenance requirements equal urine output plus obvious extrarenal losses plus insensible water loss (one third maintenance volume). Those with large surface burns, tachypnea, or fever and infants under a radiant heater have larger insensible losses. *Daily weights, input/output analysis, physical examination,* and *serum sodium levels* help determine the appropriate ongoing therapy. The child's weight should not increase. If there is a more rapid weight loss than 0.5% to 1% per day and an increase in serum sodium levels, inadequate free water has been given; an absence of weight loss and a decrease in serum sodium denotes excess free water replacement. Hyponatremia is almost always iatrogenic. Hyponatremia (<120 mEq/L) that does not respond to fluid restriction or that is accompanied by central nervous system symptoms may require hypertonic saline infusion.

When the patient is in the diuretic phase of ARF, the urinary electrolytes and volume should be measured and replaced.

Potassium

Potassium should not be given unless there is adequate urinary output. One should not underestimate the potassium load from potassium-containing antibiotics and catabolic states such as burns, trauma, sepsis, hemolysis, rhabdomyolysis, tumor lysis syndrome, and surgery. Hyperkalemia is a medical emergency requiring the halt of exogenous potassium administration, medical therapy (Table 9–15), and dialysis if the above are unsuccessful or the factors contributing to the hyperkalemia are continuing.

Calcium and Phosphorous

Hypocalcemia (decreased ionized calcium) is usually mild and managed through control of the hyperphosphatemia (dietary phosphate restriction and oral phosphate binders). Critically ill infants and children with ARF may develop severe hypocalcemia with tetany seizures or arrhythmias. These manifestations are treated with infusion of 10% calcium gluconate (100 mg/kg; maximum, 1 gm).

Acid-Base Balance

The acidosis seen in ARF is usually controlled through respiratory mechanisms; however, if alkali therapy is required, sodium bicarbonates should be given judiciously, keeping in mind the effect on hypocalemia.

Hypertension

Hypertension is a frequent problem in ARF. Asymptomatic hypertension may be treated with *sublingual nifedipine or intravenous hydralazine*. In patients who have papilledema or are encephalopathic, their pressures must be quickly reduced with intravenous *diazoxide* or a continuous *nitroprusside* infusion (Table 9–16). Diazoxide has an advantage in encephalopathic patients as it requires no special preparation. For maximal effect, the drug must be given by rapid intravenous push. Often, the hypertension in ARF is directly related to volume expansion, and dialysis may be indicated if other measures are inadequate.

Nutrition

Nutrition is an important issue, but most studies on nutrition in ARF were done with adult patients. Feeding by mouth or enterally is preferred to parenteral

Table 9–15. TREATMENT OF HYPERKALEMIA

Drug	Dose
Sodium bicarbonate	1–2 mEq/kg IV over 10–30 min
Calcium gluconate (10%)	0.5–1 mL/kg IV over 2–10 min
Glucose and insulin	Glucose 0.5 gm/kg, insulin 0.1 unit/kg IV over 30 min
Sodium polystyrene sulfonate (Kayexalate)	1 gm/kg PO or PR
Calcium polystyrene sulfonate (Resonium calcium)	1 gm/kg PO or PR

Table 9–16. TREATMENT OF HYPERTENSIVE EMERGENCIES

Agent	Dose	Onset	Complications
Sodium nitroprusside	0.5–8.0 μg/kg/min IV infusion	Within seconds	Cyanide toxicity, especially with renal failure
Diazoxide	3–5 mg/kg rapid IV push	Within minutes; peaks at 30 min	Nausea, vomiting, hyperglycemia
Labetalol	1–3 mg/kg/hr IV infusion	Within minutes	Well tolerated
Hydralazine	0.1–0.5 mg/kg IV	Within 30 min	Flushing, headache, reflex tachycardia
Nifedipine	0.25–0.5 mg/kg PO or SL	Within 30 min	Nausea, flushing
Minoxidil	0.2–1.0 mg/kg PO	Within 30 min	Hypertrichosis, fluid retention

feeding. Adequate nutrition may be difficult to obtain because of fluid restrictions without peritoneal dialysis.

DIALYSIS

Dialysis should be instituted for *uncontrollable fluid overload, acidosis,* or *hyperkalemia* and be strongly considered for *increased ventilatory difficulties* on mechanical ventilation, to *maximize nutrition,* and for an *expected long duration of ARF.* Peritoneal dialysis is the modality of choice in the critical care unit because of technical ease, especially in the very young. In many centers, continuous venovenous hemofiltration is in large part replacing the use of continuous arterial venous hemofiltration and standard hemodialysis. The technical and professional expertise of experienced dialysis staff and pediatric nephrology personnel is of utmost importance in the success of any extracorporeal program.

Prognosis

The prognosis of ARF in pediatric critical care unit patients depends on three major factors: the basic kidney condition (acute or chronic), medical or surgical disease, and involvement of other organ systems. Most ARF caused by acquired renal disease has a good prognosis; the prognosis is intermediate if associated with originally compromised kidneys or transient pulmonary insufficiency and poor if associated with multiorgan failure. In general, children with a medical reason for renal failure do better than do those who develop renal failure after surgery or secondary to trauma.

BIBLIOGRAPHY

Sehic A, Chesney RW: Acute renal failure: diagnosis. Pediatr Rev 16:101, 1995.
Sehic A, Chesney RW: Acute renal failure: diagnosis (therapy and prevention). Pediatr Rev 16:137, 1995.

9.5 **Poisoning**

CURT M. STEINHART, MD, FCCM
ANTHONY L. PEARSON-SHAVER, MD

Poisoning may be a medical emergency depending on the substance involved. Poisoning may occur after oral ingestion of a toxic agent or an inappropriate amount of a medicinal substance. Toxicity may also occur through inhalation, insufflation (snorting), transdermal absorption, or injection via the subcutaneous or intravenous route. Pediatric poisonings occur in a bimodal age distribution with the greatest incidence in toddlers and adolescents. Offending substances may be classified as medicinal or nonmedicinal.

Pathophysiology

Signs and symptoms occur primarily due to direct pharmacologic actions of the agent or agents involved. Medicinal substances create pathophysiologic derangements due to their pharmacodynamic properties and their side effects. For example, the hepatic dysfunction that occurs after large doses of acetaminophen results from its hepatic metabolism and the displacement by the salicylate of certain other protein-bound medications (see below), whereas barbiturates may cause respiratory depression as an undesirable side effect of their sedative properties.

Differential Diagnosis

At presentation, it may be known that a poisoning incident has occurred. In such circumstances, the patient or family member must be asked several questions for proper management to follow (Table 9–17). Care is then directed toward the specific agent or agents based on given answers. When there is no ingestion history, an organ system evaluation should be undertaken with an emphasis on evaluation of the respiratory, cardiovascular, and central nervous systems (Fig. 9–6). Signs and symptoms may be indicative of a specific toxic syndrome (*toxidrome*). Several well known toxidromes are given in Table 9–18.

Clinical Evaluation

Care begins with the *ABCs* of basic life support; airway, breathing, and circulatory integrity requires both initial assessment and frequent reassessment, as the patient's clinical condition may change unexpectedly. Patients with significant central nervous system depression may require that a secure airway be obtained

Table 9–17. HISTORY: IMPORTANT QUESTIONS WHEN EVALUATING POISONINGS

What toxic agents / medications were found near the patient?
What medications are in the home?
What approximate amount of the toxic agent was ingested?
   How much of the agent was available before the ingestion?
   How much of the agent remained after the ingestion?
When did the ingestion occur?
Were there characteristic odors at the scene of the ingestion?
Was the patient alert on discovery?
   Has the patient remained alert since the ingestion?
   How has the patient behaved since the ingestion?
Does the patient have a history of substance abuse?

through tracheal intubation. *This should be done expectantly rather than emergently during respiratory or cardiac arrest.* Hypoventilation caused by poisonings often requires positive pressure ventilation via a bag-valve apparatus followed by mechanical ventilation unless a specific antidote such as naloxone rapidly reverses respiratory inadequacy.

Management

When there is reasonable likelihood of opioid intoxication, 0.01 to 0.10 mg/kg *naloxone* should be given as a rapid intravenous bolus. In this manner, naloxone may be useful in aiding the diagnosis of opioid effects.

Efforts to limit absorption are often warranted. Inducement of emesis with the use of *ipecac syrup* (infants 6 to 12 months old, 10 mL; children 1 to 12 yrs, 15 mL; children 12 yrs and older, 30 mL), *gastric lavage, activated charcoal* instillation (small children, 15 to 30 gm; older children and adolescents, 50 to 100 gm; or 1 to 2 gm/kg body wt), and *whole bowel irrigation* are the primary methods to consider. Each of these interventions has inherent risks and benefits that should be analyzed before their use separately or in combination. Figure 9–7 is an algorithm to use when choosing the proper method for limiting absorption of the toxic agent. In addition, cathartics, such as *magnesium citrate* and *sorbitol*, are generally safe and often helpful.

Further therapy depends on the substance ingested. When diagnostic uncertainty remains, general supportive measures directed toward maintaining stable cardiorespiratory status often are sufficient.

Specific Agents

Certain pediatric poisonings occur with sufficient frequency to warrant specific mention: salicylates, acetaminophen, iron, tricyclic antidepressants, and some "street drugs."

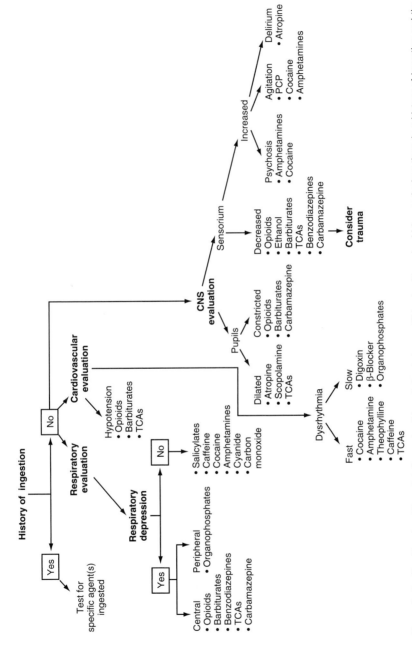

Figure 9–6. Algorithm for differential diagnosis of ingested substances. This algorithm should be used when there is a history of ingestion and the ingested substance is not known. It should be used in conjunction with a complete history, physical examination, and appropriate laboratory studies.

Table 9–18. TOXIDROMES

Syndrome	Symptom	Agents
Anticholinergic	Psychosis, tachycardia, mydriasis, vasodilation, hyperpyrexia Gastrointestinal Urinary retention, decreased salivation Decreased sweating Agitation, seizures Amnesia	Phenothiazines Antihistamines Tricyclic antidepressants Antiparkinsonian agents Anticholinergics
Cholinergic	Decreased level of consciousness Pinpoint pupils, fasciculations Salivation, lacrimation, bronchorrhea Incontinence Bradycardia	Organophosphates Carbamates Nicotine
Opioids	Depressed sensorium Hypotension Hypothermia Pinpoint pupils	Heroin Meperidine Fentanyl Morphine Lomotil Darvon
Sympathomimetic	Tachypnea, diaphoresis, agitation, hallucinations, hyperreflexia Dilated pupils Tachycardia, hypertension, dysrhythmia	Cocaine (including "crack") Theophylline Caffeine Amphetamines
Sedative/hypnotic	Depressed sensorium, hyperreflexia Depressed ventilation Dilated pupils, hypothermia Hypotension	Barbiturates Chloral hydrate Others

SALICYLATES

The characteristics of salicylate intoxication are listed in Table 9–19. Oral ingestion is most common, but transdermal absorption can occur, especially of methylsalicylate (oil of wintergreen). Peak plasma levels are usually found within the first 12 hours. Early hyperpnea resulting in respiratory alkalosis may proceed to metabolic acidosis. In severe cases, cerebral edema and increased intracranial pressure may develop. In most circumstances, forced alkaline diuresis is adequate, with frequent monitoring and treatment of electrolyte disturbances. Intravenous hydration with a solution containing 5% dextrose in 0.45% normal saline to which 77 mEq/L sodium bicarbonate has been added provides isotonic fluid replacement and urinary alkalinization. Fluid rates in excess of daily maintenance fluid requirements may be used cautiously to increase urinary clearance. In severe cases marked by very high salicylate levels (>50 μg/mL), hemodialysis may be necessary. Cerebral edema must be assessed radiographically via computed tomography scan. Loop diuretics such as *furosemide* may be useful in both aiding salicylate clearance and treating cerebral edema.

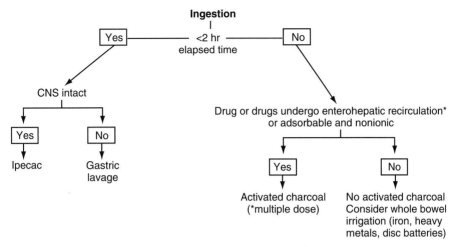

Figure 9–7. Algorithm for limiting absorption of toxins. This algorithm should be used to help determine the best method or methods to limit absorption of ingested toxic substances. Note that multiple-dose activated charcoal instillation should be reserved for agents that undergo enterohepatic recirculation.

ACETAMINOPHEN

Patients with acetaminophen intoxication may demonstrate one or more of the characteristic stages during the course of their illness (Fig. 9–8). Early symptoms may be quite mild. A serum acetaminophen level obtained 4 hours after ingestion should be plotted with the use of the Rumack-Matthew nomogram (Fig. 9–9). Serial acetaminophen level determinations are not clinically useful. *Patients with levels indicating probable toxicity should receive* N-*acetylcysteine.* An initial bolus of 140 mg/kg N-acetylcysteine should be followed every 4 hours with 17

Table 9–19. SALICYLATE INTOXICATION: FAST FACTS

Route of ingestion	Usually oral
Toxic dose	>250 mg/kg
Peak plasma level	8 to 12 hr (may be prolonged to 24 hr in very large ingestion)
Toxic level	>2 μg/mL
Symptoms	Vomiting, dehydration
	Tinnitus
	Hyperpnea (early)
	Metabolic acidosis
	Agitation, disorientation, seizures
	Respiratory failure, lethargy (late)
Treatment	Adequate hydration
	Forced alkaline diuresis
	Electrolyte replacement
	Dialysis

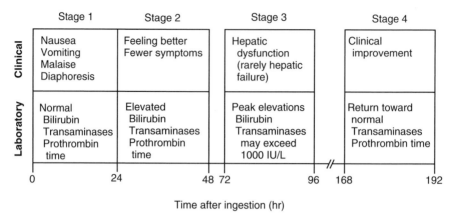

	Stage 1	Stage 2	Stage 3	Stage 4
Clinical	Nausea Vomiting Malaise Diaphoresis	Feeling better Fewer symptoms	Hepatic dysfunction (rarely hepatic failure)	Clinical improvement
Laboratory	Normal Bilirubin Transaminases Prothrombin time	Elevated Bilirubin Transaminases Prothrombin time	Peak elevations Bilirubin Transaminases may exceed 1000 IU/L	Return toward normal Transaminases Prothrombin time

0   24   48   72   96   168   192

Time after ingestion (hr)

Figure 9–8. Time-line for clinical stages of acetaminophen toxicity. Time intervals are indicative of usual time sequence, but they may vary in individual cases.

additional doses of 70 mg/kg each. Hepatic function should be assessed early and then followed daily. If no hepatic dysfunction develops within 48 to 72 hours, there is little likelihood that substantial hepatic injury will occur. Should marked hepatic failure develop, supportive management may be necessary. Fortunately, in most instances *N*-acetylcysteine administration will prevent severe hepatic injury.

IRON

Like acetaminophen, iron poisoning occurs in stages, although not all patients will manifest each stage. The initial gastrointestinal stage occurs soon after inges-

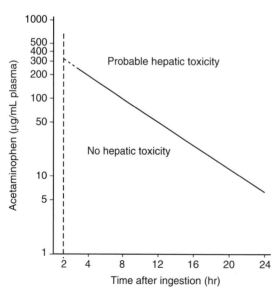

Figure 9–9. Rumack-Matthew nomogram. The serum acetaminophen level drawn 4 hours after an ingestion is most clinically useful. Levels drawn before 2 hours should not be interpreted. Patients with levels indicating probable hepatic toxicity should be administered *N*-acetylcysteine (see text). (Redrawn from Rumack BH, Matthew H: Acetaminophen poisoning and toxicity. Pediatrics 55:873, 1975.)

tion and is marked by abdominal pain and vomiting (Table 9–20) as well as by diarrhea and gastrointestinal hemorrhage. A quiescent period may begin as early as 4 hours after ingestion and continue for 48 hours. This stable period may then be followed by circulatory derangements due to volume depletion, capillary leak syndrome, hemorrhage, metabolic acidosis, and other signs of shock. Coagulopathy may enhance the bleeding diathesis, leading to further cardiovascular deterioration. Hepatic necrosis represents the fourth stage. Although rare, fulminant hepatic failure may be fatal if not reversed. Liver transplantation may be necessary to avoid death when hepatic injury becomes irreversible. A fifth stage characterized by gastrointestinal obstruction may follow as a result of scarring after corrosive injuries. This usually does not develop until several weeks elapse. Treatment is outlined in Table 9–21.

TRICYCLIC ANTIDEPRESSANTS

Tricyclic compounds produce a number of cardiovascular, respiratory, and central nervous system effects due to their complex pharmacology and uptake into the central nervous system (Fig. 9–10). Tricyclic antidepressants alter central and peripheral nervous system neurotransmitter uptake and release, leading to changes in autonomic function. *Anticholinergic symptoms,* including flushing, dry mouth, and mydriasis (pupillary dilation), occur early and are often followed by urinary retention. A *depressed sensorium* may develop. *Cardiovascular changes are "quinidine-like" and include dysrhythmias, vasodilation, and reduced cardiac output.* Dysrhythmias may appear suddenly and include premature ventricular contractions and ventricular fibrillation. Tricyclic antidepressants have a variable physiologic half-life that may be as long as 80 hours. Free drug is favored by acid pH. It is the free drug moiety that is responsible for most symptoms. Therefore, systemic

Table 9–20. FIVE CLINICAL PHASES OF IRON POISONING

1. *Gastrointestinal phase: within several hours of ingestion*
   Vomiting, diarrhea, hematochezia, abdominal pain
   Severe cases: fluid loss, bleeding, shock (hypotension, tachycardia, acidosis)
   Occasionally: fever, lethargy, coma
2. *Quiescent phase: 4–48 hr*
   Clinical improvement
   Subtle hemodynamic changes: tachycardia, decreased urine output
3. *Circulatory disturbances: 48–96 hr*
   Metabolic acidosis, hypotension, low cardiac output
   Coagulopathy and bleeding
   Multiorgan system failure
4. *Hepatic failure: 96 hr*
   May develop fulminant hepatic failure (rare)
   Mortality increases
5. *Bowel obstruction: 2–6 weeks*
   Gastric outlet or small bowel obstruction
   May develop without previous signs of circulatory or hepatic failure

Table 9–21. THERAPY FOR IRON POISONING

1. *Gastric decontamination*
   Forced emesis if within previous 2 hr
   Gastric lavage with 5% sodium bicarbonate: leave last aliquot in stomach
   No activated charcoal
2. *Secure IV line for those with symptoms*
3. *Measure initial and 4-hr serum iron levels and total iron-binding capacity*
4. *Chelate with deferoxamine for serum levels >300 mg/dL*
   Stable patients: level <500 mg/dL give 40 mg/kg IM
   Unstable, bleeding: level >500 mg/dL
      Give 20 mL/kg bolus of isotonic fluid; **then**
      Give 15 mg/kg IV over 1 hr; **then**
      Run as continuous drip at 15 mg/kg/hr
      Continue until "vin rose" color in urine disappears
5. *Monitor*
   If unstable (with IV deferoxamine)
      Systemic blood pressure
      ECG
      If hypotensive, central venous pressure
   Watch for signs of hepatic failure
      Bleeding
      Glucose imbalance
      Hyperammonemia
      Encephalopathy

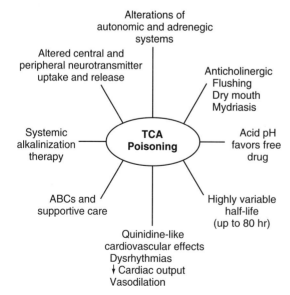

Figure 9–10. Pathophysiologic, pharmacokinetic and clinical information pertinent to acute intoxication from tricyclic antidepressants (TCA). The complex nature of this group of agents makes understanding these principles paramount for optimal patient management.

Table 9–22. STREET DRUGS

	Cocaine "Crack"	Marijuana "Mary Jane" "Weed"	Stimulants "Speed" "Black Beauties"	PCP "Angel Dust"
Route of ingestion	Inhalation, intravenous, intranasal	Inhalation (smoking), ingestion (eating, drinking)	Inhalation, ingestion (oral), intranasal, intravenous, subcutaneous	Oral ingestion, intranasal, intravenous
Central nervous system findings	Headache, dizziness, agitation, dysphoria, confusion, pupillary dilation, hyperreflexia	Confusion, short-term memory loss, pupillary constriction, nystagmus, tremor, decreased coordination, ataxia	Agitation/dilated pupils, irritability, anxiety, paranoia, hallucinations, seizures, intracranial hemorrhage, coma	Tremor, agitation, nystagmus, panic, violent behavior, delusions, dystonia
Cardiovascular findings	Tachycardia, supraventricular tachycardia, ventricular tachycardia, ventricular fibrillation, congestive heart failure, sudden death	Tachycardia	Dysrhythmias, hypertension, tachycardia	Diaphoresis, hypertension, tachycardia
Respiratory findings	Pulmonary edema, pneumothorax, bronchospasm			
Other findings	Chest pain, hyperthermia, rhabdomyolysis	Hypothermia, conjunctivitis, increased appetite, ingestion frequently complicated by other intoxicants (PCP, cocaine, alcohol)	Chest pain, abdominal pain, hyperthermia, palpitations, rhabdomyolysis	Signs and symptoms change rapidly and unpredictably
Therapy	Basic life, support, benzodiazepines for agitation/seizures, cooling and neuromuscular blockade for hyperthermia	Supportive care, benzodiazepines	Supportive care, benzodiazepines for agitation/seizures	Benzodiazepines for seizures, forced diuresis

alkalinization with the use of sodium bicarbonate should be used for any symptomatic patient. Further therapy should be supportive. Cardiovascular monitoring is warranted for 48 to 72 hours for those with mild symptoms from documented tricyclic antidepressant ingestion.

"STREET DRUGS"

With cocaine readily available, especially in the "crack" form, this widely variable group of agents produces varying degrees of toxicity. Cocaine intoxication frequently causes cardiovascular and central nervous system alterations, with many fatal cases reported. Table 9–22 lists several common illicit drugs and their symptom complexes, routes of intoxication, and recommended therapeutic interventions.

Prognosis

With attention paid to the ABCs, proper diagnosis, early supportive measures, and, in certain instances, specific pharmacologic interventions, prognosis is usually excellent. Poisoning in patients with massive overdoses and those who go undetected may be fatal. As causes of mortality, iron and tricyclic antidepressant ingestions are of particular concern.

BIBLIOGRAPHY

Lovejoy FH, Shannon M, Woolf AD: Recent advances in clinical toxicology. Curr Prob Pediatr 22:119, 1992.
Pearson-Shaver AL, Steinhart CM: Evaluation of the poisoned child. In Holbrook PR (ed): Textbook of Pediatric Critical Care. Philadelphia, WB Saunders, 1993, pp. 982–997.
Steinhart CM, Pearson-Shaver AL: Poisoning. Crit Care Clin 4:845, 1988.

9.6 Diabetic Ketoacidosis

PAUL R. ATKISON, MD, PhD, FRCP(C)

Diabetic ketoacidosis (DKA) is the result of complex metabolic derangements caused by insufficient insulin and increased levels of glucagon, catecholamines, glucocorticosteroids, and growth hormone (counterregulatory hormones). The lack of insulin may be relative or absolute. A precise biochemical definition is difficult but usually includes the following:

- *Ketones.* Serum ketone levels of >3 mmol/L or ketonuria or a positive nitroprusside reaction in a 1:2 dilution of serum.
- *Acid-Base.* Arterial (or capillary) pH < 7.3 and/or serum HCO_3^- of <15 mmol/L (or mEq/L) with a PCO_2 of <40 mm Hg. Rarely, pH may be higher, as with diuretic use, but this is uncommon in children.
- *Hyperglycemia.* Blood glucose of >15 mmol/L or 4+ glucose. *In some situations, blood glucose may be lower and even normal.*

Pathophysiology

Insulin is the primary anabolic hormone in the body, and insulinopenia results in severe metabolic and fluid disturbances, with DKA being the most serious (Fig. 9–11).

HORMONAL CHANGES IN DIABETIC KETOACIDOSIS

The physiologic effects of the hormones involved in DKA are summarized in Table 9–23. A decreased insulin level leads to increased levels of the counterregulatory hormones; these may increase further with stress. Thus, stress may cause a relative insulin deficiency. The net effect will be an increase in plasma glucose, leading to osmotic diuresis and hypovolemia, which will further increase catecholamine levels. *Hypovolemia is therefore an important factor in the evolution of DKA.* Hyperglycemia exacerbates the insulinopenia by increasing insulin resistance and decreasing any residual insulin secretion.

Figure 9–11. Metabolic consequences of the hormonal changes in diabetic ketoacidosis.

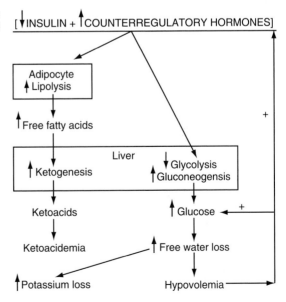

Table 9–23. SUMMARY OF THE PHYSIOLOGIC EFFECTS OF THE MAJOR HORMONES IN DKA ON CARBOHYDRATE, FAT, AND PROTEIN METABOLISM

Hormone	Substrate		
	Glucose	*Fat*	*Protein*
Insulin	↑ Glycogen synthesis ↓ Gluconeogenesis ↑ Glucose utilization	↑ Lipogenesis ↓ Lipolysis	↑ Protein synthesis
Glucagon	↑ Glycogenolysis ↑ Gluconeogenesis	↑ Lipolysis ↑ Ketogenesis (liver)	
Catecholamines	↑ Glycogenolysis	↑ Lipolysis	
Growth hormones, glucocorticoids	↑ Gluconeogenesis	↑ Ketogenesis (liver)	

METABOLIC CONSEQUENCES OF ALTERED HORMONAL STATE

The metabolic consequences of DKA are summarized (see Fig. 9–11) and elaborated below.

Hyperglycemia. Absent or decreased insulin with increased counterregulatory hormones results in increased glycogenolysis, gluconeogenesis, and decreased glucose utilization. Hyperglycemia causes an osmotic diuresis, resulting in hypovolemia, which in turn will decrease renal output and thereby decreasing renal glucose clearance. This will further exacerbate the hyperglycemia. In some situations, DKA may develop with normal glycemia to moderate hyperglycemia (e.g., fasting or minimal insulin).

Ketones. Concomitantly, lipolysis accelerates increasing plasma free fatty acids. These in turn are metabolized in the liver to ketone bodies at a rate that exceeds the capacity to metabolize them. Most of the ketone bodies are ketoacids, resulting in ketoacidemia.

Acid-Base Disturbances. Increased ketoacidemia results in an anion gap metabolic acidosis, which may be exacerbated by lactic acidosis from hypovolemia. In addition, it is clear that many patients with DKA will have varying degrees of coexistent hyperchloremic metabolic acidosis at presentation, and most will develop a degree of hyperchloremic metabolic acidosis during treatment. Usually, this is not a concern, and it will resolve on its own within a few days. *The degree of acidosis is not related to the severity of hyperglycemia. The acidemia takes longer to correct and requires continuing insulin therapy.*

Electrolyte Disturbances. *Potassium* is always depleted, and patients will have lost 3 to 5 mEq/kg. However, the initial serum K^+ is often increased due to acidosis, possible glucagon-stimulated hepatic K^+ release, decreased renal clearance due to azotemia, and decreased insulin-stimulated hepatic uptake of K^+. Once therapy for DKA begins, the serum K^+ will decrease as the acidemia resolves. Insulin increases the cellular uptake of K^+, and fluid therapy will increase renal loss.

Sodium is usually decreased at the outset due to dilution from glucose. It is important to calculate the true sodium; *if the patient is hypernatremic, then fluid replacement should be more gradual and the serum sodium should be reduced gradually.*

Phosphate is always depleted, although usually this is not clinically important unless it is very low. Provision of phosphate in the therapeutic regimen (as potassium phosphate) provides an alternative to chloride, thus decreasing the degree of hyperchloremia during therapy. *The disadvantage of phosphate therapy* is its precipitation with calcium, causing hypocalcemia. This may be exacerbated in the presence of hypomagnesemia, which will interfere with calcium mobilization. Therefore, if phosphate is used, it should be infused at a slow rate.

Magnesium and *calcium* are also depleted; however, they usually do not present a problem except as noted above, and replenishment will occur through normal diet.

Differential Diagnosis

The diagnosis of DKA should not be difficult except in children with new-onset diabetes. *Septicemia, pneumonia, uremia, methanol ingestion, or acetylsalicylic acid toxicity are other diagnoses that should be considered. Alcoholic ketoacidosis may occur in adolescents.*

CAUSES OF DIABETIC KETOACIDOSIS

Determining the cause of DKA is critical in management; causes include the following:

- New-onset diabetes
- Infection
- Intentional omission of insulin, particularly in adolescents
- Accidental omission as might occur with the use of subcutaneous insulin pumps; inappropriate decreases in insulin on sick days
- Concurrent steroid use or Cushing disease
- Hyperthyroidism
- Menstrual cycles are associated with increased risk of DKA, probably due to hormonal changes

Diagnosis

The diagnosis of DKA can often be made at the bedside. An appropriate history of diabetes with polyuria, polydipsia, and polyphagia along with weight loss will usually suggest the diagnosis. The presence of Kussmaul respirations and the typical odor of acetone in conjunction with an elevated blood glucose measurement and ketonuria will confirm the diagnosis. In a patient already receiving insulin, a blood sugar level of <15 mmol/L does not rule out the diagnosis. A lower-than-anticipated ketone measurement as measured with a urine test strip may reflect a high β-hydroxybutyrate concentration relative to acetoacetate acid. A serum measurement will clarify this.

Treatment

The following elements (summarized in Table 9–24) are essential to the successful treatment of DKA.

- General principles of resuscitation (i.e., ABCs)
- Fluid

Table 9–24. SUMMARY OF MANAGEMENT OF DKA

Treatment	Management
ABCs	Protect the airway Treat shock Determine underlying cause
Fluid	*Initial* 10 mL/kg normal saline in 1 hr (20 mL/kg rapidly if in shock) This may be repeated as necessary *Subsequent* Assume 10% dehydration Fluid replacement should be gradual (24–48 hr) **Maximum fluid administration 4 L/m²/day (including initial boluses)** Normal saline used from 1 to 6 hr; then 50% normal saline Continue intravenous fluids until oral fluids are well tolerated and the metabolic defects are corrected
Insulin	*Initial* IV: 0.1 unit/kg/hr CZI by continuous infusion IM: Load with 0.15 unit/kg IV and 0.15 unit/kg IM; then 0.1 unit/kg/hr IM *Subsequent* Double if no improvement in glucose or pH by 3 hr Maximum glucose decline: 3 to 5 mmol/L/hr At 15 mmol/L glucose, add dextrose to intravenous solutions (up to 12.5%) as needed to maintain plasma glucose at 12–15 mmol/L Continue insulin regimen until the acidemia is corrected (pH > 7.3 and/or $HCO_3^- > 18$) Start subcutaneous insulin with a 1-hr overlap in the intravenous/intramuscular insulin
Potassium	Monitor ECG If the K^+ is <3.5 mEq/L, add 40 to 60 mEq/L; if 3.5 to 5, add 30 mEq/L; if >5.0, then hold K^+ replacement After 3–5 hr, half of K^+ replacement as K^+ phosphate
Bicarbonate	Only use bicarbonate (HCO_3^-) for pH <7.0 Increase pH to 7.1 or final bicarbonate to 12 mEq/L [mEq HCO_3^- = 12-measured $HCO_3^- \times 0.6 \times$ body weight (in kg)] Add HCO_3^- slowly maximum 50 mEq/500 mL IV solution (over 2–3 hr) Maximum HCO_3^- should be 50 mEq/500 mL IV solution

- Insulin
- Potassium and electrolyte replacement
- Bicarbonate
- Frequent clinical and laboratory monitoring

Initial Resuscitation. The *airway* should by secured in patients who present in coma with vomiting and/or hypoventilation (due to severe acidosis). Shock must be treated with fluid boluses as indicated below. Once these urgent problems have been addressed, attention can be focused on the metabolic derangements.

Fluid. Treatment of severe hypovolemia should be initiated before making detailed calculations of fluid deficits. Fluids will not improve the acidosis with the exception of a coexistent lactic acidosis. Recommendations for an initial fluid vary; however, both lactated Ringer's and isotonic saline are acceptable.

Initial. Initial treatment should be 10 mL/kg normal saline over 1 hour (20 mL/kg rapidly for shock). This may be repeated as necessary.

Subsequent Fluid Management

- Assume 10% dehydration (may be 15% in an infant).
- Water loss usually exceeds electrolyte loss due to osmotic diuresis.
- Fluid replacement should be gradual and uniform to minimize rapid changes in serum osmolarity, which may be associated with cerebral edema (see below).
- Hyperosmolarity and hypernatremia require slower fluid replacement (up to 48 hours).
- *Maximum fluid administration should not exceed 4 L/m²/day (including initial boluses).*
- The fluid of choice over the first 6 hours is normal saline.
- Maintenance fluids are included in the usual way.
- In general, urinary losses should not be replaced unless excessive.
- The intravenous fluids may be switched to 45% saline after 4 to 6 hours.
- Continue administering intravenous fluids until the patient is tolerating oral fluids well and the metabolic defects are corrected (see below).

Insulin. The initiation of insulin therapy is not urgent, and there are some advantages to waiting 1 to 2 hours. The serum glucose will decrease as a result of fluid therapy due to dilution of the serum glucose, increase in the renal glucose clearance, and decrease in the counterregulatory hormone levels. Finally, improvement in peripheral perfusion will mobilize any subcutaneous insulin. Therefore, temporary withholding of insulin may stabilize the glucose and result in a more predictable decline in serum glucose once insulin therapy begins. Intravenous or intramuscular insulin is acceptable; however, the use of intravenous insulin may have advantages. Intramuscular insulin may be inappropriate due to poor or erratic absorption in a setting of shock. *Subcutaneous insulin has no role in DKA.*

Initial Insulin Dosing

- *Intravenous.* The intravenous dosage is 0.1 unit/kg/hr by continuous infusion with a separate infusion pump. Prepare by diluting 1 unit regular

(CZI) insulin/10 mL of normal saline and run at a rate equal to the patient's body weight in kg/hr = 0.1 unit/kg/hr.
- *Intramuscular*: The intramuscular route should not be used initially in the presence of shock or other contraindications such as a coagulopathy. The *loading dose* is 0.15 unit/kg IV or 0.15 unit/kg IM; thereafter, 0.1 unit/kg/hr IM can be administered.

Subsequent Insulin Management

- The glucose will require 1 to 2 hours to begin to decline, and pH will take 1 to 3 hours before improvement is seen.
- If no improvement in either parameter is seen by 3 hours, then the dose of insulin should be doubled.
- Glucose should decrease no faster than 3 to 5 mmol/L/hr; if it is faster, then decrease the insulin by one half or add glucose to the intravenous line.
- Correction of the glucose will generally take 4 to 6 hours to obtain a glucose of 15 mmol/L.
- pH will generally take longer (8 to 12 hours).
- Initially, the glucose should be monitored every hour.
- Once the blood glucose falls to ≈15 mmol/L, this should be maintained by adding up to 12.5% dextrose to the intravenous solutions. Higher glucose may result in more rapid correction of the ketogenesis.
- *The intravenous or intramuscular insulin regimen is continued until the acidemia is corrected. pH should be >7.3 and/or the bicarbonate should be >18 mmol/L. This is primary in treating DKA; correction of glucose is secondary.*
- *Subcutaneous insulin* should be restarted by allowing a 1-hour overlap with intravenous or intramuscular insulin.
- In an established diabetic, the previous dose (if appropriate) should be used; in the new diabetic, start with 0.3 to 0.5 unit/kg/day with two thirds administered in the morning and one third administered in the evening. Increase the dose as necessary to 1 unit/kg/day.

Electrolytes. Potassium is the main electrolyte abnormality. The initial K^+ may be elevated, and a good urine output should be present before K^+ is included in the intravenous solutions. The amount of replacement should be guided by the serum K^+.

- If the K^+ is <3.5 mEq/L, add 40 to 60 mEq/L. If ECG changes are present, this may require K^+ bolusing, which should not exceed 1 mEq/kg/hr.
- If the K^+ is 3.5 to 5, add 30 mEq/L.
- If the K^+ is >5.0, then hold K^+ replacement.
- After 3 to 5 hours, one half of the K^+ replacement may be given as potassium phosphate. Phosphate may precipitate with calcium, resulting in hypocalcemia; therefore, the calcium should be monitored.

Bicarbonate Therapy. The guidelines vary widely for bicarbonate use in DKA. Severe acidemia (pH <7.0) may cause problems; however, caution should be exercised with bicarbonate therapy due to potential adverse effects. Increasing the pH with bicarbonate will further decrease serum potassium levels, decrease tissue delivery of oxygen, and increase the hypophosphatemia. A change in serum pH that is too rapid may cause a paradoxic decrease in cerebrospinal fluid pH due to the differential permeability of carbon dioxide and bicarbonate at the blood-brain barrier. Also, bicarbonate will increase the sodium load during therapy. Furthermore, ketoacids are a source of bicarbonate and are converted during therapy. Thus, a small predicted correction through the addition of bicarbonate may result in a too-rapid correction of pH as additional bicarbonate is formed from ketoacid precursors.

Therefore, bicarbonate infusions should be used only for severe acidemia with pH <7.0 and only to increase to pH ≤7.1 or increase the final bicarbonate concentration to 12 mEq/L as determined by the following formula:

Bicarbonate (mEq) = (12 − measured bicarbonate) × 0.6 × body weight (kg)

The bicarbonate should be added slowly (over 2 to 3 hours) with no more than 50 mEq/500 mL IV solution unless there are significant adverse affects from the acidemia, in which case a bolus of bicarbonate may be required.

Careful Clinical Monitoring. Successful management of patients with DKA requires careful and frequent monitoring and reassessment. Neurologic status and vital signs should be monitored every 20 to 30 minutes during the initial hours of therapy and then every hour. A flow sheet should be established to monitor the clinical signs and essential laboratory investigations (Table 9–25).

Complications

There are several complications of DKA, including cerebral edema, adult respiratory distress syndrome, coagulation abnormalities, rhabdomyolysis, and mu-

Table 9–25. SAMPLE FLOW SHEET FOR CLINICAL MONITORING OF PATIENTS WITH DKA

	Hours of Treatment												
	0	*1*	*2*	*3*	*4*	*5*	*6*	*7*	*8*	*9*	*10*	*11*	*12*
Neurologic signs													
Vital signs													
Glucose								X		X		X	
pH		X		X		X		X	X	X		X	X
Pco$_2$		X		X		X		X	X	X		X	X
HCO$_3^-$		X		X		X		X	X	X		X	X
Anion gap		X		X		X		X	X	X		X	X
Lactate		X	X	X	X	X	X	X	X	X	X	X	X
K$^+$, Na$^+$, Cl$^-$								X		X		X	
Ca^{2+}, Mg^{2+}, PO$_4^{2-}$		X	X	X	X	X	X	X	X	X	X	X	X
β-Hydroxybutyrate	X	X	X	X	X	X	X	X	X	X	X	X	X
ECG							X	X	X	X	X	X	X

Continue until patient's metabolic status is corrected. Note that neurologic and vital signs are checked every 30 min until stable; otherwise, each parameter is monitored at the times indicated by the empty boxes. The duration and frequency of monitoring must be individualized.

cormycosis. The most important of these is *cerebral edema,* which is an infrequent but serious complication of DKA and is more common in children than in adults. In particular, this is most often seen in young children with new-onset diabetes and in adolescent females. The mortality rate is 50% to 90%. It usually occurs 4 to 24 hours after the initiation of therapy, when the patient's biochemistry is improving. Signs and symptoms include the following:

- Decreasing level of consciousness
- Headache that is often sudden and severe
- Increased combativeness or disorientation
- Change in vital signs
- Visual disturbances
- Pupillary disturbances
- Papilloedema
- Seizures

Frequent neurologic monitoring may allow early identification of and intervention in patients who are developing cerebral edema. *If these signs develop, the patient should receive mannitol (1 gm/kg) and an urgent computed tomography scan.* The presence of cerebral edema may require further neuroresuscitative measures, including hyperventilation and fluid restriction. *Fluid therapy should be decreased until cerebral edema resolves, and then further rehydration should be continued at a slower rate.*

The cause of cerebral edema is unknown, although at least one study has suggested that it is more likely to occur in patients who have had DKA present for longer periods of time and in patients with elevated serum osmolality. Thus, it is prudent to prolong fluid rehydration in these patients.

Summary

Successful management of DKA requires an understanding of the many abnormalities that are present and meticulous attention paid to detail. In particular, the patient requires frequent reassessment in terms of his or her clinical and biochemical status. Complications are infrequent, but if they occur, a favorable outcome may depend on early recognition and treatment.

BIBLIOGRAPHY

Bello FA, Sotos JF: Cerebral oedema in diabetic ketoacidosis in children. Lancet 336:64, 1990.
Fleckman AM: Diabetic ketoacidosis. Endocr Metab Clin North Am 22:181, 1993.
Krane EJ: Diabetic ketoacidosis: biochemistry, physiology, treatment and prevention. Pediatr Clin North Am 34:933, 1987.
Rosenbloom AL, Schatz DA: Diabetic ketoacidosis in childhood. Pediatr Ann 23:285, 1994.

9.7 Inherited Metabolic Disease

JONATHAN B. KRONICK, MD, PhD, FRCPC

Children admitted to the pediatric intensive care unit (PICU) with inborn errors of metabolism (IEM) are an uncommon but challenging group of patients. Most children presenting to the PICU with an undiagnosed IEM will present with symptoms and signs that are more commonly associated with other diagnoses. Because the sooner an IEM is recognized and appropriately managed, the better is the likelihood of a good outcome, it is essential that the physician has a *high index of suspicion for IEM*. This chapter discusses the approach to recognizing unsuspected IEM in the PICU and to initiating appropriate management until specialist consultation can be obtained.

Definition

IEM are disorders that are inherited in a mendelian or mitochondrial fashion in which the genetic mutation results in a metabolic or biochemical abnormality that leads to disease. Discussion is limited to IEM that can present acutely and therefore may require care in the PICU.

Pathophysiology

IEM usually result from a heritable deficiency of enzyme activity that affects a crucial step in intermediary metabolism. The normal metabolic pathway leading to the enzymatic conversion of a substrate to a product is blocked, either partially or completely, resulting in disease. Deficient enzyme activity may lead to disease due to substrate or alternate metabolite accumulating in toxic quantities, to a deficiency of an essential product, or to a combination of both of these mechanisms (Fig. 9–12). Classically, IEM present acutely in the neonatal period; however, it is now well recognized that many IEM with variable phenotypes can initially present well after the neonatal period.

Children with IEM may have a long period of apparent good health before sudden catastrophic deterioration. Metabolic decompensation and sudden illness are often precipitated by an otherwise trivial intercurrent infection, a change in diet, or fasting. Also, sudden increases in substrate availability (such as a high-protein meal in a child with a urea cycle defect) leading to a rapid increase in toxic substrate accumulation (e.g., ammonia) can lead to sudden severe illness in a previously well child.

NORMAL

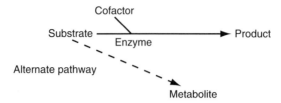

INBORN ERROR OF METABOLISM (deficiency of enzyme)

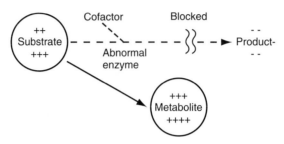

Disease may be due to toxic substrate and/or metabolite accumulation, product deficiency, or a combination of the above.

Figure 9–12. Paradigm of possible mechanisms of disease in an inborn error of metabolism.

Differential Diagnosis

Children presenting to the PICU with an unsuspected IEM generally have nonspecific symptoms that are more commonly due to infectious, traumatic, or toxic etiologies. It is only after these more common causes are eliminated from the differential diagnosis that an IEM is considered. It is therefore important that the clinician has a high index of suspicion and carefully considers factors that may be clues to the presence of a previously unrecognized IEM.

HISTORICAL CLUES

Previous episodes of a similar acute illness in the affected child or a family history of a similar illness is suggestive. The presence of *consanguinity* suggests autosomal recessive inheritance, whereas a history of affected males on the maternal side suggest X-linked inheritance. Maternal inheritance suggests a mitochondrially mediated disorder. The association of symptoms with changes in diet, fasting, or the presence of a peculiar odor suggests an IEM. The *dietary history* should be obtained in detail. Subtle findings, such as the child who self-selects a low-protein diet, may be a clue to an IEM in which protein metabolism is abnormal. Burgundy-colored urine should raise the possibility of acute intermittent porphyria.

PHYSICAL EXAMINATION CLUES

Most IEM do not have unique findings on physical examination; however, the presence of an *unusual odor* on the child's breath, in the urine, or the cerumen should suggest an IEM (probably an organic acidopathy). *Hepatosplenomegaly* may be associated with a storage disorder, *hypotonia* with metabolic myopathies, *ocular findings* such as cataracts in galactosemia, dislocated lens in homocystinuria, and occasionally *dysmorphic features* in peroxisomal disorders and pyruvate dehydrogenase deficiency.

CLINICAL PRESENTATION

Examples of common acute presentations of selected IEM are given in Table 9–26. The most common type of presenting symptom is neurologic, with abnormalities of level of consciousness with or without seizures being the most frequent. A child with an acute encephalopathy in the absence of trauma, exogenous intoxication, or infection should be suspected of having a possible IEM. Acute or acute-on-chronic muscle weakness, neuropathy, and stroke are also recognized presentations of IEM. Shock and acute cardiac failure can be due to an IEM, particularly the organic acidopathies and mitochondrial myopathies. Gram-negative sepsis associated with shock is a well-known presentation of infants with galactosemia. Severe myopathy leading to respiratory failure has been associated with disorders involving carnitine and the respiratory chain, whereas near-miss sudden infant death syndrome has been most frequently associated with medium-

Table 9–26. ACUTE PRESENTATIONS OF UNSUSPECTED METABOLIC DISEASE

Presentation	Example
Neurologic	
Coma	Urea cycle, organic acidopathy
Seizures	Organic acidopathy
Stroke	Mitochondrial encephalopathy lactic acidosis and strokes (MELAS)
Weakness	Porphyria, tyrosinemia, oxphos
Cardiovascular	
Shock	Adrenoleukodystrophy, oxphos, adrenogenital syndrome
Cardiomyopathy	Glycogen storage, oxphos, organic acidopathy
Sepsis	Galactosemia
Respiratory	
Aborted sudden infant death syndrome	Medium-chain acyldehydrogenase deficiency, organic acidopathy
Severe myopathy	Carnitine, oxphos
Gastrointestinal	
Liver failure	Wilson disease, galactosemia, tyrosinosis
Pancreatitis	Organic acidopathy

Oxphos, disorders of oxidation phosphorylation.

chain acyl-CoA dehydrogenase deficiency as well as other less frequent IEM. Acute liver failure and pancreatitis have been associated with a variety of IEM.

BIOCHEMICAL CLUES

When other causes have been excluded, certain findings on routine biochemistry should suggest the possibility of an IEM (Table 9–27). Hypoglycemia can be due to many causes other than IEM; however, it is a frequent finding in disorders affecting mitochondrial function and both gluconeogenesis and glycogen synthesis. Metabolic acidosis associated with an elevated anion gap is a frequent finding in many IEM (Fig. 9–13). Lactic acidosis that is not secondary to inadequate tissue oxygen delivery is often a nonspecific biochemical marker of an IEM (Fig. 9–14). Hyperammonemia in the absence of liver failure strongly suggests a possible IEM. Isolated hyperammonemia unassociated with other metabolic abnormalities, such as acidosis, ketosis, or hypoglycemia, strongly suggests a disorder of one of the five steps of the urea cycle (Fig. 9–15). Electrolyte disturbances may suggest an IEM, particularly the combination of hyponatremia and hyperkalemia in a dehydrated infant (salt-losing adrenogenital syndrome). The presence of ketonemia and ketonuria can be a normal finding in the fasting state; however, in a setting otherwise suggesting an IEM, ketosis may be of significance. Ketosis in the neonatal period is very strongly suggestive of an IEM. On rare occasions, acute pancytopenia has been associated with organic acidopathies.

LABORATORY INVESTIGATIONS

Table 9–28 outlines the approach to investigating a child with a suspected IEM. When screening investigations (see above) or the clinical picture is suggestive of an IEM, additional secondary investigations are indicated. Additional, more-specific investigations should be done in consultation with a metabolic specialist and may require the use of laboratories in specialized institutions. In some cases, a specific diagnosis can be tentatively made on the basis of the secondary investiga-

Table 9–27. ROUTINE BIOCHEMICAL FINDINGS THAT MAY BE CLUES TO A POSSIBLE INBORN ERROR OF METABOLISM

Finding	Example
Hypoglycemia	Respiratory chain disorders, glycogen storage disease
Anion gap metabolic acidosis	Organic acidopathy
Lactic acidosis	Respiratory chain disorder
Hyperammonemia	Urea cycle defect
Hyponatremia/hyperkalemia	Adrenogenital syndrome
Ketonemia/ketonuria	Organic acidopathy
Pancytopenia	Organic acidopathy

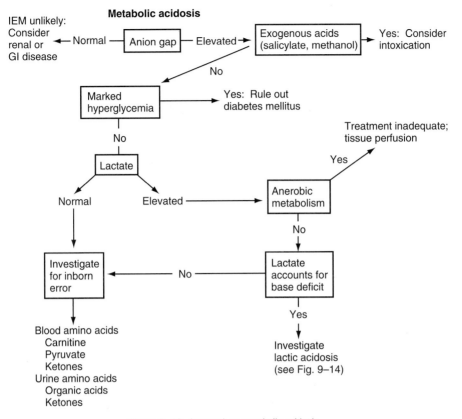

Figure 9–13. Approach to metabolic acidosis.

tions outlined; however, it is frequent that tertiary investigations must be undertaken either to confirm the diagnosis or, in particularly challenging cases, to reach a probable diagnosis. The approach to investigation of an elevated anion gap metabolic acidosis, lactic acidosis, and hyperammonemia is outlined (see Figs. 9–12 through 9–14). In all situations, it is strongly recommended that when an IEM is being seriously considered, specialist consultation should be obtained for both investigation and management of the patient.

Management

Children with acute decompensation of IEM require *appropriate supportive care,* including *treatment of precipitating factors* such as infections as well as any complications that arise (Table 9–29). Many IEM presenting with acute neurologic symptoms are associated with *raised intracranial pressure,* and this serious complication must be recognized and managed appropriately.

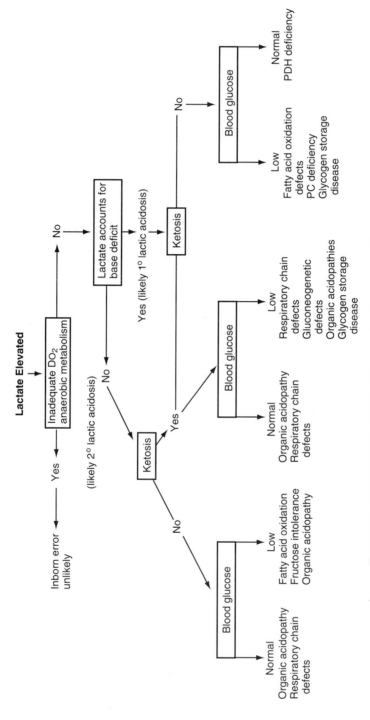

Figure 9–14. Approach to lactic acidosis. PDH, pyruvate dehydrogenase; PC, pyruvate carboxylase.

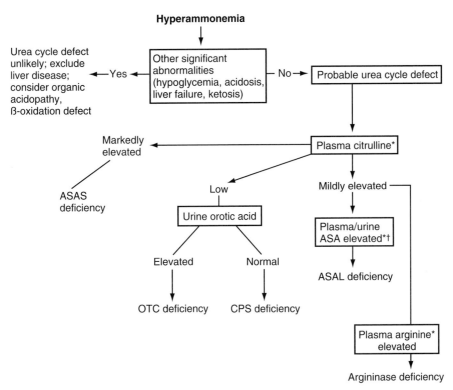

Figure 9–15. Approach to hyperammonemia. ASAS, argininosuccinic acid synthetase; OTC, ornithine transcarbamylase; CPS, carbamyl phosphate synthetase; ASAL, argininosuccinic acid lyase; ASA, argininosuccinic acid. *Citrulline, arginine, and ASA measured by plasma amino acids. †ASA measured by urine amino acids.

The principles of managing an acute metabolic decompensation include efforts to minimize toxic substrate/metabolite accumulation and replacement of any deficient metabolic product (see Fig. 9–12 and Table 9–29). It is essential to prevent catabolism by providing adequate glucose and, usually, lipid calories to minimize the metabolic flux through the affected biochemical pathway. In selected disorders (e.g., maple syrup urine disease, urea cycle defects), special dietary and parenteral nutrition formulas are available to enhance caloric and nutrient intake. Efforts must be made to remove any source of exogenous substrate such as protein in the diet or in parenteral nutrition. In addition, efforts must be undertaken to rapidly and effectively remove accumulating toxic substrate or metabolites. Exchange transfusion has been used; however, dialysis, preferably hemodialysis, may be the most effective method of removing toxic substrates such as ammonia, lactic acid, or other organic acids. In selected disorders, specific metabolic strategies can be used to remove toxic accumulations, such as the use of sodium phenylacetate and sodium benzoate in patients with hyperammonemia. Situations in which replacement of deficient product is available are limited; however, many disorders are

GENERAL CRITICAL CARE

Table 9–28. APPROACH TO INVESTIGATIONS OF POSSIBLE INBORN ERRORS OF METABOLISM

Screening	Secondary*	Tertiary†

Glucose, electrolytes, blood gas, lactate, ammonia, complete blood count, urine ketones	Blood
	    Amino acids, lactate-to-
	        pyruvate ratio, carnitine,
	        β-hydroxybutyrate,
	        acetoacetate
	Urine
	    Organic acids, amino
	        acids, orotic acid
	Cerebrospinal fluid
	    Amino acids, lactate
		Enzyme assay, tissue biopsy molecular studies, very long-chain fatty acids, free fatty acids, loading studies

*Actual investigations will depend on clinical and laboratory findings. Additional investigations may be indicated in selected cases.
†In conjunction with metabolic disease specialist.

Table 9–29. GENERAL PRINCIPLES OF TREATMENT OF THE ACUTELY ILL CHILD WITH A POSSIBLE INBORN ERROR OF METABOLISM

Objective	Examples
Appropriate general supportive care: ABCs, and so on	Intermittent positive pressure ventilation, inotropes
Treat precipitating factors	Antibiotics, antipyretics
Treat complications (↑ ICP, seizures)	Control ICP, anticonvulsants
Minimize toxic substrate/metabolite accumulation:	
Prevent catabolism	Antipyretics: high glucose infusion with or without lipid infusion Withhold protein or other substrate source
Remove exogenous substrate Enhance substrate/metabolite elimination	
General	Exchange transfusion, dialysis, hemofiltration
Specific	Phenylacetate plus sodium benzoate (↑ NH₄); carnitine (MCAD)
Replace deficient product	
General	Glucose for hypoglycemia
Specific	Arginine (CPS, OTC)
Enhance residual enzyme activity: cofactor/vitamin therapy	Thiamine, riboflavin, biotin, pyridoxine, coenzyme Q, and so on

When a specific diagnosis is known, therapy must be tailored appropriately.
ICP, intracranial pressure; NH₄, ammonia; MCAD, medium chain acyl-CoA dehydrogenase deficiency; CPS, carbamoyl phosphate synthetase deficiency; OTC, ornithine transcarbamoylase deficiency.

Table 9–30. PERIMORTEM PROTOCOL

Samples To Be Obtained in Patient Dying of Suspected Inherited Metabolic Disease*	
Essential	*Optional*
Plasma/serum	Cerebrospinal fluid
Urine	Other tissues
Skin fibroblast culture	
White blood cells for DNA	
Liver	
Muscle	

*To be done in consultation with a metabolic disease specialist. Samples obtained will depend on the disorders being considered and previous investigations. Samples intended for possible enzymatic study or analysis of potentially unstable metabolites should be obtained as soon as possible and rapidly frozen in liquid nitrogen.

associated with hypoglycemia, and therefore glucose administration is essential in the vast majority of IEM. In selected specific disorders, product replacement is of benefit, including the use of arginine or citrulline supplements for some disorders of the urea cycle. Occasional IEM are responsive to vitamin or cofactor therapy that results in rapid biochemical and often clinical improvement. A variety of cofactors have been found to be of benefit, including thiamine, riboflavin, biotin, pyridoxine, and vitamin B_{12}. Cofactor therapy should be undertaken only with advice from a metabolic specialist.

Unfortunately, there are occasions when children present with fulminant metabolic decompensation secondary to an IEM and die before a definitive diagnosis is reached. Under these circumstances, it is imperative that appropriate samples be obtained to facilitate later diagnosis, reproductive counseling, and possible treatment for other affected family members. Table 9–30 outlines investigations that can be done before or immediately after death to obtain appropriate samples for later analysis.

Prognosis

The prognosis of children presenting acutely to the PICU with an IEM depends primarily on three factors: (1) the specific IEM involved, (2) the complications that arise, and (3) the rapidity with which a diagnosis is made and appropriate therapy is instituted. Children whose IEM is diagnosed and treated promptly have the best chance for a good outcome.

BIBLIOGRAPHY

Cunniff C, Cormack JL, Kirby RS, Fiser DH: Contribution of heritable disorders to mortality in the pediatric intensive care unit. Pediatrics 95:678, 1995.

Kronick JB, Scriver CR, Goodyer PR, Kaplan PB: A perimortem protocol for suspected genetic disease. Pediatrics 71:960, 1983.

Ozand PT, Gascon GG: Organic acidourias: a review. J Child Neurol 6:196, 288, 1991.
Saudubray JM, Charpentier C: Clinical phenotypes: diagnosis/algorithms. *In* Scriver CR, et al. (eds): The Metabolic and Molecular Basis of Inherited Disease. New York, McGraw-Hill, 1995, pp. 327–400.

9.8 Acute Pain Management

ALLAH B. HAAFIZ, MD
NIRANJAN KISSOON, MD, FCCM, FRCPC

Pain is defined by the International Association for the Study of Pain as *"an unpleasant sensory and emotional experience associated with actual or potential tissue damage, or described in terms of such damage."* Pain is a common accompaniment of many acute medical and surgical conditions. Although greatly helpful in the localization and diagnosis of disease, there are no physiologic advantages of pain. Instead, it contributes to the unfavorable pathophysiologic, emotional, and psychologic effects of the underlying disease. Moreover, relief of pain rather than definitive therapy is often the most important concern of the child. Despite its common occurrence and importance, children's pain is still widely underestimated and undertreated.

The common painful conditions encountered will vary depending on whether the patient is being treated in the critical care or emergency setting (Table 9–31). Regardless of the setting, appropriate pain assessment and relief are important for any child. Nonpharmacologic techniques like explanation, reassurance, distraction, and hypnosis can decrease the anxiety and improve cooperation. However, pharmacologic measures are the cornerstone of acute pain management. The drugs commonly used in pain management may be classified as an analgesic or a sedative depending on the primary effect. An *analgesic* relieves or reduces pain without an intentional sedative effect. *Sedatives,* on the other hand, induce a state of decreased awareness of the environment or pain perception. Application of clinical, pharmacologic, and technical knowledge should be in keeping with the guidelines of the American Academy of Pediatrics and the Pediatric Committee of the American College of Emergency Physicians. Discussion in this chapter is limited to clinical issues related to acute pain in an intensive care or emergency department setting.

Pathophysiology

The appreciation of pain sensation depends on nociceptive impulses, sensed by free nerve endings and a plexiform network of fibers and transmitted to the brain. These receptor nerve endings are present in virtually every tissue of the

Table 9–31. DIFFERENTIAL DIAGNOSIS OF ACUTE PAIN IN THE EMERGENCY
DEPARTMENT AND INTENSIVE CARE SETTINGS

Trauma (Major and Minor)
Lacerations
Bruises
Fractures
Major trauma (e.g., motor vehicle accident)

Postoperative
Congenital heart disease
Major developmental anomalies
Neurosurgical procedures
Major trauma

Medical Conditions
Vaso-occlusive sickle cell crisis
Pneumonia (pleuritic chest pain)
Meningitis (headache)
Otitis media (otalgia)
Peritonitis

Iatrogenic
Diagnostic procedures
   Lumbar puncture
   Bone marrow aspiration
   Venipuncture
Ancillary and therapeutic procedures
   Central venous and arterial lines
   Pleural and pericardial tube placements
   Pleural, pericardial, or peritoneal paracentesis
Enlarged, undetected urinary bladder
   Related to medications (e.g., anticholinergics, morphine)
   Central nervous system diseases
Gastric dilatation

The differential diagnosis of acute pain is infinite; only common conditions are outlined.
Postoperative pain is usually seen in the critical care unit, whereas other conditions are common in
   both the critical care and emergency setting.

body. Sharp and localized pain is transmitted by myelinated A delta fibers, whereas
unmyelinated C fibers transmit dull and diffuse pain. Products of tissue injury
such as serotonin, histamine, and bradykinin activate both types of fibers. The
pathway of somatic pain perception is depicted in Figure 9–16.

PLASTICITY OF NOCICEPTIVE SYSTEM

Modulation of pain starts at the entry of signals to the posterior horn of the
spinal cord. Multiple peripheral and descending inputs determine attenuation or
amplification of discharge patterns of dorsal horn cells. Selective activation of
abundant opioid receptors (Fig. 9–17) in this area "filters" central transmission of
nociceptive signals. Cortical influence on pain perception has dynamic implications. Biofeedback, hypnosis, and other psychotherapies help to decrease perception and response to pain.

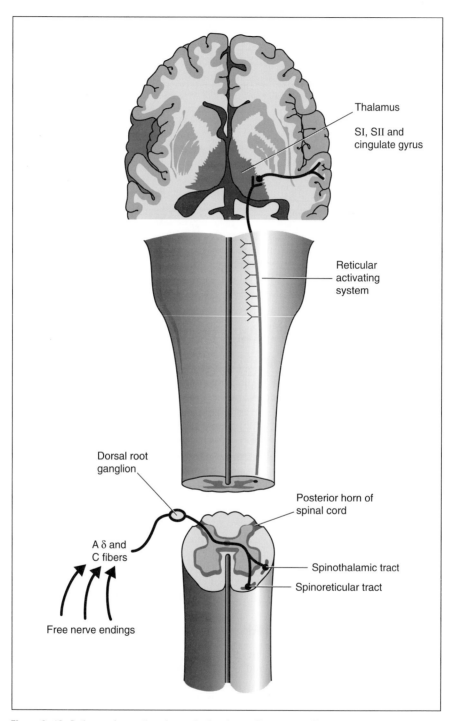

Figure 9–16. Pathway of somatic pain conduction from afferent nerve fibers to somatosensory cortex (SI and SII) in the parietal lobe and the cingulate gyrus of cerebral cortex.

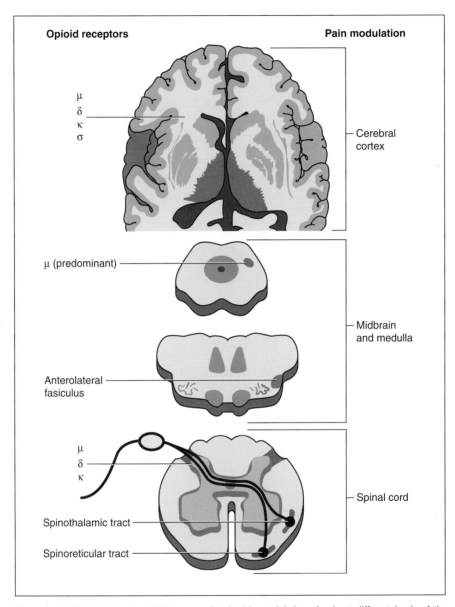

Figure 9–17. Distribution of opioid receptors involved in modulation of pain at different levels of the CNS from the spinal cord to the cerebral cortex. The μ receptors in the cortex are predominately μ_1. The different physiological and therapeutic effects produced by the activation of the opioid receptors are: μ_1, analgesia; μ_2, respiratory depression, physical dependence; κ, mild sedation, myosis; δ, analgesia, euphoria, physical dependence, respiratory depression; and σ, hallucination, depression.

NEUROENDOCRINE EFFECTS

Pain is associated with a dramatic stress-release response manifested by increased pancreatic, steroid, and pituitary hormones. As a result, the metabolic homeostasis is disrupted, with a trend to a negative nitrogen balance. An increased level of catecholamines in conjunction with a catabolic state (e.g., severe trauma) predisposes the patient to dysrhythmias, impaired immunologic function, metabolic acidosis and thromboembolic complications.

Differential Diagnosis

The etiology of acute pain in a patient in the emergency department or intensive care unit is usually obvious from the underlying condition. The most common scenarios requiring pain management in acute care settings are outlined in Table 9–31.

Although the causes of acute pain are fairly obvious, a common pitfall is the tendency of medical personnel to concentrate on the underlying disease and ignore the role of pain in the patient's comfort and his or her perception of the disease and therapy.

Laboratory Investigations

The cause of acute pain is usually obvious. Investigations should be focused to establish the underlying disease or its complication. However, pain should be in the differential diagnosis as a clinical entity in the event of an unexplained acute manifestation of sympathetic discharge such as tachycardia and hypertension. In addition, restlessness, hyperglycemia, and profuse sweating may also be manifestations of pain. Inadequate and inappropriate analgesia should be considered when these symptoms occur in patients already receiving analgesics.

Evaluation of Pain

The assessment of pain should be an integral component of a patient's evaluation. Pain is a multifaceted experience modified by a myriad of environmental and internal factors. Accordingly, optimum assessment of the degree of pain requires incorporation of subjective, behavioral, and physiologic responses. These responses are the function of age and cognitive level of the child, type of pain experienced, and the situation in which the pain occurred. There is no single clinical or laboratory technique available to quantify the degree of pain. Important components of the assessment of pain are outlined in Table 9–32.

Physiologic parameters like elevated heart rate and blood pressure are nonspecific indicators, and their relation to the intensity and duration of pain is not established. However, pain should be a serious consideration in the evaluation of an unexplained tachycardia or hypertension. The results of behavioral assessment tools such as Children's Hospital of Eastern Ontario Pain Scale (CHEOPS) or of

Table 9–32. METHODS OF DIRECT AND INDIRECT ACUTE PAIN ASSESSMENT

Physiologic Parameters
Heart rate
Blood pressure
Transcutaneous oxygen saturation
Palmar sweat response
Endorphin levels

Behavioral Assessment
Facial expressions
Cries
Body movements
Children's Hospital of Eastern Ontario Pain Scale (CHEOPS)
Observational Scale of Behavioral Distress

Direct Report Techniques
Pain questionnaires
Visual-Analogue Scales (VAS)
Pain thermometers
Interval scales (faces, poker chips)

Projective Methods
Drawings
Cartoons

The physiologic parameters (heart rate, respiratory rate, TSao$_2$ [transcutaneous oxygen tension], and palmar sweat response) should be assessed in all patients as part of the general examination. Behavioral assessment, direct report techniques, and projective methods represent more detailed assessments and should be adopted after appropriate inservice training.

direct reporting techniques such as visual-analogue scales (VASs) are a function of age and require in-depth training and appreciation of their usefulness before widespread use can occur in clinical practice.

PITFALLS OF ACUTE PAIN ASSESSMENT AND MANAGEMENT

As opposed to adults, children receive much less attention and treatment for pain. This differential attitude stems from lack of information and training and unfounded concepts of health care personnel about children's pain perception. Pain evaluation of infants is particularly difficult because of their inability to verbalize and a lack of clear, consistent, and reproducible assessment tools. These difficulties should increase the sensitivity of physicians in recognizing and treating the pain effectively as an issue equally important as the primary disease or condition.

Management

Acute pain relief is important because it is associated with deleterious physiologic, psychologic, and pathologic effects. Prompt attention to acute pain ensures patient satisfaction and can improve physiologic functioning. For example, the relief of pleuritic pain can improve tidal volume. Similarly, immunologic and metabolic derangements can be minimized and therefore lead to decreased complications and hasten recovery.

EMERGENCY DEPARTMENT

A multitude of conditions in which pain is a major factor (see Table 9–31) are seen in children who present to emergency departments. Diagnostic and therapeutic procedures are contributors to acute pain in the emergency setting. Therefore, pain control measures should be promptly instituted once relative cardiorespiratory stability is achieved. Although nonpharmacologic techniques facilitate cooperation, most acute nociceptive conditions require additional pharmacologic interventions. This may be due in part to the child's high level of anxiety and the lack of adequate time to prepare a child for the procedure.

Choice and route of the agent are dictated by *severity of pain, depth of sedation required,* and *general condition of the patient* (Table 9–33). Minor pain (e.g., acute pharyngitis, musculoskeletal pains) can be treated with *acetaminophen, aspirin,* or *ibuprofen*. Combinations of acetaminophen or aspirin with *codeine* or its semisynthetic analgesics, *hydrocodone* and *oxycodone*, are appropriate options

Table 9–33. COMMON CLINICAL EMERGENCY DEPARTMENT SCENARIOS ASSOCIATED WITH ACUTE PAIN AND APPROPRIATE CHOICE OF ANALGESICS

Pain Control Measure	Condition	Agent
Analgesia without sedation	Minor trauma	Acetaminophen*
	Abrasion	(PO/PR, 10–15 mg/kg)
	Contusion	
	Sprain	Ibuprofen
	Nondisplaced fracture	(PO, 5–10 mg/kg)
	Infections	Aspirin*
	Otitis media	(PO/PR, 10–15 mg/kg)
	Otitis externa	
	Pharyngitis	
Sedation without analgesia†	Improve cooperation	Chloral hydrate, midazolam,
	Computed tomography scan	diazepam
	Laceration repair under local anesthesia	
Sedation and analgesia†	Painful procedures	
	Complex laceration repair	Morphine and midazolam
	Foreign body extraction	
	Fracture reduction	Fentanyl
	Wound debridement	Morphine
	Abscess drainage	

*Also available as a combination with codeine, hydrocodone, and oxycodone. Combination with these opioids enhances potency and provides some sedation. Aspirin is used less frequently because of safer alternatives and its association with Reye syndrome.
†Routes, doses, and pharmacologic properties are outlined in Table 9–34 and 9–35.

for outpatient management of mild to moderate pain. Moderate to severe pain should be managed by parenteral routes, with more potent agents like opioids. *Parenteral opioid analgesics* should be liberally used in the emergency department for moderate to severe pain associated with fractures, burns, and invasive procedures. Competitive inhibition by *naloxone* makes opioids ideal for use in this setting because undesirable effects may be easily reversed. However, the effect of naloxone lasts for only half an hour, and the patient should not be discharged soon after its use. *Fentanyl* is rapidly acting, more potent than morphine and meperidine, and causes less respiratory depression. Lower doses of fentanyl should be used when combined with benzodiazepines to avoid respiratory depression. A rapid bolus of fentanyl may cause chest wall rigidity, which is only partially reversed by naloxone. The characteristics of individual analgesics and sedatives are summarized in Tables 9–34 and 9–35, respectively. Patient evaluation, technical equipment, skills, monitoring, and discharge should be done according to established criteria of the Pediatric Committee of American College of Emergency Physicians.

LOCAL ANESTHETICS

Local anesthetics are commonly used to facilitate laceration repair and for noninvasive maneuvers such as closed fracture reduction. Although a variety of agents and methods can be used, *lidocaine* is the standard for infiltrative anesthesia. However, topical agents are being used with increasing frequency. A comparison of commonly used agents is outlined in Table 9–36. To avoid iatrogenic pain, infiltration should be done after rubbing the skin and then inserting the smallest needle through the margins of the wound with gentle pressure. Buffering the solution with *bicarbonate* decreases the pain associated with infiltration at the cost of shelf-life of the solution to 1 week. The dose of lidocaine can be increased (to 7 mg/kg) if combined with *epinephrine* for vasoconstrictive effect. However, lidocaine should not be combined with epinephrine when used in areas supplied by end arteries (e.g., pinna of ear, penis, and digits). Lidocaine also is very effective for regional nerve block, which may be used instead of local infiltration. Regardless of the technique used, 10 to 15 minutes should be allowed for onset of anesthesia.

Topical application of anesthetic agents does not give a uniform anesthetic effect. The most commonly used topical anesthetic is *TAC* (0.5% tetracaine/0.05% epinephrine/11.8% cocaine). TAC may produce adequate local anesthesia when used for laceration of scalp, face, and wounds on the extremities. However, 10% to 25% of patients may require the addition of lidocaine infiltration. Because of the vasoconstrictive properties of epinephrine and cocaine, TAC should not be used in areas supplied by end arteries. TAC is contraindicated on extensively abraded skin and any of the mucosal sites. Significant absorption can occur through these sites, leading to disorientation and seizures. *EMLA,* an eutectic mixture of pilocaine 2.5% and lidocaine 2.5%, is effective as a local anesthetic for lumbar and venipuncture. However, at least 60 minutes of application is required to produce local anesthetic. The long interval for onset of action precludes its widespread use in acute care settings when the procedure or pain relief is required urgently. It has not yet been approved as an anesthetic agent for laceration repair.

Table 9-34. PROPERTIES OF PHARMACOLOGIC AGENTS USED FOR ACUTE PAIN MANAGEMENT

Drug	Route and Dose (mg/kg)	Therapeutic Potentials	Onset and Duration (hr)	Advantages	Disadvantages
Morphine*	IV/IM/SC, 0.1–0.2 (10 mg maximum)	Analgesic, sedative, euphoric, anxiolytic	Rapid (3–4)	Potent sedative and analgesic; no myocardial depression; clearance unaffected by hepatic or renal disease	Nausea and vomiting, respiratory depression, hypotension
Fentanyl†	IV/IM (0.01 mg maximum)	Analgesic, sedative, anxiolytic, euphoric	Rapid (0.5–0.8)	100-Fold more potent than morphine; no hemodynamic compromise	Chest wall rigidity, seizures, facial puritis
Meperidine‡	IV/IM/PO, 1.0 (100 mg maximum)	Sedative, analgesic	Rapid (2–3)	Well absorbed through enteral route	Disorientation, tremors, convulsions, small therapeutic index
Ketorolac tromethamine§	IV/IM, 0.5 (30 mg maximum)	Analgesic	6	Adjunct to opioids to decrease their requirement; effective in postoperative pain	Platelet dysfunction, gastrointestinal bleeding, decreased glomerular filtration rate, bronchospasm
Ketamine‖	IV, 1.0; IM, 3–5; PO, 6–10		Rapid (20–30 min)	Rapid analgesia and amnesia, lack of significant respiratory depressant effect, preserves protective reflexes, bronchodilatation and improved pulmonary compliance	Unpleasant recovery with dreams and hallucinations, increase in salivary and bronchial secretions, may increase intracranial pressure
Nitrous oxide¶	Inhalation, 30–50%		Rapid (3–5 min)	Quick recovery, minimal effects on respiratory and cardiovascular system when used on short-term basis	Environmental contamination, potential abuse, diffusional hypoxia

*†‡Opiates.
§Nonsteroidal anti-inflammatory agent.
‖Dissociative anesthetic.
¶Inhalational anesthetic.
*†‖In the critical care unit, may be administered through continuous infusion to ensure optimal levels and pain control.

PEDIATRIC INTENSIVE CARE UNIT

Ideally, undertreatment of pain should not occur in the critical care unit because of the availability of skilled staff, technical facilities, and controlled cardiorespiratory conditions. However, patients in this setting are likely to have complex hemodynamic alterations requiring pharmacologic support with multiple medications. Typically, analgesia with or without sedation is required in intensive care for conditions outlined in Table 9–31. In addition, sedation and analgesia may be necessary to facilitate the patient's cooperation and, therefore, synchrony during mechanical ventilation.

The duration of desired sedation and analgesia varies according to the intended therapeutic end point. The intravenous route of administration is preferred because the dose can be titrated according to the effect. There is no single, ideal agent available. The selection of the agent is made according to required duration and its inherent potential to facilitate or aggravate the patient's underlying cardiorespiratory status. The credibility of a sedative and analgesic in general is judged by the following features (see Tables 9–34 and 9–35, respectively):

- Rapidity of onset, and predictable duration of action
- Instantaneous dissipation of effect when discontinued
- Choice of multiple routes of administration
- Lack of effect on cardiorespiratory function
- Lack of interaction with other drugs
- Wide therapeutic index

Adequate analgesia not only satisfies the patient but also precludes deterioration of the hemodynamic status by avoiding swings in cardiorespiratory function and potential metabolic derangements associated with neuroendocrine stimulation. *Opioid analgesics* are commonly used in intensive care settings as continuous infusion, on demand, or on a fixed-interval basis. They are frequently administered in collaboration with sedatives to provide optimal and titratable continuous relief of pain. *Fentanyl* is widely used; however, *morphine* is cost effective in patients with stable cardiovascular function. *Opioids* are also commonly used for sedation in children <1 year old, after which *benzodiazepines* are relatively safe for respiratory function. If regularly used for more than 1 week, the doses should be tapered to avoid withdrawal symptoms such as agitation, tachycardia, diarrhea, and sweating. *Ketamine* is an especially good choice for patients with reactive airway disease. Nitrous oxide and other inhalational gases (e.g., enflurane and isoflurane) are rarely used in intensive care units because of logistic difficulties. Table 9–37 outlines the sedative and analgesics commonly administered through continuous infusion.

Postoperative Pain Management

Adequate analgesia is an important part of postoperative management. It should be part of the continuum of preemptive and intraoperative analgesia. Preemptive analgesia is the administration of preoperative analgesia, which facilitates the use of much smaller doses during and after the procedure. The choice of a pharmacologic agent is made by considering its potential to modulate physiologic

Table 9-35. PHARMACOLOGIC PROPERTIES OF SEDATIVES USED IN EMERGENCY DEPARTMENT AND INTENSIVE CARE SETTING

Drug	Route and Dose (mg/kg)	Pharmacokinetics	Advantages	Disadvantages
Benzodiazepines Diazepam	IV, 0.05–0.2; PR, 0.5	Metabolism: hepatic Elimination half-life: 12–24 hr *n*-Desmethyldiazepam is an active metabolite	Most commonly used as sedatives, selective anterograde amnesia, flumazenil is selective antagonist	No intrinsic analgesic effect, physical dependence with prolonged use, abstinence syndrome if discontinued abruptly, dose-related respiratory inhibition
Midazolam (twofold to fourfold more potent than diazepam)	IV, 0.01–0.7; PO/IN/PR, 0.3–0.7; SL, 0.2	Metabolism: hepatic Elimination half-life: 2–4 hr Prolonged use may lead to accumulation of active metabolite		
Lorazepam	IV/IM, 0.02–0.05	Metabolism; hepatic Elimination half-life: 4–12 hr		
Chloral hydrate	PO/PR, 50–100	Active compound is trichloroethanol	Good for less-emergent procedures not requiring IV access (e.g., radiographic studies)	Disagreeable taste, long onset of action, not recommended for <3 mon

Barbiturates				
Thiopental*	IV, 3–5	Metabolism: hepatic Excretion: renal Elimination half-life: 7.6–10.6 hr Significant tissue redistribution	Rapid, pleasant induction and fast recovery; effective when narcotics and benzodiazepines fail to produce sedation; ideal for brief procedures; decrease cerebral oxygen demand and intracranial pressure; potent anticonvulsant properties	Dose-related respiratory depression, antianalgesic properties at low plasma levels, trigger hypotension in hypovolemic states, no antagonist available
Methohexital*	IV, 1; PR, 18–25	Elimination half-life: 1.8–6 hr		
Pentobarbital (effect lasts 2–6 hr)	IV/IM, 2–5	Elimination half-life: 15–48 hr		
Propofol	IV, 0.25–0.13	No active metabolite	Rapid onset, quick recovery; antiemetic properties; decreased intracranial pressure	Hypotension, opisthotonic posturing and seizures, dose-related respiratory depression
Etomidate	IV, 0.2–0.5	Metabolism: hepatic	Rapid onset, ultrashort duration of action	Respiratory depression, myoclonic jerks, not approved for <12 years old

Preferred route is listed first.

*Ultrashort-acting barbiturates. Their effects last <10 min because of tissue redistribution. Repeated administrations can lead to significant accumulation of the drug.

Table 9–36. COMPARISON OF LOCAL ANESTHETICS IN COMMON CLINICAL USE

Agent	Concentration (%)	Maximum Dose (mg/kg)	Duration of Action	Relative Potency
Lidocaine*	0.5–2	4	Short	3
Procaine	0.5–2	15	Short	1
Mepivacaine	1	5–7	Long	2.4
Bupivacaine	0.25–0.75	7	Intermediate	8
Tetracaine	1–2	2	Short	8

*Buffering with bicarbonate (lidocaine to bicarbonate, 10:1) decreases pain felt on administration. Combination of epinephrine decreases blood loss and doubles the total safe dose.

parameters such as pulmonary vascular resistance, cerebral blood flow, hemodynamic status of the patient, and whether the patient is ventilated. Postoperative continuous infusion of an *opioid* titrated to the level of patient's comfort is the best technique to ensure adequate analgesia. However, the use of a *PCA* (patient controlled analgesia) *device* for an older child who is not drowsy or sedated is equally effective and acceptable. Synthetic opioids such as *fentanyl, sufentanil,* and *alfentanil* are particularly safe for postoperative cardiac patients who have relatively compromised cardiovascular status and are prone to develop pulmonary vasospasms.

Pain Management during a Procedure

All procedures should be done under proper sedation and analgesia. *Ketamine* or *midazolam* and *fentanyl* are appropriate for short procedures such as endotracheal intubation, whereas *morphine infusion* is a better choice for ongoing sedation and analgesia for a child who requires multiple interventions and mechanical ventilation. Careful cardiorespiratory monitoring is also essential for a patient who

Table 9–37. SEDATIVES AND ANALGESICS COMMONLY USED AS CONTINUOUS INFUSION IN THE INTENSIVE CARE UNIT

Morphine	10–30 µg/kg/hr
Fentanyl	2–4 µg/kg/hr
Lorazepam	0.025 mg/kg/hr (2 mg maximum)
Midazolam	0.05–0.2 mg/kg/hr
Ketamine*	0.5–1 mg/kg/hr
Pentobarbital*	1–2 mg/kg/hr
Propofol†	0.01–0.05 mg/kg/min

*Infusion should be preceded by a bolus dose of 1–2 mg/kg.
†The dose for continuous infusion is not yet established. The suggested dose of initial trials is given.

is breathing spontaneously. This assumes greater importance when collaborations of sedatives and potent analgesics are used simultaneously.

Summary

Pain is a common accompaniment of conditions treated in the acute care setting and requires individualized potent pharmacologic interventions. Although novel therapeutic modalities exist, underestimation of pain results in underuse of these techniques. Prompt and appropriate treatment of pain can decrease patient suffering and minimize unfavorable pathophysiologic alterations. The proliferation of literature during the past decade on pediatric pain management is an encouraging trend.

BIBLIOGRAPHY

American Academy of Pediatric, Committee on Drugs, Section of Anesthesiology: Guidelines for monitoring and management of pediatric patients during and after sedation for diagnostic and therapeutic procedures. Pediatrics 89:1110, 1992.
Anand KJS, Carr DB: The neuroanatomy, neurophysiology, and neurochemistry of pain, stress and analgesia in newborns and children. Pediatr Clin North Am 36:795, 1989.
Glebe-Gage D, McGrath P, Kissoon N: Children's response to painful procedures in the emergency department. *In* Bond MR, Charlton JE, Woolf CJJ (eds): Proceedings of the 6th World Congress on Pain. New York, Elsevier Science Publishers, 1991, pp. 441–446.
McGrath PA: Evaluating a child's pain. J Pain Symptom Manage 4:197, 1989.
Sacchetti A, Schafermeyer R, Gerardi M, et al: Pediatric analgesia and sedation. Ann Emerg Med 23:237, 1994.
Tobias JD, Rasmussen GE: Pain management and sedation in the pediatric intensive care unit. Pediatr Clin North Am 41:1269, 1994.
Yaster M, Deshpande JK: Management of pediatric pain with opioid analgesics. J Pediatr 113, 1988.

9.9 Burn Injury

CHRISTOPHER G. SCILLEY, MD, FRCSC

The successful management of burn victims requires a timely and methodical assessment of problems and the establishment of treatment priorities. This chapter will review many of the problems encountered in the acutely burned patient and outline the guidelines for management.

Pathophysiology

The four major categories of burns are thermal, chemical, electrical, and radiation. Thermal injuries predominate in children, with scald injuries being more common in children <5 years old and flame injuries being more common in children >5 years old.

BURN WOUND

The burn wound is composed of three zones of injury:

- *Zone of Necrosis/Coagulopathy.* Tissue has been irreversibly destroyed by injury.
- *Zone of Stasis/Ischemia.* Located adjacent to the zone of necrosis, this tissue has been damaged, circulation is abnormal but has the potential to recover or go on to necrosis depending on the severity of injury and treatment.
- *Zone of Hyperemia/Inflammation.* Tissue is essentially uninjured but undergoes vascular changes in response to mediators released from damaged tissue.

BURN SHOCK

Many factors contribute to the development of burn shock. Skin damage results in the *loss of barrier function* with increased insensible fluid loss. Chemical mediators (leukotrienes, prostaglandins, oxygen radicals, histamine) increase *permeability,* especially in the area of injury and, to a lesser extent, systemically. This increase in permeability results in the *loss of plasma* from the intravascular space to the interstitial space. The *fall in colloid oncotic pressure* secondary to protein loss is the major cause of systemic edema. Cell membrane sodium pump dysfunction results in the *intracellular accumulation of sodium and water.* In burns of >40% body surface area (BSA), *myocardial depression* may occur as a result of changes in resting cell membrane potential, increased myocardial stiffness, and direct depression by chemical mediators. The fluid losses peak at 8 to 12 hours after the burn and then begin to reverse. In burns >40% BSA, fluid loss may be ongoing for 36 to 48 hours.

INHALATION INJURY

Direct Thermal Injury. Direct thermal injury results in damage to the mucosa and underlying tissues above the level of the cords. The resulting edema *may progress to airway obstruction* within hours of injury.

Chemical Injury. Smoke contains a variety of chemical agents that are toxic to the cells of the lower airways. Water-soluble compounds produce inflammation, ulceration, bronchorrhea, and bronchospasm in the upper airway, trachea, and large bronchi. Lipid-soluble compounds penetrate to the more distal airways, where they cause full-thickness mucous membrane loss, denaturation of alveolar surfactant, and alveolar capillary damage, leading to pulmonary edema. Mild injury predisposes to *pneumonia* secondary to airway obstruction, which is usually manifest at 3 to 10 days after the burn. In severe injury, *adult respiratory distress syndrome* may develop within 24 to 48 hours.

Carbon Monoxide. CO_2 produced by the incomplete combustion of carbon-containing compounds competes with O_2 for hemoglobin binding sites, shifts the oxyhemoglobin dissociation curve to the left, resulting in *decreased O_2 delivery to the tissues,* and binds intracellular mitochondrial cytochrome oxidase enzymes, *impairing cellular metabolism.*

    Impaired Chest Wall Compliance. Circumferential deep/full-thickness torso burns produce *decreased chest wall compliance.* Decrease in functional reserve capacity produces atelectasis and ventilation/perfusion mismatch. The work of breathing is increased, with an increased risk for developing respiratory failure. In ventilated patients, high ventilation pressures may be needed, exposing the patient to complications of barotrauma.

Clinical Evaluation

A thorough history and physical examination are essential to determine a complete definition of the extent of the injury. However, because a burn injury can be an acutely life-threatening situation, early emphasis on managing the airway, breathing, and circulation is essential.

HISTORY OF INJURY

The following historical data are essential: time since injury, loss of consciousness, circumstances (closed space, home/work, associated trauma/explosion), and prehospital care. The following patient history items are also essential: medications, allergies, tetanus toxoid status, and any pre-existing illness.

In the pediatric population, the question may arise of possible *abuse.* This possibility should be considered in the following situations: accident occurring when the child is alone, an injury attributed to the actions of a sibling, historical details that are unclear, previous accidental injury, history incompatible with injury or motor development of child, delay in presentation for treatment, unstable family situation, or presentation for care by someone other than the parent or guardian.

Physical Assessment and Management

AIRWAY AND BREATHING

Immediate evaluation should include signs of respiratory distress (e.g., respiratory rate, in drawing), airway obstruction (e.g., stridor, hoarseness), lower airway distress (e.g., wheezing), and the presence of burns on the face, neck, and torso.

The provision of basic airway maneuvers should include the following:

- 100% humidified O_2
- Suctioning
- Head elevation
- Proper positioning if child is unconscious

Upper Airway Injury

It is essential to identify very early patients who are at high risk for upper airway obstruction (Table 9–38). The high-risk patients should be considered for immediate intubation (see Chapter 2).

The largest-caliber endotracheal tube should be used as changing the tube later in the presence of edema is not without risk. The endotracheal tube should not be cut at the lips or nares because swelling will render it too short. *Patients with an inhalation injury who are not at high risk of early obstruction should be observed closely and may be managed without intubation* (Table 9–38).

Suspect CO_2 poisoning when there is a closed space burn, decreased level of consciousness, and facial burns. Confirm through determination of carboxyhemoglobin levels. Remember that levels measured in the emergency department may have been significantly lowered by prehospital treatment with O_2. Administer 100% O_2 and intubate if there is impaired level of consciousness. Hyperbaric O_2 should be considered if levels are >30% to 40% and the patient's condition permits.

Lower Airway Injury

The onset of lower airway disease usually occurs after 24 to 48 hours unless the injury is very severe. *Fiberoptic bronchoscopy is the gold standard for diagnosis for lower airway injury.* Patients who demonstrate mucosal inflammation, ulceration, and sloughing are at increased risk. Parenchymal damage can be demonstrated with a xenon scan within 48 hours after injury showing areas of decreased gas washout consistent with airway obstruction. It is important to remember that lower airway pathology may develop with or without upper airway obstruction. Both groups of patients are at risk and should be monitored with the use of clinical evaluation, chest radiography, and arterial blood gases. Prophylactic antibiotics have no role in treatment, and systemic steroids may increase mortality without proven benefit. Fluid resuscitation should not be restricted as hypovolemia and decreased perfusion may accentuate lung injury. Fluid resuscitation should be titrated carefully to avoid overresuscitation or underresuscitation in these patients.

Table 9–38. HIGH-RISK PATIENTS SHOULD BE INTUBATED IMMEDIATELY, WHEREAS LOW-RISK PATIENTS SHOULD BE OBSERVED CLOSELY

High Risk	Low Risk
Decreased level of consciousness	Small superficial facial/neck burns
Deep burns of face/neck	Carbonaceous sputum
Edema/sloughing of mucosa in upper airway	Increased respiratory rate
Stridor, hoarseness	Wheezes on auscultation
Supraclavicular indrawing	Absence of slough of mucosa in upper airway
Respiratory distress (Pao₂ <60 mm Hg; Pco₂ >55 mm Hg)	Satisfactory arterial blood gases

Patients with inhalation injury who do not develop adult respiratory distress syndrome are at risk for pneumonia 3 to 10 days after the injury. Treatment consists of appropriate antibiotics and ventilatory support. The diagnosis of decreased chest wall compliance in patients with severe torso burns may be difficult. Escharotomy of the circumferential deep chest wall burns should be considered early in patients at high risk for pulmonary problems.

CIRCULATION

Burn patients are different in that heart rate and blood pressure may not always accurately reflect volume status due to excess catecholamine release. Renal perfusion (0.5 to 1 mL/kg/hr for patients <30 kg, 30 to 50 mL/hr for patients >30 kg) is the best measure of volume status. Burns >20% BSA are at an increased risk of burn shock.

renal output
① .5-1 cc/kg/hr — <30 kg
② 30-50 cc/° — >30 kg

Fluid Resuscitation

Two large-bore intravenous lines must be inserted; the intraosseous route may be used. If the child is hemodynamically unstable, administer 10 to 20 mL/kg of an isotonic solution and repeat if necessary until stable.

Parkland Formula. The Parkland formula is 4 mL/kg body wt/% burn within first 24 hours.

Parkland (4cc/kg) / % burn in 1st 24°

- Add this the fluid based on this formula to daily maintenance fluid for 24 hours.
- In the first 8 hours, give one half of the total amount of fluid; give the remainder over the next 16 hours.
- Fluid should be crystalloid (lactated Ringer's or normal saline).
- The adequacy of fluid resuscitation should be based primarily on urine output (>1 mL/kg/hr). Heart rate, peripheral perfusion, and blood pressure may not always be reliable. Acid-base status and lactate may also assist in fluid management. It is important to remember that these are only guides. Infusion rates should be adjusted depending on the response of the patient.
- Some patients are at *increased risk for altered fluid needs:* patients with pre-existing cardiac or renal disease, inhalation injury, diabetes, electrical injury, or burns of >80% BSA. These patients and those not responding to fluid resuscitation may require invasive monitoring (central venous pressure, pulmonary capillary wedge pressure).

Inotropic Support. Patients with burns of >30% to 40% BSA may clinically demonstrate evidence of myocardial depression. These patients may require inotropic support in the form of *dopamine* or *dobutamine. Digoxin* should be avoided because rapid fluid and electrolyte shifts may increase the risk of toxicity.

Colloid Replacement. Colloid replacement therapy may be used at 8 to 12 hours because permeability changes may begin to reverse. Fresh frozen plasma may be used for patients with coagulation abnormalities.

Other Organ Systems

All other organ systems should be thoroughly reviewed. Burns of >20% to 30% BSA frequently result in gastric dilation requiring nasogastric tube insertion. Extremities should be evaluated for compartment syndrome. Assess the level of consciousness and occurrence of transverse myelitis (early and late), which may occur after electrical burns.

Laboratory Investigations

In severely burned patients, a series of investigations are required for the diagnosis of complications and monitoring (Table 9–39).

Assessment and Care of Burn Wounds

- All clothing and debris should be removed from the patient.
- *Estimate BSA burn:* The rule of 9s does not apply to children <10 years old (Fig. 9–18).
  - □ See Lund and Browder chart (Fig. 9–18).
  - □ Include only partial- or full-thickness injury, not erythema.
  - □ If chart is not available, the patient's palm equals 1% BSA.
  - □ Accurate assessment of BSA is critical to allow accurate estimation of fluid resuscitation.

BURN DEPTH

- Full-thickness injury is obvious: white, yellow, charred, leathery, waxy feel.
- Distinguishing superficial from deep partial-thickness injury may be difficult.
- Assess capillary refill.
  - □ Most useful
  - □ Present in superficial injury
  - □ Absent or sluggish in deeper injury

Table 9–39. SUGGESTED INVESTIGATIONS IN SEVERE BURNS

Complete blood cell count	Electrolytes
Blood urea nitrogen, creatine	Prothrombin and partial thromboplastin times
Protein, albumin	Blood sugar
Urinalysis	Magnesium, calcium, phosphorus
Liver function tests	Group and reserve
Arterial blood gases	Chest radiograph
CO levels	Drug screen
Urine myoglobin	ECG

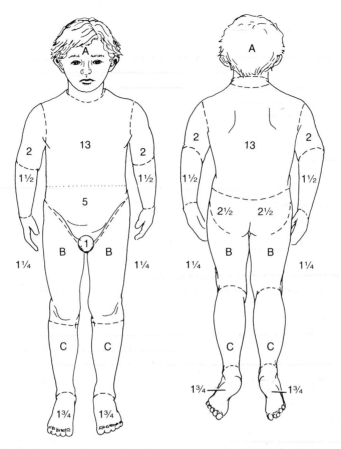

Figure 9–18. The Lund and Browder Chart is more accurate for children than is the rule of nines. (From: Reisdorff BJ, Roberts MR, Wiegenstein JG: Pediatric Emergency Medicine. Philadelphia, WB Saunders, 1993.)

■ Burn injury tends to progress over 24 to 48 hours, so what appeared superficial at the initial assessment may ultimately become deep partial or full thickness.

MANAGEMENT

1. Neutralize source of burn injury.
   ■ Remove all clothing and debris that may still be causing injury.
   ■ Cool the wound.
      □ Advantages: Provides analgesia, minimizes depth of injury, best done immediately (little benefit 1 hour after injury)
      □ Disadvantages: Increased heat loss, hypothermia (shivering), increased O_2 consumption, increased risk if used for burns of >10% to

15% BSA, vasoconstriction may occur (causing decreased blood flow and extending tissue damage)
2. Avoid excess heat loss.
   - Treat in warm environment: 25°C to 30°C.
   - Do not cool burns of >10% to 15% BSA.
   - Keep patient covered.
3. Clean the wound.
   - Remove debris and blisters.
   - Wash with dilute cleansing solution (chlorhexidine).
4. Prevent infection.
   - Administer tetanus immunization.
   - Administer systemic antibiotics; there is no role for antibiotics prophylactically.
   - The exception is a short course of penicillin G in patients at high risk of group B β-hemolytic *Streptococcus* infection.
   - *Topical antibiotics:* The goal is not to sterilize the wound but rather to minimize the number of bacteria colonizing the wound. The topical agents should be applied twice daily, and the wound should be protected with an absorptive dressing. The agents to be used are listed (Table 9–40).
5. Facilitate wound closure.
   - Superficial partial-thickness burns will heal in 2 to 3 weeks with dressing changes.
   - Excision and skin grafting are usually done by 48 hours for deep partial- and full-thickness burns.

Complications

Compartment Syndrome. This usually occurs in circumferential full-thickness extremity burns; however, it may also occur in unburned extremities or in extremities with partial-thickness, noncircumferential injuries. It is important to

Table 9–40. TOPICAL ANTIBIOTICS

Drug	Characteristics
Silver sulfadiazine	Most commonly used
Side effects	Leukopenia (transient), allergies (rare)
Mafenide acetate	
Advantage	Readily penetrates avascular eschar
Side effects	Carbonic anhydrase inhibitor that produces metabolic acidosis, pain, allergy (5%)
Silver nitrate (aqueous 0.5%)	
Side effects	Leaches sodium, potassium, magnesium, chloride, calcium; stains black everything it touches
Ointments	Superficial burns only; Bacitrin, Polysporin, Neosporin

maintain a high index of suspicion because it may not manifest until resuscitation is well under way (6 to 8 hours). Diagnosis can be made by assessing for pain, pulseless, pallor, paresthesia, paralysis, firmness of compartment, and direct measures of compartment pressures of >30 mm Hg.

Treatment. Escharotomy must be conducted along midlateral lines of the extremity, which must extend down to the underlying fascia; however, if there is no response, then fascia must also be released. This must also be extended into unburned tissue or proximal extremity. After this, wounds are dressed with topical antibiotics.

Myoglobinuria. This occurs most commonly in electrical current flow injury. Myoglobin crystallizes in the renal tubules, leading to tubular obstruction. This clinically manifests as red to tea-colored urine and can be confirmed through measurement of myoglobin levels.

Treatment. It is essential to maintain a high urine output (100 to 200 mL/hr), often with the use of an osmotic diuretic (*mannitol*). Alkalinization of the urine through systemic sodium bicarbonate is necessary to increase excretion and discourage crystal formation. Dialysis may be necessary in refractory cases. If the source of myoglobin is identified, aggressive surgical debridement is needed.

Hypermetabolic State. This is usually established by 3 to 5 days after the injury and results in catecholamine release, which is proportional to burn size up to 60% BSA. Thereafter, there is little increase. This is often ongoing until after the wounds have healed.

Treatment. The treatment goal is to prevent >10% decrease in preburn weight. These needs can often be met with use of the enteral route. The need can be estimated using the Curreri formula modified for children: kcal/day = 60 × wt (kg) + (35 × % BSA). The composition includes fats (15%), protein (20% to 25%), and carbohydrates (60% to 75%). During this phase, it is useful to monitor weight (twice weekly), calorie count (daily), urinary nitrogen, and indirect calorimetry where available.

$$Kcal/day = (60 \times kg) + (35 \times \% BSA)$$

Prognosis

Death from burn injury of <30% BSA in the pediatric population is unusual. The LD_{50} in patients 0 to 20 years old is ≈50% to 65% BSA. The presence of inhalation injury significantly increases the mortality for any burn. With improved survival comes an increase in the number of complications, with 40% BSA burn patients experiencing an average of six major complications during hospitalization.

Successful management of the burn patient requires constant vigilance and aggressive treatment extending through the acute resuscitation phase until discharge from hospital.

BIBLIOGRAPHY

Bostwick JA (ed): The Art and Science of Burn Care. Rockville, MD, Aspen Publishers, 1987.

Demling RH: Burns and environmental injury. In Hall JB, Schmidt GA, Wood LDW (eds): Principles of Critical Care. New York, McGraw-Hill, 1992, pp. 797–827.

Krob MJ, Deppe SA, Thompson DR: Burn injury. In Civelta JM, Taylor RW, Kirby RR (eds): Critical Care, 2nd ed. Philadelphia, JB Lippincott, 1992, pp. 781–787.

9.10 Guidelines for Nutritional Support of Critically Ill Children

DAVID M. STEINHORN, MD

Nutritional support of the critically ill patient signifies the provision of nutrient substrates to patients during an interruption in the normal process of ingestion, absorption, or utilization of foodstuffs. Nutrients may be classified as *macronutrients* (proteins, carbohydrate, and fats) or *micronutrients* (electrolytes, minerals, trace elements, and vitamins). Nutritional support also involves monitoring the patient's response to the prescribed regimen to demonstrate a beneficial response and the absence of evolving complications. Nutritional support is an essential component in the overall management of all hospitalized patients regardless of the diagnosis or degree of stress. Potential benefits of nutritional support include sparing of lean body mass, improved healing and immunity, maintenance of gut mass and function, and reduced overall morbidity. Potential risks include metabolic derangement (hyperammonemia, uremia, acidosis), bowel injury (perforation, necrotizing enterocolitis), line infections (associated with parenteral nutrition), aspiration of formula, and wastage of materials.

Pathophysiology

During periods of high physiologic stress, nutrients are handled differently than during periods of health; thus, major differences exist between simple fasting in a healthy individual and the physiologic response to stress, as summarized in Table 9–41.

Urinary urea excretion in critically ill children is comparable to that in critically ill adults; however, the percentage of urinary nitrogen excreted as urea varies widely, from 45% to 87% of the total nitrogen. This finding supports the current practice of using *total urinary nitrogen* in determining nitrogen balance in critically ill children. Plasma amino acid analysis of critically ill children indicates that children at high levels of physiologic stress may have a depressed level of plasma branched-chain amino acids, similar to that of physiologically stressed adults. When resting energy expenditure is measured through indirect calorimetry, it is found to be lower during acute, critical illness than predicted based on standard tables or nomograms. Data from parenterally fed children in the pediatric intensive care unit suggest that nitrogen may be more efficiently retained when commercially available parenteral amino acid solutions containing at least *30% branched-chain amino acids* are infused; however, data are not available supporting improved outcome and reduced morbidity in *nonneonates* based on these more

Table 9–41. COMPARISON OF NUTRIENT METABOLISM IN STARVATION VERSUS SEPSIS/TRAUMA

	Starvation	Sepsis/Trauma
Protein breakdown	+	+ + +
Hepatic protein synthesis	+	+ + +
Ureagenesis	+	+ + +
Gluconeogenesis	+	+ + +
Energy expenditure	Reduced	Increased
Mediator activity	Low	High
Hormone counterregulatory capacity	Preserved	Poor
Utilization of ketones	+ + +	+
Loss of body stores	Gradual	Rapid
Primary fuels	Fat	Amino acids, glucose, triglycerides

Adapted from Barton R, Cerra FB: The hypermetabolism. Multiple organ failure syndrome. Chest 96:1153, 1989.

costly formulations. Physiologic stress is associated with high levels of endogenous epinephrine, cortisol, glucagon, and growth hormone. While insulin production is intact, levels of blood glucose are often elevated because the high levels of catabolic (stress) hormones produce a breakdown in peripheral tissue with increased central glucose synthesis. Additional factors affecting the utilization of nutritional substrates during critical illness include altered hormonal receptor physiology during acidosis, effects of peptide mediators (e.g., tumor necrosis factor, interleukin-1) on substrate flux, effects of endotoxin and mediators on intermediary metabolism, and side effects of various drugs (e.g., glucocorticoids). Outcome studies of the role of nutrition support in reducing morbidity or duration of hospitalization have not been performed in critically ill children.

Protein-calorie malnutrition has been documented in children cared for in the pediatric intensive care unit. Pre-existing or chronic malnutrition implies a long-standing, inadequate intake of protein and calories, leading to a height that is lower than predicted for age. Recently acquired or acute malnutrition implies an adequate nutrient intake to have achieved a stature appropriate for chronologic age but recent loss of body stores from imbalance in nutrient supply versus utilization. It is reflected in a low weight for height (Table 9–42).

Clinical Evaluation

On admission to the pediatric intensive care unit, all patients should have an initial evaluation of their nutritional status (see Table 9–43). The determination of triceps skin-fold and midarm circumference has a relatively high degree of error in infants and in the presence of edema. Capillary leak syndrome, seen frequently in critically ill patients, leads to a decrease in the levels of most serum proteins; however, baseline serum transferrin, albumin, and total protein levels may provide

Table 9–42. SEVERITY OF PROTEIN-CALORIE MALNUTRITION IN THE PEDIATRIC INTENSIVE CARE UNIT

Acute			Chronic	
PCM Grade	*Patients (%)*	*Nutritional Risk*	*PCM Grade*	*Patients (%)*
0 (>0.9)*	64	Normal	0 (>0.95)†	53
1 (0.8–0.9)*	18	At risk	1 (0.9–0.95)†	30
2 (0.7–0.8)*	15	At risk	2 (0.85–0.89)†	10
3 (<0.7)*	3	Malnutrition	3 (<0.85)†	6

*Index$_{(weight/height)}$ = (actual weight/50th percentile‡ weight for height).
†Index$_{(height/age)}$ = (actual height/50th percentile‡ height for age).
‡See standard growth chart.
PCM, protein-calorie malnutrition.

an indication of the recent nutritional status. A brief evaluation of the skin and hair as part of the global first examination of the newly admitted patient reveals signs of micronutrient deficiency. Evaluation of cellular immunity may be screened through determination of the total lymphocyte count and the presence of a response to routine skin testing (Fig. 9–19).

ADMISSION ASSESSMENT

Follow the axiom that "If you don't look, you won't see" (see Table 9–43).

NUTRITIONAL SUPPORT

Begin nutritional support as soon as stable using the gastrointestinal tract whenever possible and supplementing with peripheral or central parenteral nutrition

Table 9–43. ASSESSMENT OF NUTRITIONAL STATUS ON ADMISSION

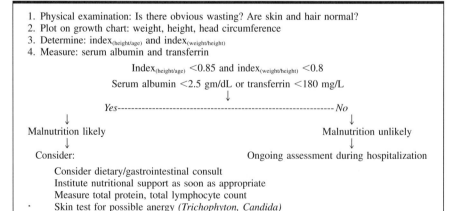

1. Physical examination: Is there obvious wasting? Are skin and hair normal?
2. Plot on growth chart: weight, height, head circumference
3. Determine: index$_{(height/age)}$ and index$_{(weight/height)}$
4. Measure: serum albumin and transferrin

Index$_{(height/age)}$ <0.85 and index$_{(weight/height)}$ <0.8

Serum albumin <2.5 gm/dL or transferrin <180 mg/L
↓
Yes---No
↓   ↓
Malnutrition likely   Malnutrition unlikely
↓   ↓
Consider: Ongoing assessment during hospitalization

  Consider dietary/gastrointestinal consult
  Institute nutritional support as soon as appropriate
  Measure total protein, total lymphocyte count
  Skin test for possible anergy (*Trichophyton, Candida*)

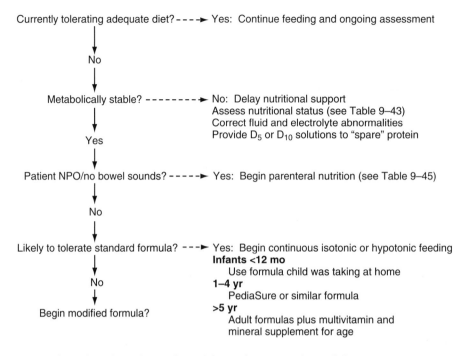

Currently tolerating adequate diet? ----▸ Yes: Continue feeding and ongoing assessment

No

Metabolically stable? --------▸ No: Delay nutritional support
Assess nutritional status (see Table 9–43)
Correct fluid and electrolyte abnormalities
Provide D_5 or D_{10} solutions to "spare" protein

Yes

Patient NPO/no bowel sounds? -----▸ Yes: Begin parenteral nutrition (see Table 9–45)

No

Likely to tolerate standard formula? ---▸ Yes: Begin continuous isotonic or hypotonic feeding
Infants <12 mo
Use formula child was taking at home
1–4 yr
PediaSure or similar formula
>5 yr
Adult formulas plus multivitamin and
mineral supplement for age

No

Begin modified formula?

Short bowel syndrome, fat malabsorption, severe heart failure:
Infants (<1yr):
Begin drip feeds at 1 mL/kg/hr
Use medium-chain triglyceride fortified formula, e.g., Pregestimil, Portagen.
Consult dietitian as needed.

Older children:
May use adult formula such as Tolerex, Osmolyte, Reabilan, Isocal.
Initial rate: 1 mL/kg/hr up to a maximum of 20 mL/hr to start.
Advance as tolerated

Children with inborn error of metabolism:
Contact metabolism service or dietitian.

Figure 9–19. Algorithm for nutritional support guidelines.

when enteral intake is inadequate. In practice, initiating feedings during the second hospital day are feasible in most patients. Bolus feedings may be less preferable, especially in patients with respiratory distress. Transpyloric feeding when possible via weighted Silastic catheters should be used to minimize the risk of gastroesophageal reflux and aspiration. Initial enteral nutrition support for most stressed infants and children should be a lactose-free or elemental formula, i.e., casein hydrolysate with some portion of the fat as medium-chain triglycerides, such as Pregestimil (<1 year), PediaSure (1 to 5 years), or Osmolyte or Tolerex (>5 years). Normal quantities of protein should be provided unless hyperammonemia or severe azotemia necessitates limiting protein intake. *Infants <6 months old* should receive isotonic or hypotonic feedings initially until tolerance has been demonstrated. Young children *1 to 5 years old* should receive PediaSure or a dilute adult formula with appropriate supplements of vitamins and trace elements. Critically ill children >*5 years old* usually tolerate enteral formulas developed for adult patients with supplementation of vitamins and micronutrients as needed for age. Enteral formulas should be initially hypotonic to minimize the possibility of diarrhea from excess osmotic load to the gut and to facilitate absorption (Table 9–44). Infusion rates are begun conservatively at 1 mL/kg/hr with a stepwise increase every 4 to 6 hours as tolerated up to the desired final rate. Once an acceptable rate is achieved, tonicity may be increased as tolerated. Blue food coloring may be added to formula to detect subclinical evidence of gastroesophageal reflux. Recovery of glucose is a sensitive indicator of pulmonary aspiration of formula.

ENERGY REQUIREMENTS

Follow the axiom that "More is not always better." Target goals for nonprotein calories (kcal/kg/day) during the acute phase (first 3 to 5 days) and the convalescent phase (after 5 days) are 50 to 80 and 80 to 120 for young children (<10 kg), 45 to 65 and 75 to 90 for children 1 to 7 years old, and 30 to 50 and 30 to 75 for children >7 years old, respectively.

Nutrient requirements are different during the acute phase of critical illness compared with the later convalescent phase. Calorie requirements during *acute* critical illness are generally lower than during the subsequent hypermetabolic phase of critical illness. The resting energy expenditure may be derived by measuring the minute oxygen consumption and carbon dioxide production (see

Table 9–44. SIGNS OF ENTERAL FEEDING INTOLERANCE

Problem	Possible Reason	Possible Remedy
Diarrhea, malabsorption	Delivery too fast	Decrease delivery rate
	Hypertonicity	Dilute formula
	Mucosal injury	Total parenteral nutrition, continuous low-rate drip to allow bowel recovery
	Substrate intolerance	Use more elemental formula, especially disaccharide-free formula with medium-chain triglycerides
Gastric retention	Hypertonic formula	Decrease osmolarity, dilute
	High long-chain fat content	Change to medium-chain triglyceride–containing formula
	Hypodynamic gut	Positioning right-side down, consider prokinetic agent: Cisapride, Reglan
Abdominal distension	Ileus, constipation	Rule out surgical abdomen and constipation, add bulking agent or stool softener

Table 9–45. INITIAL TPN ORDERS

1. Determine acceptable daily fluid intake	
2. Initial solution to contain:	

Dextrose:	10–15% advance to caloric goal	Na$^+$	3–4 mEq/kg/day
Protein:	1–2 gm/kg/day	K$^+$	2–3 mEq/kg/day
Fat emulsion: 1 gm/kg/day		Ca^{2+}	0.5–2.0 mEq/kg/day
Acetate: Cl$^-$ (initially 1:1) balance to desired		PO$_4$	0.5–1.0 mM/kg/day
acid-base effect			
Vitamins, trace elements as per pharmacy norms		Mg^{2+}	0.5 mEq/kg/day

Consider adding 3–6 mEq/kg/day if aggressive diuresis is under way **and** urine output is high

Example: 80 (mL/kg/day) $\times$ 0.15 (D$_{15}$) $\times$ 3.4 (kcal/gm   = 41 kcal/kg/day
   dextrose)
                1 gm/kg/day of 20% fat emulsion   = 10 kcal/kg/day
                                   Total   = 51 nonprotein kcal/kg/day
   1.5 (gm/kg/protein) $\div$ 4 6.2 (gm protein/gm nitrogen)   = 0.242 gm nitrogen/kg/day
51 (nonprotein kcal/kg/day) $\div$ 0.242 (gm nitrogen/kg/day)   = 210 (calorie to nitrogen
                                                 ratio)

equation); however, uncuffed endotracheal tubes are a potential source of error in young children

$$kcal/kg/day = 2.49 \times \dot{V}_{O_2} + 1 \times \dot{V}_{CO_2}$$

where $\dot{V}_{O_2}$ and $\dot{V}_{CO_2}$ are measured in mL/kg/min.

Carbohydrates

Children usually can tolerate and use *6 to 9 mg/kg/min of glucose,* which has a caloric density of 3.4 kcal/gm. Rates of glucose infusion over 12 to 14 mg/kg/min are likely to lead to fatty infiltration of viscera, hyperglycemia, and excess CO_2 generation. Unless unavoidable hyperglycemia occurs, insulin usually is not used to manage hyperglycemia because it may promote hepatic steatosis, excess carbon dioxide production, and electrolyte imbalance. Approximately *30% to 50%* of the total caloric intake should be derived from carbohydrates.

Fat

A maximum of *20% to 30%* of the caloric intake should be derived from fat. Intravenous fat should be infused as a 20% emulsion in infants to provide a concentrated calorie source (2 kcal/mL) as well as to supply essential fatty acids and lipids critical to central nervous system development and cell membrane repair. Intravenous fat emulsions are usually administered over 16 to 20 hr/day, allowing a $\geq$4-hour lipid-free period to demonstrate adequate lipid clearance. A typical maximum for intravenous fat emulsion is *2 to 3.5 gm/kg/day.* Patients on enteral feedings may tolerate medium-chain triglycerides after bowel injury or with right-sided heart failure better than long-chain fats. Medium-chain triglycerides are absorbed directly into the portal circulation, avoiding the complex absorptive process needed to digest long-chain fats.

AMINO ACID SOLUTIONS

Follow the axiom that "Spare the lean tissue—improve the child!" Protein requirements (in gm/kg/day) during the acute phase (first 3 to 5 days) and convalescent phase (after 5 days) are 1.0 to 2.0 and 2.0 to 3.0 for infants and children <7 years old and 1.0 to 1.5 and 1.5 to 2.5 for children >7 years old, respectively.

Standard amino acid solutions are commonly used for pediatric parenteral nutrition and are usually well tolerated. Advanced hepatic and renal failure requires input from the subspecialties managing those patients; however, meticulous attention to nutritional needs will minimize morbidity. Amino acid solutions developed for neonates, e.g., Trophamine, which contains taurine, tyrosine, cysteine, and histidine, may provide an advantage for select newborns and young infants with biliary disease or sepsis or under high physiologic stress. This effect derives from the increased branched-chain and age-essential amino acid content and a reduction in nonessential amino acid loading. The higher amino acid requirements associated with the hypermetabolism of critical illness suggest the need for a nonprotein calorie-to-nitrogen ratio of 125 to 175:1 during acute critical illness.

$$\text{Calorie-to-nitrogen ratio} = \text{calories}_{(\text{glucose} + \text{fat})} \div (\text{gm of protein}/6.2)$$

MONITOR NUTRITIONAL SUPPORT

Follow the axiom that "Just look! In the land of the blind, the Cyclops is king!"

For clinical support, monitor intake/output hourly and then each shift when stable, vital signs every shift, weight and calories, protein intake, calorie-to-nitrogen ratio daily and urine glucose twice a shift until stable; Na^+, K^+, Cl^-, HCO_3^- glucose, Ca^{2+}, blood urea nitrogen, and creatine twice daily until stable and then weekly or as needed; triglycerides, ALT, bilirubin, PO_4, complete blood cell count, and platelets daily until proper dose is established and then weekly; and transferrin and albumin weekly.

Triglyceride levels must be monitored to document clearance of lipids (see Energy Requirements). New onset of hyperlipidemia, hyperglycemia, and glycosuria may be an early sign of sepsis and warrants investigation.

MICRONUTRIENTS

Follow the axiom that "You can't see them, but they're in there working."

For children weighing <3 kg, copper, zinc, manganese and chromium requirements are 20, 300, 10, and 0.2 gm/kg/day; children weighing 3 to 25 kg, 20, 100, 10, and 0.2 gm/kg/day; and children weighing >25 kg, 0.5, 2.5, 0.25, and 10 mg/day.

Although the requirements for trace elements, vitamins, and minerals are probably increased during critical illness, the current practice is to provide normal recommended amounts guided by plasma (Ca^{2+}, Mg^{2+}, PO_4) or when unusual losses occur (Zn^{2+} with biliary or gastrointestinal fistula).

STANDARD NUTRITIONAL ASSESSMENT

This should be considered for each patient after the initial stress phase of critical illness. End-organ response to nutritional support is monitored by assessing whether serum transferrin is rising or falling and whether genuine weight gain is occurring in convalescing patients.

In the event of failure of response to nutritional support, a more detailed examination is necessary, including the measurement of albumin, total protein, and transferrin; a 24-hour urine collection for nitrogen balance determination; and, if possible, measurement of energy expenditure. Total urinary nitrogen should be used to determine nitrogen balance in critically ill children. As long as cardiopulmonary function is stable and lactic acidosis is not present, indirect calorimetry (see Energy Requirements) can provide practical information regarding overall energy expenditure and substrate utilization.

Total caloric intake during recovery is adjusted to provide 15 to 25 gm of weight gain per day in the neonate or 0.5% increase in daily body weight in the older infant and child.

When fluid volume is restricted, the parenteral nutrients should be concentrated in a volume that is 50% to 60% of the total daily volume allotment. The balance of the fluid volume is made up of a standard glucose and electrolyte solution, the volume and composition of which can be adjusted to compensate as needed for ongoing changes in blood chemistry. The infusion rate of the latter solution can be adjusted to restrict or liberalize total fluid intake, permitting the more costly parenteral nutrition to run uninterrupted and deliver the intended quantity of nutrients.

BIBLIOGRAPHY

Alexander JW, MacMillan BG, Stinnett JD, et al: Beneficial effects of aggressive protein feeding in severely burned children. Ann Surg 192:505, 1980.

Heird WC: Parenteral support of the hospitalized child. *In* Suskind RM, Lewinter-Suskind L (eds): Textbook of Pediatric Nutrition, 2nd ed. New York, Raven Press, 1993, pp. 225–238.

Pollack MM, Wiley JS, Kanter R, et al: Malnutrition in critically-ill infants and children. JPEN 6:20, 1982.

Steinhorn DM, Green TP: Severity of illness correlates with alterations in energy metabolism in the pediatric intensive care unit. Crit Care Med 19:1503, 1991.

Wesley JR: Nutrient metabolism in relation to the systemic stress response. *In* Fuhrman BP, Zimmerman JJ (eds): Pediatric Critical Care. St. Louis, Mosby, 1992, pp. 755–774.

Wesley JR, Coran AG: Intravenous nutrition for the pediatric patient. Semin Pediatr Surg 1:212, 1992.

10

Organ Transplantation

10.1 Pediatric Heart Transplantation

ALAN H. MENKIS, MD, FRCS(C)
RICHARD J. NOVICK, MD, MSc, FRCS(C), FACS
F. NEIL McKENZIE, MB, ChB, FRCS(C)

Since the modern era of transplantation began in the early 1980s with the widespread availability and use of cyclosporine, heart transplantation has become the preferred therapy for end-stage heart failure due to cardiomyopathy and for certain structural congenital heart defects in children. It is well known that Barnard performed the first successful heart transplantation on December 3, 1967. What is not widely known is that on December 7, 1967, Dr. Adrian Kantrowitz performed a heart transplantation in a 17-day-old newborn with tricuspid atresia. This patient, however, died several hours after transplantation. This germinal interest in pediatric transplantation was enhanced by the Baby Fay xenograft experiment by Dr. Leonard Bailey in 1984. Approximately 20 years earlier, Dr. James Hardy had attempted a xenograft from a chimpanzee to a human in a man with end-stage heart failure who could not be separated from cardiopulmonary bypass. The heart ultimately was too small and terminally failed several hours after implantation.

The number of pediatric heart transplantations performed worldwide has been proportionately stable compared with the total number of heart transplantations for the past 10 years. There have been approximately 3000 heart transplantations performed annually for the past several years, and approximately 300 of these are performed in individuals from 0 to 18 years old (Fig. 10–1). The greatest number of transplantations were performed in patients 6 to 18 years old; however, the greatest growth rate in pediatric heart transplantation has occurred in the <1-year-old age group; the first one was performed in 1984, and currently ≈100 to 120 are performed annually (Fig. 10–2).

Approximately one third of the pediatric transplants reported by the Registry

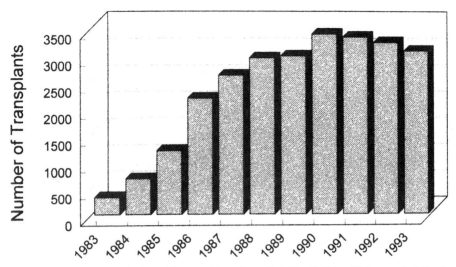

Figure 10–1. International Society of Heart and Lung Transplantation Registry 1994. Journal of Heart and Lung Transplantation Vol 13, No 4.

of the International Society for Heart and Lung Transplantation since 1984 have been in infants <1 year old.

The actuarial 1-year survival rate for pediatric heart transplant recipients by age group is as follows: <1 year old, 66%; 1 to 5 years, 72%; and 6 to 18 years,

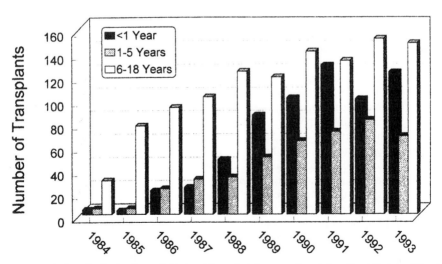

Figure 10–2. Age distribution for pediatric heart transplantation over time. International Society of Heart and Lung Transplantation Registry 1994. Journal of Heart and Lung Transplantation Vol 13, No 4.

82%; at 2 years, the rates are 64%, 70%, and 77%, respectively. The older age group has a statistically significant better survival ($p < .05$) than the two younger age groups.

There are approximately 70 centers in North America that list babies as potential recipients for heart transplantation. A shortfall in the availability of donor organs is the most important factor in the mortality of patients listed for transplantation. The mortality rate for patients on waiting lists may exceed 30%, particularly for infants and neonates. This is much higher than the expected mortality associated with the heart transplantation procedure.

According to the International Society for Heart and Lung Transplantation Registry data, the indications for pediatric heart transplantation by age group are as follows: <1 year old, 79.8% congenital heart disease, 13.5% cardiomyopathy, 1.5% retransplantation, and 5.3% other; 1 to 5 years old, 45.2% congenital heart disease, 47.5% cardiomyopathy, and 3.6% each for retransplantation and other; and 6 to 18 years old, 63.2% cardiomyopathy, 25.9% congenital heart disease, 7.8% other, and 3.1% retransplantation.

Donor Selection

The cause of death for infant cardiac donors has primarily been sudden infant death syndrome and birth asphyxia, followed by traumatic causes such as head trauma and child abuse. In children, the primary causes relate to motor vehicle accidents and violence causing head injury.

The first criterion is that the donor must be declared brain dead (see Chapter 8.5).

In addition, the donor must have a negative screen for human immunodeficiency virus and hepatitis B and C. Normal heart function should be confirmed by echocardiography. Shortening fraction should be >0.25 with no significant valvular or structural lesions. The ECG should reveal no active ischemia or infarct process. The donor must be ABO identical or compatible with the recipient. The appropriate size match is dependent on the recipient pulmonary vascular resistance (PVR). For a normal low PVR, the donor may be >20% smaller than the recipient. Donors may be ≥300% larger than the recipient by body weight.

The donor heart function must also be assessed with respect to the need for inotropic agents. In the presence of adequate filling pressures, inotropic support in excess of the equivalent of 15 μg/kg/min dopamine warrants careful consideration. In assessing a potential donor heart that had less-than-optimal cardiac function or requires excessive inotropic support, the projected ischemic time enters into the decision-making process. The better the donor heart function is on minimal inotropic agents, the longer the projected ischemic time that would be acceptable. *Total ischemic times of <4 hours* are generally considered optimal: however, successful outcomes have been reported with ischemic times of >8 hours.

The condition of the prospective recipient is an important consideration in assessing the suitability of a particular donor. If the recipient's condition is poor to a point where survival until another donor is identified would be unlikely, then a less-than-optimal donor might be an acceptable compromise.

Donor Operation

Multiorgan retrieval is the expectation that the heart; possibly the lungs, liver, and kidneys; and possibly the small bowel and pancreas will be retrieved from each donor. Coordination, therefore, is essential among two or more retrieval teams. A balance must be struck between infusion of excessive volume to enhance preload to maintain blood pressure, which may result in deterioration of lung function due to pulmonary edema, and the excessive use of vasopressors, which may induce ischemia in the heart or ischemia and/or vasospasm in the abdominal viscera. Nevertheless, a concerted effort should be made to minimize inotropic support at the time of harvesting. There are a variety of satisfactory cardioplegic agents; however, the important elements remain constant regardless of the agent used: hypothermic diastolic arrest and the use of a low cardioplegia perfusion pressure, particularly in the very small donor heart. Avoidance of hypothermic injury to the heart is achieved by not allowing the myocardial temperature to drop below 4°C. The amount of donor inferior and superior vena cavae, aorta, and pulmonary artery that are retrieved is dependent on the presence and type of structural congenital heart disease in the prospective recipient. The donor heart is removed with inflow occlusion, followed by aortic cross-clamping and administration of cold cardioplegia (most often crystalloid) into the aortic root. If additional lengths of superior vena cava and/or innominate vein are required, the superior vena cava is not ligated but instead is temporarily clamped, and the inferior vena cava is opened at the cavoatrial junction to prevent distention of the heart. The aorta is then clamped, and cardioplegia is administered. Topical cooling with cold crystalloid is also used.

The donor cardiectomy is carried out by completing the incision at the inferior cavoatrial junction followed by intrapericardial transection of the pulmonary veins. The left and right main pulmonary arteries are then transected. An appropriate amount of superior vena cava and/or innominate vein is retained before transection. The aorta is then transected, usually at the ascending aorta; however, in certain circumstances, the aortic arch must be retained (e.g., if the recipient has hypoplastic left heart syndrome).

Mechanical Circulatory Support: Bridge to Transplant

Since the mechanical pump was introduced in 1954 by Dr. John Gibbon, surgeons have used cardiopulmonary bypass for short periods of time to support inadequate ventricular function after cardiac surgery. This concept evolved into the development of other devices such as pneumatic and centrifugal ventricular assist devices and the total artificial heart as well as the intra-aortic balloon pump, which could be used for prolonged periods of support. The use of these devices was extended into the transplant population as a bridge to transplant. The use of mechanical circulatory support devices in children has been restricted primarily due to size limitation. In patients <10 years old, the intra-aortic balloon pump has been of little benefit. The implantable devices such as a total artificial heart and left ventricular assist devices have also not been particularly useful in small individuals. The most appropriate devices at this time for children remain extracorporeal ventricular assist devices or extracorporeal membrane oxygenation (see Chapter 6).

Recipient Selection

The indication for pediatric heart transplantation remains *end-stage congestive heart failure* due to cardiomyopathy where the expectation of survival beyond 1 year is limited. There are certain *structural congenital heart* diseases that are associated with limited survival, such as hypoplastic left heart syndrome. These indications are not without controversy. In general, the indication for transplantation due to cardiomyopathy is well accepted. However, the therapeutic alternatives for hypoplastic left heart syndrome vary among countries and centers and include (1) termination of pregnancy after intrauterine diagnosis of hypoplastic left heart syndrome, (2) palliative treatment only after birth and diagnosis of hypoplastic left heart syndrome, (3) Norwood's multistage repair, and (4) orthotopic transplantation.

The diagnosis and investigation of prospective recipients for heart transplantation include history and physical examination with specific emphasis on the presence and degree of both left and right heart failure. It is primarily on this basis that an estimation of duration of survival is based. Clinical and laboratory evidence of significant comorbidity, particularly neurologic status and evidence of hepatorenal dysfunction, is important. These are both contraindications to transplantation. Should there be an irreversible neurologic deficit, then the potential for useful rehabilitation after transplantation is limited. In addition, the presence of *hepatorenal dysfunction* may be made considerably worse after transplantation due to exposure to cardiopulmonary bypass and hepatotoxic and nephrotoxic drugs, particularly cyclosporine. *Active sepsis* and *uncontrolled malignancy* are contraindications to transplantation. Assessment of PVR is of critical importance. *A PVR of >6 Wood Units or a transpulmonary gradient of >15 to 20 mm Hg* after a challenge with oxygen, inotropic agents, vasodilators, and nitric oxide are strong relative contraindications to transplantation.

The degree of immunologic stimulation in the recipient may also have a bearing on the outcome. Panel-reactive antibodies (PRA) are preformed antibodies that react to a general pool of donor lymphocytes. This occurs particularly in children who have had prior surgical procedures and blood transfusions. If the PRA is >25%, the child has a significant likelihood of dying of causes related to rejection within 5 years. Conversely, if the PRA is <5%, this likelihood is <15%.

Surgical Management

The surgical management of the recipient for heart transplantation is influenced by several factors. The first factor is the size of the recipient. In some institutions, neonates are subjected to circulatory arrest for a portion of the transplantation procedure, whereas other centers prefer bicaval cannulation with moderate hypothermia and continuous low-flow cardiopulmonary bypass. With larger infants and children, bicaval cannulation with moderate hypothermia is the standard.

The operative techniques are tailored to the recipient's anatomy and the presence of prior palliative procedures. There is no situation from the point of view of native recipient anatomy or prior surgery that anatomically contraindicates transplantation. Circumstances that require special considerations include (1) prior palliation, either shunts or baffles such as the Fontan, Senning, and Mustard procedures; (2) abnormalities of systemic venous anatomy; and (3) situs inversus.

The basics of planning the transplantation procedure in the presence of prior palliation or structural congenital heart disease include the following considerations: (1) extended lengths of donor tissues, specifically, vena cava, innominate vein, aorta, pulmonary artery, and inferior vena cava; (2) atrial septation; (3) baffle removal or incorporation into the transplant; and (4) complete orthotopic transplantation.

The greater the extent of anatomic abnormalities, native or iatrogenic, the greater is the indication for performing a complete orthotopic transplantation to simplify the procedure. Specifically, individual anastomoses of the superior and inferior vena cavae, left and right pulmonary venous confluences, and potentially left and right pulmonary artery anastomoses may be fashioned as opposed to construction of complex baffles and diversions. After the recipient cardiectomy has been performed and the individual structures (specifically, the right and left superior venae cavae, if present; inferior vena cava; pulmonary arteries; and right and left pulmonary veins with a retained cuff of recipient left atrium) are trimmed back to near the pericardial reflection, the donor heart can be directly anastomosed to these structures with additional lengths of superior vena cava, pulmonary artery, and, potentially, inferior vena cava from the donor (Fig. 10–3).

The donor organ must be also carefully inspected for the presence of a patent foramen ovale to prevent right-to-left shunting after transplantation.

Resuscitation of the donor heart during the transplant procedure includes (1) readministration of cardioplegia, (2) adequate de-airing maneuvers, (3) an adequate period of reperfusion before separation from cardiopulmonary bypass, and (4) in the presence of an elevated PVR or right heart dysfunction in the donor organ, therapy directed at lowering PVR and stimulating myocardial contractility while maintaining adequate tissue perfusion pressure.

Postoperative Care

MONITORING

Continuous monitoring of cardiac function includes blood pressure, central venous pressure, and, if indicated, pulmonary artery pressure. Continuous monitoring of oxygenation and ventilation includes O_2 saturation and noninvasive CO_2 monitoring (e.g., end-tidal CO_2). *Serial investigations* to monitor cardiac, respiratory, and hematologic functions and immunosuppressive therapy are necessary (Table 10–1). Routine body fluid cultures are essential for early diagnosis of sepsis.

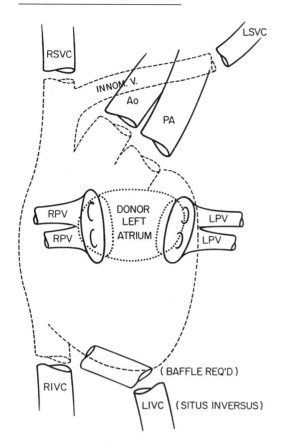

Figure 10–3. Possible connections for orthotopic heart transplantation in structural congenital heart disease. Donor heart -------; recipient structure.

Table 10–1. POSTOPERATIVE MONITORING

Continuous	Blood pressure, central venous pressure, pulmonary artery pressure
	Oxygen saturation, end-tidal CO_2
	Urinary output
Serial	Electrolytes, arterial blood gases, glucose q4h
	CBC, lactate, INR, PTT q8h
	Alkaline phosphatase, aspartate aminotransferase, bilirubin, creatine kinase, calcium, magnesium, albumin, urea, creatinine q12h
	Serology (cytomegalovirus, Epstein-Barr virus, herpes, toxoplasma, mycoplasma) every Monday and Thursday
	Urine and blood for culture and sensitivity every Monday and Thursday
Daily T cell subsets (CD_3) while on OKT3	Daily chest radiograph while on ventilator
	Daily echocardiogram and EKG $\times$ 7 days then every Monday and Thursday

FLUIDS

Fluids are restricted for the first 24 to 48 hours to *60% maintenance* due to the expected generalized capillary leaks and renal dysfunction. If the patient is clinically hypovolemic, a colloid transfusion (e.g., 5% albumin or fresh frozen plasma [FFP]) is recommended.

VENTILATION

It is recommended that patients should be fully ventilated during the initial postoperative phase. Because many patients demonstrate high PVR, it may be necessary to maintain *hyperoxia and hypocarbia*. This will likely lower PVR and improve the right ventricular function. It may also be necessary to use other non*selective pulmonary vasodilators* (e.g., nitroglycerin, nitroprusside, prostaglandin E, amrinone) if there is evidence of significant right ventricular dysfunction. In some cases, *nitric oxide* should be considered (especially with refractory pulmonary hypertension and impaired right ventricular function).

INOTROPIC SUPPORT

Impaired myocardial function in the transplant organ is a multifactorial problem and begins with the donor around the time of brain death, when there are massive hormonal fluctuations. The effect of donor hypertension and hypotension may also be important, as well as the duration and magnitude of inotropic support in the donor and ischemic injury in the donor or as it relates to inadequacies of myocardial preservation after donor organ retrieval. The nature of the primary cause of death in the donor may also have considerable bearing on myocardial function after transplantation. Blunt trauma such as might occur in motor vehicle accidents may give rise to myocardial contusions. CO_2 poisoning is also associated with myocardial necrosis. Considerably worse myocardial function may be seen after a period of ischemia followed by transplantation.

For a complete description of all inotropic agents, refer to Chapter 7.5.

One unique characteristic of transplanted hearts is the tendency for *exquisite sensitivity to catecholamines,* possibly due to the fact that these hearts are now denervated. For example, the recipient may be critically dependent on a very low dose of dopamine (2 to 4 mg/kg/min) without which hypotension would result. Conversely, slightly higher doses might result in hypertension.

Immunosuppression

There are a variety of successful protocols for immunosuppression after heart transplantation. The major therapeutic choices revolve around the following options:

- Use of cyclosporine versus the use of FK506
- Use of cytocytic induction (e.g., OKT3, RATG), in part to avoid cyclosporine-related nephrotoxicity early after surgery

- Use of maintenance steroids: this remains somewhat controversial. Groups that advocate a "steroid-free" protocol cite the avoidance of steroid-associated complications as a benefit. However, cumulative doses of steroids given for acute rejection episodes are similar to total doses found in maintenance steroid protocols.

The immunosuppression protocol that we use includes the following: (1) no preoperative immunosuppression; (2) administration of *methylprednisolone intraoperatively* (10 mg/kg); and (3) *postoperative methylprednisolone* (1 mg/kg IV; steroid is tapered rapidly to 0.2 mg/kg/day at 3 months after transplantation), *OKT3* (1 to 5 mg IV daily to maintain CD_3 levels at 0 for 1 week), introduction of *cyclosporine* on the second or third day after surgery to maintain monoclonal whole-blood radioimmunoassay at approximately 450 ng/mL, and *azathioprine* (2 to 4 mg/kg) introduced after discontinuation of OKT3.

ACUTE REJECTION

Treatment includes optimization of cyclosporine dose for *mild rejection.* Increase oral steroids to 1 mg/kg/day for 3 days and rapidly taper to the baseline dose within 1 to 2 weeks for *moderate rejection. Moderate rejection with hemodynamic compromise* and *severe rejection* are treated with intravenous steroids (5 to 10 mg/kg IV for 3 days with rapid tapering). OKT3 can also be used for *severe rejection.* Conversion to FK506-based immunosuppression, methotrexate, or total lymphoid irradiation may be options for *resistant rejection.*

REJECTION MONITORING FOR INFANTS IS PRIMARILY NONINVASIVE

Monitor for (1) tachycardia, presence of a third heart sound, dysrhythmias, tachypnea, other signs of distress or irritability, poor feeding, crackles and wheezes on auscultation, hepatomegaly, fever, or a change in feeding, sleeping, or activity patterns; (2) ECG changes, reduction in combined voltages, supraventricular dysrhythmias, ventricular dysrhythmias, or heart block; and (3) echocardiographic changes, increasing wall thickness of the posterior wall and septum, decreasing systolic and diastolic function, pericardial effusion, and decrease in left ventricular shortening fraction.

Whenever possible, even in the very young and very small, endomyocardial biopsy remains the gold standard for rejection monitoring.

Graft coronary artery disease is the major factor in limiting long-term survival of heart transplant recipients. The etiology of this condition is uncertain, but several factors have been implicated, including endothelial injury at the time of brain death or retrieval, chronic cellular rejection, hyperlipidemia, cytomegalovirus infection, and chronic vascular rejection.

The vascular abnormalities are represented by intimal thickening with a normal media. This condition is best identified early in its course with the use of intracoronary ultrasound. There is some evidence that calcium antagonists and possibly captopril may help prevent this condition.

Infection

Infection prophylaxis is an important consideration, with concentration on three specific areas: prophylaxis of routine postoperative infections by standard perioperative antibiotic prophylaxis, prophylaxis against cytomegalovirus infection with cytomegalovirus immunoglobulin and high-dose acyclovir, and chronic antibiotic prophylaxis directed at opportunistic bacterial infections with chronic cotrimoxazole prophylaxis.

Summary

There have been many innovations in pediatric transplantation in the past 5 years. These innovations have influenced the management of pediatric patients. More young children and infants with structural congenital heart disease are receiving transplants. It is possible to use increasingly more sophisticated mechanical circulatory support systems both before and after transplantation. Intraoperative and postoperative management of right ventricular failure and pulmonary hypertension has taken a major step forward with the introduction of inhaled nitric oxide therapy. Immunosuppressive agents continue to evolve. Cyclosporine, steroids, and azathioprine continue to be the mainstay of immunosuppression; however, FK506 and newer agents, such as mycophenolate mofetil and monoclonal and polyclonal cytolytic agents, may allow continuous improvement in management of acute and chronic rejection.

The quality of life that these children enjoy is excellent. Most children are discharged from hospital within a few weeks after transplantation, and most subsequent monitoring involves outpatient visits. The most serious problem facing pediatric heart transplantation is the critical shortfall of donor organs. If all potential organ donors were identified to organ procurement agencies, this would go a long way to addressing that critical need. This requires the coordinated efforts of health care professionals, legislators, and a concerned public to ensure that the needs of children with end-stage heart disease can be fulfilled.

BIBLIOGRAPHY

Bailey LL, Grundry SR: Hypoplastic left heart syndrome. Pediatr Clin North Am 37:137, 1990.
Hosenpud JD, Novick RJ, Breen TJ, Daily OP: The Registry of the International Society for Heart and Lung Transplantation: eleventh official report–1994. J Heart Lung Transplant 13:561, 1994.
Kirklin JK, Naftel DC, Kirklin JW, et al: Pulmonary vascular resistance and the risk of heart transplantation. J Heart Transplant 7:331, 1988.
Menkis A, McKenzie N, Novick R, et al: Special considerations for cardiac transplantation in congenital heart disease. J Heart Transplant 9:602, 1990.
Pennington DG, Noedel N, McBride LR, et al: Heart transplantation in children: an international survey. Ann Thorac Surg 52:710, 1991.

10.2 Postoperative Management of the Liver Transplant Recipient

ANN THOMPSON, MD, FAAP
JERRIL GREEN, MD

Advances in immunosuppression, organ preservation, surgical technique, and postoperative intensive care management have made liver transplantation standard therapy for most end-stage liver disease in children. *Indications* for pediatric liver transplantation include extrahepatic biliary atresia (accounting for about 50% of transplants), intrahepatic cholestasis, inborn errors of metabolism, toxin-mediated and infectious hepatitis, and liver tumors. These patients benefit from a multidisciplinary approach to their care, from evaluation for transplantation through a prolonged follow-up period.

Preoperative Management of the Liver Transplant Recipient

The intensivist faces the gamut of multiple organ system pathology related to liver failure. *Altered mental status, pulmonary vascular and parenchymal disorders, abdominal distention,* and *malnutrition* all contribute to the need for mechanical ventilation. *Profound coagulopathy* may require continuous treatment with blood products. *Hepatic encephalopathy* will at times be associated with increased intracranial pressure (ICP) that requires medical management. *Renal failure* may require dialysis or continuous hemofiltration. *Metabolic acidosis* may be intractable in the moribund patient, and require continuous alkali infusion or renal replacement therapy. *Nutritional support* and *pain control* are also issues for the intensivist.

Postoperative Management of the Liver Transplant Recipient

PULMONARY MANAGEMENT

Essentially all children require mechanical ventilation after liver transplantation. Those who are greater than one year of age are usually weaned from mechanical ventilation and extubated within one to four days. However, infants less than one year frequently need more prolonged ventilator support, particularly those with severe growth failure, minimal muscle mass, and severe abdominal distention.

Ventilator management follows conventional guidelines. Adequate oxygenation is essential to graft survival. *Inspired oxygen (FIO₂) should be sufficient to maintain an arterial PO₂ of >70 mm Hg, or an oxygen saturation (SaO₂) >92%. Positive end-expiratory pressure (PEEP) of 4–6 cm H₂O is routine, unless an FIO₂ of greater than .60 is required: then the PEEP should be increased to 8–10 cm H₂O or higher, as needed.* However, to the extent that airway pressure is transmitted to the pleural space, increasing PEEP may increase the central venous pressure (CVP), and decrease perfusion pressure across the transplanted liver. Most patients who benefit from increased airway pressure have significant parenchymal disease, and transmit rather little of the pressure to the pleural space, but in each case improved oxygenation should be evaluated with liver perfusion in mind. *Ventilation to maintain PCO₂ of 35–45 mm Hg is usually possible with effective tidal volumes of 8–12 mL/kg or peak inspiratory pressures of 20–35 mm Hg and a ventilator rate of 15–20 breaths/minute.* Intermittent arterial blood gas monitoring particularly to determine blood pH, along with pulse oximetry and end-tidal CO₂ monitoring is desirable.

A variety of complications may make respiratory management more difficult. *Atelectasis, pulmonary edema, and pleural effusions are common.* Effective pulmonary toilet with airway suctioning, appropriate positioning, and chest physiotherapy is indicated. *Diaphragmatic excursion is frequently restricted* in infants and small children by ascites, relatively large grafts, ileus, intra-abdominal bleeding, or by phrenic nerve injury. Chronic malnutrition with muscle weakness may prolong weaning from mechanical ventilation.

Anatomic arteriovenous intrapulmonary fistulas resulting from chronic liver failure cause a decrease in oxygenation that is minimally responsive to manipulation of mechanical ventilation. In most cases this problem is recognized preoperatively. However, if chest radiographs do not reveal other causes of hypoxemia, and increasing FIO₂ or mean airway pressure is ineffective, the possibility of intrapulmonary shunting should be considered. In some cases significant hypoxemia must be tolerated, and will resolve only slowly over a period of many months.

Pulmonary infection caused by bacterial, viral, fungal and other pathogens requires escalation in treatment similar to that required by other patients with these disorders. Bronchoalveolar lavage is appropriate early in the course of respiratory dysfunction. Decreasing or discontinuing immunosuppression may be necessary. (See Infectious Disease section.)

CARDIOVASCULAR MANAGEMENT

The goal of cardiovascular management is to assure a cardiac output that provides adequate tissue perfusion, and in this setting, promotes graft survival. *Evidence of adequate tissue perfusion includes urine output of at least 1–2 mL/kg/ hour, warm distal extremities with easily palpable distal pulses, capillary refill of no more than one to two seconds, normal or improving mental status, and absence of metabolic acidosis. Of particular importance is adequate perfusion of the newly transplanted liver. As a general rule, the difference between mean arterial pressure (MAP) and CVP should be greater than 60 mm Hg.* Low MAP or high CVP may compromise graft perfusion and function and may increase the risk of vascular thrombosis. *Poor tissue perfusion should be recognized before hypotension and hemodynamic instability occur. Causes include inadequate replacement of intraoperative fluid or blood loss, on-going hemorrhage, sepsis, or severe graft failure. Hypotension and/or persistent metabolic acidosis are ominous signs and demand immediate evaluation and treatment.* In the early postoperative course and in patients who remain coagulopathic, significant bleeding must be excluded immediately. Treatment should be directed toward restoration of adequate circulating volume using crystalloid, 5% albumin, or blood products (depending on hematocrit and coagulation profile). Vasoactive agents should be added for hypotension which persists in spite of volume replacement when surgical bleeding has been excluded or corrected.

Another common hemodynamic problem after liver transplantation is hypertension. Contributing factors include fluid overload, inadequate analgesia or sedation, and side effects of steroids, cyclosporine, and tacrolimus. Careful use of narcotics while monitoring respiratory status is the preferred method for sedation and pain relief. If the fluid intake and output record is consistent with fluid overload, the CVP is high, or significant edema is present, fluid restriction and diuretic administration may be indicated. Care must be taken not to cause hypovolemia with these measures. Cyclosporine or tacrolimus may be the etiology of hypertension even with nontoxic drug levels. Regardless of the cause, hypertension can be severe and requires urgent treatment. Table 10–2 *lists antihypertensive drugs and doses commonly used in children.*

FLUID AND ELECTROLYTES

As discussed above, ensuring adequate circulating volume is essential to hemodynamic stability and graft survival. *Warm distal extremities with easily palpable pulses, normal capillary refill, normal urine output, and a CVP of 4–10 cm H$_2$O suggest adequate circulating volume. Intravenous fluids should be run at half to full maintenance rate depending on volume status. Concentrations of glucose and electrolytes are based on serum values, but 5% dextrose in .2–.45% sodium chloride (NaCl) is usually acceptable. Drainage from wounds, enterostomies, and the like should be replaced completely with isotonic crystalloid or colloid initially and then adjusted as volume and electrolyte status dictate.* Third space losses along with drain and wound output may quickly result in hypovolemia.

Electrolyte abnormalities are common in the early postoperative period. If graft viability is questionable, serum potassium must be followed closely because

Table 10–2. ANTIHYPERTENSIVE DRUGS

Drug	Dose
Nifedipine	0.25–0.5 mg/kg PO or SL q4–6h
Hydralazine	0.1–0.5 mg/kg IV q4–6h
Sodium nitroprusside	0.1–10 μg/kg/min
Labetalol	0.25–1.5 mg/kg q10min, then q6h
Diazoxide	3–5 mg/kg/dose rapid IV bolus

graft necrosis can be associated with the rapid onset of severe, life-threatening hyperkalemia which must be managed aggressively. More commonly diuretic therapy and alkalosis are associated with *hypokalemia.* It is very well-tolerated in most cases but should be treated when severe (e.g., <2–2.5 mEq/L). In patients with good graft function and urine output, potassium chloride (KCl) can be added to maintenance fluids or administered as concentrated infusions (0.3 mEq/kg/hour for 2–3 hours).

Hyponatremia may result from excess free water administration and/or diuretic therapy. *Hypernatremia* is usually the result of large volumes of crystalloid and colloid given as replacement fluid or sodium bicarbonate treatment of metabolic acidosis. In cases of graft failure with hyperammonemia treated with lactulose, hypernatremia may be secondary to free water loss. Chelation of calcium secondary to administration of citrated blood products can cause *hypocalcemia.* Treatment is with calcium chloride (CaCl) 10–20 mg/kg via a central vein as needed. Use of calcium gluconate is less desirable as it must be metabolized by the liver. *Hypomagnesemia* also occurs, especially with tacrolimus. Treatment is with magnesium sulfate 25–50 mg/kg/dose.

ACID-BASE BALANCE

Respiratory alkalosis and metabolic acidosis are common in severe liver disease. In most patients these acid-base abnormalities resolve rapidly after successful transplantation. *Persistent metabolic acidosis is an ominous finding that often reflects sepsis, rejection, or graft necrosis.* While appropriate evaluation is underway, acidosis may be treated with sodium bicarbonate. More commonly, massive transfusion, fluid restriction, diuretics, and gastrointestinal tract drainage lead to metabolic alkalosis with sometimes dramatic compensatory respiratory acidosis. Patients may demonstrate remarkable hypercarbia without any evidence of respiratory distress. In these children mechanical ventilatory support is best weaned based on pH, oxygenation, and respiratory effort. In most cases alkalosis resolves spontaneously as long as adequate potassium and chloride are provided. In a few instances treatment with acetazolamide or administration of arginine or ammonium hydrochloride may be worthwhile to hasten resolution.

HEMATOLOGIC PROBLEMS

While less common now than in the past, major intraoperative blood loss may occur, requiring massive transfusion. This is likely to result in anemia, leukopenia, thrombocytopenia, hypothermia, persistent alkalosis (as citrate is metabolized), hypocalcemia, and hyperkalemia. *A falling hemoglobin associated with hemodynamic instability, especially in the early postoperative period, requires that surgical bleeding be excluded as a cause. Anemia should be corrected slowly when the hemoglobin drops below 8 to 10 gm. Over-transfusion and a higher hemoglobin may increase the risk of vascular thrombosis.* Leukopenia resolves spontaneously over 24 to 48 hours. *Thrombocytopenia should be treated only if the platelet count drops below 20,000/mm³ or if there is active bleeding. Again, overly zealous replacement may increase the risk of vascular thrombosis.*

The coagulopathy of severe liver disease resolves briskly as graft function improves, usually within days after transplantation. *Treatment of the coagulopathy with fresh frozen plasma (FFP) is indicated only in the case of active bleeding, or in the event of graft failure. Aggressive use of FFP may increase the risk of vascular thrombosis.*

INFECTIOUS DISEASE ISSUES

Most patients receive 1 to 5 days of *prophylactic antibiotics* after transplantation, for example, ampicillin and cefuroxime. Early in the postoperative period bacterial infections are most common. Skin flora and enteric organisms are the most common offenders. *Broad spectrum antibiotics, for example, vancomycin and ceftazidime are indicated when bacterial infection is suspected.* Intravenous and urinary catheters increase the risk of bacterial infection and should be removed as soon as is prudent. Another pathogen which may cause disease early and then at any time post-transplant is *Pneumocystis carinii. Prophylaxis against Pneumocystis carinii* with trimethoprim/sulfamethoxazole (5 mg/kg q12h IV) should begin immediately after surgery.

Viral infections increase in incidence 1 to 2 months after transplantation. The most common is cytomegalovirus (CMV), but Epstein-Barr virus (EBV), herpes simplex virus (HSV), respiratory syncytial virus (RSV), and adenovirus also occur. *Prophylaxis against CMV* with gancyclovir (1 mg/kg/day) is commonly used, and serves to prevent development of disease during the period of maximal immunosuppression and to decrease the severity of disease if it does occur. In addition to acute infection with EBV, *post transplant lymphoproliferative disorder (PTLD)* is associated with new or reactivated EBV infection. Along with supportive care, PTLD is treated by reducing or discontinuing immunosuppression.

Fungal infections may occur at any time in immune suppressed patients but, aside from infection with candida species, they are more common months after transplantation in this population. Treatment with broad spectrum antibiotics increases the risk of fungal infection. Infection with candida species is most common but aspergillosis, mucormycosis, and other infections also occur. Oral rinse with Mycostatin will decrease the risk of yeast infection. While candida species can be cultured from routine blood and body fluid cultures, other fungi, especially aspergillus, usually require tissue biopsy and/or culture for diagnosis. *Treatment with amphotericin B (1 mg/kg/day) should begin early, while awaiting cultures, if fungus is suspected.* Other antifungal agents such as fluconazole and itraconazole may increase both tacrolimus and cyclosporin levels.

NEUROLOGIC COMPLICATIONS

Hepatic encephalopathy usually resolves within the first two days following transplantation. With graft failure, however, encephalopathy progresses, associated with *cerebral edema, increased intracranial pressure (ICP), and death.* ICP monitoring may be useful for distinguishing pure metabolic derangements from the secondary effects of intracranial hypertension and for guiding therapy. However, in the presence of a coagulopathy, the risk of bleeding complications is high, and the benefits of ICP monitoring must be balanced against this risk. Depressed neurologic function may also occur due to delayed clearance of anesthetic agents, intracranial hemorrhage, thromboembolism, and cerebral edema.

Central nervous system (CNS) infections are not common early after transplantation but should be considered as a late cause of altered mental status. *Seizures in transplant recipients are usually the result of electrolyte abnormalities, hypoglycemia, and toxic effects of cyclosporine and tacrolimus.* On rare occasions, they are the result of CNS infection, hemorrhage, or other structural abnormalities. Post transplant lymphoproliferative disease may occur in the CNS and may present with seizures or with focal neurologic symptoms. Anticonvulsants such as phenytoin, phenobarbital, and carbamazapine, may decrease levels of both tacrolimus and cyclosporin. These levels should be monitored closely and adjusted accordingly when treating seizures in transplant patients.

RENAL COMPLICATIONS

In the presence of a well-functioning graft, hepatorenal syndrome from the preoperative period usually resolves briskly. However, decreased renal function may be a problem in the postoperative period even when renal function was normal before transplantation. *Causes include toxic effects of cyclosporine and tacrolimus, decreased cardiac output from either hypovolemia or myocardial dysfunction, perioperative ischemia, tense abdominal distention, and graft dysfunction.* It is essential to assess the patient's intravascular volume status, using primarily physical criteria (e.g., perfusion and central venous pressure, blood pressure, and heart rate) because chemical indicators of renal function such as BUN, creatinine, and serum electrolytes may be confused by diuretic therapy, chronic malnutrition, and cyclosporin or tacrolimus. Meticulous attention to daily weight, and intake and output is also essential.

When renal failure occurs despite adequate circulating blood volume, low dose dopamine (0.5–3 µg/kg/min) may improve renal blood flow. Dosing for all nephrotoxic medications should be adjusted for renal failure. Dialysis or hemofiltration may be required, but its need is an ominous sign.

HEPATIC COMPLICATIONS

Hepatic complications involve the transplanted liver and/or its vascular and biliary structures (Table 10–3). Primary nonfunction, infection, rejection, and vascular insufficiency have many similarities. *Primary nonfunction* is characterized by rapidly worsening, markedly abnormal liver function, oliguria, hyperkalemia, hypoglycemia, metabolic acidosis, and encephalopathy progressing to coma. The only effective treatment is aggressive supportive care until a new organ becomes available for retransplantation. Rejection, infection, and vascular occlusion are all characterized by fever, malaise, and worsening graft function, and liver biopsy is commonly necessary to differentiate them.

Vascular occlusion occurs most frequently in the hepatic artery but may affect the portal vein as well. *Hepatic artery thrombosis* occurs most often in small patients. About one third of cases are asymptomatic. Alternatively, liver function may deteriorate acutely and progress to complete graft failure and necrosis. Fever and sepsis secondary to enteric organisms, or bacteremia with essentially un-

Table 10–3. EVALUATION OF POST-TRANSPLANT LIVER DYSFUNCTION

Criterion	Infection	Rejection	Vascular Occlusion	Harvesting Injury	Biliary Obstruction
Fever	+	+	±	–	–
Bilirubin	Normal to mild ↑	Mild to severe ↑	Mild to severe ↑	Mild to moderate ↑	Mild to moderate ↑
AST/ALT	Mild to moderate ↑	Mild to severe ↑	Mild to severe ↑	Mild to severe ↑	Mild ↑
γGT	↑	↑	↑		↑↑
Prothrombin time	Normal to mild ↑	Mild to severe ↑	Mild to severe ↑	Mild to moderate ↑	Normal to mild ↑
WBC count	Mild to moderate ↑	Mild to moderate ↑	Normal to mild ↑	Normal to mild ↑	Normal to mild ↑
Cultures	+	–	±	–	–
Ultrasound	Abscess	Echogenicity ↑	Occluded vessel, infarction	–	Dilated biliary structures
Computed tomography scan	Abscess	–	Occluded vessel, infarction, biliary or bowel disruption	–	Dilated biliary structures
Angiography	Parenchymal defect	–	Occluded vessel	–	–
Biopsy	Inflammatory infiltrate, inclusion bodies, positive cultures	Periportal, mononuclear infiltrate; single hepatocyte necrosis	Massive necrosis	Diffuse zonal necrosis	Dilated ducts

Table 10–4. COMMON IMMUNOSUPPRESSIVE AGENTS

Agent	Indication	Side Effects
Corticosteroids	Rejection prophylaxis and treatment of acute rejection	Infection, sodium and water retention, hypertension, altered glucose metabolism, adrenal suppression, muscle weakness, personality changes
Cyclosporine	Rejection prophylaxis and treatment of acute rejection	Infection, nephrotoxicity, hypertension, hepatotoxicity, tremors, seizures, gingival hypertrophy, hirsutism, lymphoproliferative disease
Tacrolimus	Rejection prophylaxis and treatment of acute rejection	Infection, nephrotoxicity, neurotoxicity, hyperglycemia, gastrointestinal symptoms, hypertension, PTLD
Azathioprine	Rejection prophylaxis	Infection, myelotoxicity, nausea, vomiting, mucosal ulcerations
OKT3	Treatment of acute rejection	Infection, lymphopenia, anaphylaxis, pulmonary edema, PTLD
Lymphocyte immune globulin	Treatment of acute rejection	Thrombocytopenia, lymphopenia, anaphylaxis, serum sickness, increased blood urea nitrogen and creatinine

changed liver function may result from abscess formation within a region of hepatic necrosis. Bile leak and peritonitis due to bile duct ischemia may also occur. *Portal vein thrombosis* may present with graft necrosis, ascites or bowel wall edema, or as bleeding esophageal varices. Diagnosis of vascular thrombosis may be made with abdominal ultrasound with Doppler. If flow in these vessels is not detected, angiography is indicated to confirm the diagnosis. In infants and small children prophylaxis against vascular thrombosis is routine, including dextran 40 (5 mL/hour IV for 5 days), heparin (5 units/kg IV q12h), and/or Persantine.

Acute rejection is typically characterized by fever, malaise, anorexia, and increasing bilirubin and transaminases including γGT. As viral hepatitis and systemic sepsis may have similar presentations and liver biopsy may be required to guide therapy. In patients who become seriously ill, supportive care and broad spectrum antibiotics are indicated while the diagnostic evaluation proceeds. *When acute rejection is confirmed, intensified immunosuppression is indicated including increased corticosteroids, cyclosporine or tacrolimus, and addition of muromonab (OKT3) if the rejection is refractory to other measures.*

GASTROINTESTINAL ISSUES

Bleeding may occur at any point along the GI tract. Early upper GI bleeding may be from nasal vessels, gastric erosions, or gastric perforation, and early lower GI bleeding is likely to be from intestinal anastamoses in patients with Roux-en-Y choledochoenterostomies. Postoperative bleeding from esophageal varices suggests portal vein thrombosis. Most GI bleeding will resolve spontaneously with supportive care, including correction of coagulopathy. If persistent, surgical intervention may be required. *Stress ulcer prophylaxis is routinely provided with H_2 blockers, specifically ranitidine (0.75–1.5 mg/kg/dose IV q6–8h), antacids (to keep the gastric pH 5), or sucralfate.*

NUTRITION

Many liver transplant recipients have longstanding malnutrition that may inhibit their post-transplant recovery. As soon as electrolytes are stable, parenteral nutrition should be started. *Calories administered may be based upon actual measured requirements, for example, O_2 consumption, CO_2 production, and urine nitrogen excretion, or on usual nutritional guidelines (100 Cal/kg for children under 10 kg, or 1500 Cal/ m^2). Calories should be distributed approximately as 8–10% protein, 50–55% carbohydrate, and 30–40% fat.* There are no data currently to support use of special parenteral or enteric formulas in these patients. Excessive carbohydrate loads should be avoided if CO_2 retention is a concern. Administered calories should be increased when metabolic requirements increase, for example, fever, major surgery, or sepsis. When enteral feeding can be tolerated, often by the third or fourth post-operative day, an age-appropriate diet should gradually replace parenteral nutrition (over 2–4 days).

IMMUNOSUPPRESSION

While all patients receive immunosuppression following liver transplantation, protocols vary from one institution to another. *In general, immediately after transplantation, treatment begins with two or three drugs including corticosteroids and either cyclosporine or tacrolimus.* Cyclosporine and tacrolimus-based regimens produce similar patient and graft survival. However, tacrolimus treated patients have less acute rejection and less refractory or corticosteroid-resistant rejection. Tacrolimus may however have a higher incidence of complications. Some protocols add a third agent, commonly azathioprine (Table 10–4). *Rejection,* varying in severity, is common and is treated with intensified immunosuppression, usually including increased corticosteroids and increased doses of cyclosporine or tacrolimus (Table 10–4). In patients with rejection unresponsive to these steps, addition of OKT3 or anti-lymphocyte globulins may be necessary. In the short term, these agents are associated with systemic symptoms of cytokine release, including fever, chills, stridor, pulmonary edema, and hypotension, which are treated as in anapylactic reactions. In the long term, OKT3 in particular, appears to be associated with a higher incidence of PTLD. Improvements in immunosuppression and measures to inhance immunotolerance will likely account for improved transplant outcomes in the future.

BIBLIOGRAPHY

Afessa B, et al: Pulmonary complications of orthotopic liver transplantation. Mayo Clin Proc 68:427, 1993.

Becht MB, et al: Growth and nutritional management of pediatric patients after orthotopic liver transplantation. Gastroenterol Clin North Am 22:367, 1993.

Busuttil RW, McDiarmid S, Klintmalm GB: The U.S. Multicenter FK506 Liver Study Group: a comparison of tacrolimus (FK506) and cyclosporine for immunosuppression in liver transplantation. N Engl J Med 331:1110, 1994.

Kocoshis SA, Tzakis A, Todo S, Reyes J, Nour B: Pediatric liver transplantation: history, recent innovations, and outlook for the future. Clin Pediatr (Phila) 32:386, 1993.

Rosenthal P, Podesta L, Sher L, Makowka L: Liver transplantation in children. Am J Gastroenterol 89:480, 1994.

10.3 Pediatric Renal Transplantation

DOUGLAS G. MATSELL, MD, CM, FRCPC

Renal transplantation is considered to be the optimal form of renal replacement therapy for children with end-stage renal disease (ESRD). Over the past 25 years, major advances in technical expertise and immunosuppression have occurred and are reflected in the dramatic improvement in clinical outcome of transplant recipients over years of follow-up.

The incidence of ESRD for children in the United States between the ages of 0 and 19 years is ≈11 per 1 million population per year; in Canada, it is estimated to be ≈8 per 1 million population for the ages of 0 to 14.

The etiology of ESRD is varied in this population, with glomerulonephritis being the most common category of renal disease necessitating transplantation. However, when considered as a single group, the most common causes of renal failure in children undergoing transplantation are congenital lesions, including renal dysplasia and obstructive uropathy (Table 10–5).

Both living-related donor (LRD) and cadaveric renal transplantations are performed, with improved outcomes in the LRDs. In North America, LRD kidneys account for 43% of all transplants in children, although the Canadian experience greatly favors the use of cadaver donors, for unknown reasons. Among recipients of cadaver kidneys, 74% of grafts survived at 1 year and 62% survived at 3 years. For LRD kidneys, 89% survived at 1 year and 80% survived at 3 years. At all ages, pediatric renal transplant recipients have lower mortality rates than dialysis patients of the same age, and there exist few contraindications to transplantation in children with ESRD.

Clinical Management of the Renal Transplant Patient

SELECTION OF THE DONOR

Related Donors

Relatives who have ABO compatibility with the recipient are tissue typed. The potential donor whose HLA-A, -B, -C, and -D/DR antigens most closely match is further evaluated (Table 10–6).

Table 10–5. ETIOLOGY OF ESRD IN CHILDREN UNDERGOING TRANSPLANTATION IN NORTH AMERICA FROM 1987 THROUGH 1992

Diagnosis	%
Aplastic/dysplastic kidneys	17
Obstructive uropathy	17
Focal segmental glomerulosclerosis	12
Reflux nephropathy	5
Systemic immunologic disease	5
Chronic glomerulonephritis	4
Congenital nephrotic syndrome	4
Membranoproliferative glomerulonephritis (I and II)	3
Prune belly syndrome	3
Medullary cystic disease	3
Hemolytic uremic syndrome	3
Polycystic kidney disease	3
Cystinosis	3
Familial nephritis	2
Other	16

Revised from Yadin O, Grimm P, Ettenger R: Renal transplantation in children. *In* Holliday MA, Barratt TM, Avner ED (eds): Pediatric Nephrology. Williams & Wilkins, Baltimore, 1994, pp. 1390–1418.

Cadaveric Donors

The ideal cadaveric donor is a young person with normal vital signs before death who is free of infection and malignancy and has died in-hospital after hours of observation. The potential cadaveric donor is evaluated with a complete blood count, coagulation parameters, serum electrolytes, urea, and creatinine. The donor should be free of infection, malignancy, and preexisting renal disease. Before brain death, the potential donor should have blood samples taken for ABO and potential tissue typing to minimize cold ischemia time of the kidney. On declaration of

Table 10–6. EVALUATION OF POTENTIAL RELATED RENAL TRANSPLANT DONORS

General	Laboratory	Special Radiology
History and physical examination	Complete blood count	Renal arteriogram
Blood pressure determinations	PT/PTT/INR	
Chest X-ray	Serum electrolytes	
ECG	Liver function tests	
Intravenous pyelogram	Serum urea, creatinine, 24-hour urine	
	Serum calcium, phosphorus	
	Urinalysis, urine culture	
	Viral titers (CMV, EBV, HSV)	

brain death and after appropriate consent is given, a forced diuresis is achieved with saline, mannitol, and furosemide.

Removal of the kidney or kidneys is often performed in conjunction with the harvesting of other organs. The renal blood vessels are isolated and dissected with attention paid to the renal arterial anatomy. The ureter is dissected at the level of the bladder. The most common preservation for the kidney is simple hypothermic storage, which is limited to 36 hours of preservation. The kidneys are externally cooled, and the renal artery is flushed with a solution of sodium and potassium concentrations similar to intracellular values. The organ is then stored on ice in a sterile fashion.

Before transplantation, an appropriate cross-match must be performed to identify any recipient preformed antibodies to the donor T lymphocytes. This procedure usually takes several hours and occurs during organ preservation.

RENAL TRANSPLANTATION

Anesthesia

Anesthetics excreted solely by the kidney should be avoided. Before surgery, the recipient's hematocrit should be >30%, and excessive ultrafiltration during pretransplantation dialysis should be avoided.

Intraoperative Management

Hypothermia should be avoided by maintaining the ambient temperature at >32°C and placing the patient on warming blankets. At the time of revascularization, the kidney is warmed with saline. Arterial blood pressure is monitored through an arterial catheter; central venous pressure is monitored through a Hickman catheter into the right atrium. This dual-lumen catheter should be large enough to permit hemodialysis postoperatively if needed. At the time of induction of anesthesia, an intravenous prophylactic antibiotic is given, and a Foley catheter is inserted. The bladder can be filled with a neomycin solution (0.1%), and the catheter should be clamped.

Surgical Aspects

The surgical approach may vary according to the preferences of the surgeon and the size of the recipient. In children weighing <15 to 20 kg, a transperitoneal approach through a midline incision is performed. In larger children, the graft can be placed in the retroperitoneal iliac fossa. The right iliac fossa is preferred, using a right or left kidney, because dissection of the right fossa is simpler. For the anastomosis, the distal aorta, vena cava, and common iliac vessels are identified and dissected free. Perivascular lymphatics are ligated. The renal vessels are anastomosed with the external iliac vessels using an end-to-side anastomosis. Alternatively, the arterial anastomosis may be performed using the distal hypogastric artery or the aorta. The ureter is tunneled into the bladder, and a ureteroneocystostomy is performed. The kidney is then placed in the right retroperitoneal space. Before releasing the vascular clamps, the child should be transfused to raise the central venous pressure to 10 to 12 cm H_2O. In addition, a bolus of sodium bicarbonate should be administered.

Post-transplant and Intensive Care Unit Support

Fluid and Electrolytes. The most important goal of postoperative care is the maintenance of a generous intravascular volume to ensure proper perfusion of the transplanted kidney. Attempts should be made to maintain the *central venous pressure at >10 cm H_2O,* although if the graft is nonfunctioning, this may result in pulmonary edema from fluid overload.

In younger children and in patients who in addition have had nephrectomies, *third-space losses* may be significant. These should be accounted for and replaced with blood or colloid to maintain an adequate or slightly elevated blood pressure without causing congestive heart failure or pulmonary edema.

Urine output in the immediate postoperative period is replaced isovolumetrically with crystalloid in the form of 5% dextrose in 0.45% normal saline. This should be done at least hourly to avoid volume depletion. In a graft that is functioning well, a forced diuresis will occur, and after the first 24 hours, urine replacement can be decreased decrementally.

Hyperglycemia will often occur with this aggressive fluid replacement, necessitating a decrease in or discontinuation of glucose in the replacement fluid.

Life-threatening *hypokalemia* and *hypocalcemia* can develop, and serum electrolytes should be monitored and replaced appropriately.

Hypertension. Hypertension commonly occurs in the recovery phase and is related in part to the generous intravascular volume. *Mild hypertension* is tolerated.

More *severe hypertension* (>95% for age and height) should be treated with a combination of calcium channel–blocking agents (nifedipine 0.25 mg/kg/dose PO), diuretics (furosemide 1.0 to 2.0 mg/kg/dose IV), or a β-blocker (labetalol 1 to 3 mg/kg/hr IV).

The child with a *delayed functioning graft* will often become fluid overloaded, which should be treated with furosemide (1 to 2 mg/kg IV initially).

As graft function and fluid balance improve, the *antihypertensive medications* should be weaned and discontinued if possible.

Renal Function. Parameters of renal function to be monitored in the immediate postoperative period include urine output, serum urea and creatinine, serum and urinary electrolytes, serum calcium, and phosphorus. Within the first 24 hours of transplantation, a nuclear renal scan (^{99m}Tc-diaminotetraethylpentacetic acid [^{99m}Tc-DTPA]) is recommended—earlier in the case of a nonfunctioning or poorly functioning graft. The renal scan will provide information concerning the vascular anastomosis, renal parenchymal function (i.e., acute tubular necrosis), and ureteral patency.

Complications. The most serious complication of renal transplantation is failure of the graft to initiate or maintain renal function. In the early postoperative period, the graft may never function, have delayed onset of function, or fail after a brief period of function. The causes include acute tubular necrosis, hyperacute rejection, and technical complications (i.e., renal artery/vein occlusion, urinary obstruction). Other complications include postoperative bleeding, upper gastrointestinal bleeding, bowel obstruction, and infection (Fig. 10–4).

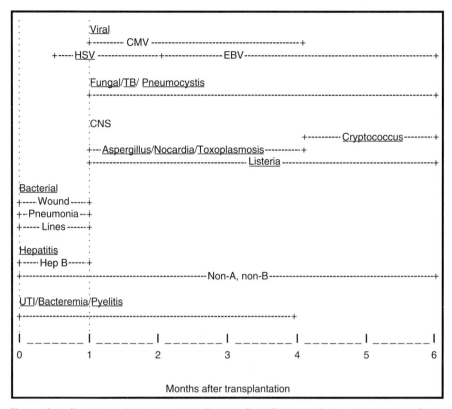

Figure 10–4. Chronology of Infections in the Pediatric Renal Transplant Patient. (Adapted from Rubin RH, Wolfson JS, Cosimi AB, et al: Infection in the renal transplant patient. Am J Med 70:405, 1981.)

IMMUNOSUPPRESSION AND CHEMOPROPHYLAXIS

Immunosuppressive strategies vary from center to center; however, most include induction with an antilymphocyte/blast globulin preparation (ALG or ATG) and subsequent triple therapy immunosuppression with corticosteroids, azathioprine, and cyclosporin A. More recent experience has been reported with the use of the drug FK-506 as single therapy.

The dosing schedule usually begins with intravenous ALG or ATG during the first 2 weeks post-transplant at a dosage of 10 to 20 mg/kg/day before the initiation of oral cyclosporin A therapy. Cyclosporin A is started when renal function has reached an acceptable level (serum creatinine <175 μmol/L) at a dosage of 5 to 15 mg/kg/day. Younger children and infants require a larger starting dose and, often, a TID dosing schedule to achieve desirable serum trough concentrations of 200 to 300 ng/mL in the immediate postoperative period. These higher and more frequent dosing requirements are due to age-related decreased absorption and increased metabolism of the drug. Caution should be exercised during concurrent administration of other medications because several of these will increase or decrease the metabolism of cyclosporin A (Table 10–7). If the child is not able to take oral cyclosporin A, then a 24-hour intravenous infusion may be started, usually requiring a dose reduction.

Prednisone or its equivalent is started in the immediate postoperative period at a dosage of 2 mg/kg/day, to be tapered quickly in the first month to 0.3 to 0.5 mg/kg/day. Azathioprine is also administered from the time of transplantation (at a dosage of 1 of 2 mg/kg/day) and requires close monitoring of the complete blood count.

Cytomegalovirus Prophylaxis

Infection after transplantation in pediatric patients accounts for approximately half of morbidity and mortality. Cytomegalovirus (CMV) is the principal infectious agent. In an attempt to prevent CMV infection in the transplant recipient, three agents have been used: CMV hyperimmune intravenous immunoglobulin, polyvalent immunoglobulin, and acyclovir. Administration of the intravenous immunoglobulin preparations does not prevent the CMV infection; however, they have been shown to attenuate the CMV syndrome. The use of prophylactic acyclovir decreases the incidence of CMV infection, specifically in the seronegative recipient of a transplant from a seropositive donor.

Prognosis

Several pretransplant and post-transplant factors influence the outcome of the renal transplant (Table 10–8). In the past 10 years, results in all age groups of childhood transplants are improving. Historically, transplantation in the child <2 years old was associated with an unacceptable mortality rate. Recent data demon-

Table 10–7. DRUG INTERACTIONS WITH CYCLOSPORIN A

Drugs that Decrease Cyclosporin A Levels	Drugs that Increase Cyclosporin A Levels
Anticonvulsants	*Antibiotics*
Phenytoin	Erythromycin
Carbamazepine	Ciprofloxacin
Phenobarbital	*Calcium Channel Blockers*
Antituberculous Agents	Verapamil
Isoniazid	Diltiazem
Rifampin	Nicardipine
Other	*Antifungals*
Mineral oil, cholestyramine	Ketaconazole
	Fluconazole
	Other
	Methylprednisolone, metoclopramide, ethinylestradiol, levonorgestrel

Table 10–8. FACTORS INFLUENCING TRANSPLANT OUTCOME IN CHILDREN

Recipient age
Donor age
HLA compatibility
Recipient immunoresponsiveness
Recurrence of primary kidney disease
De novo glomerulonephritis
Malignancy

strate a 1-year renal survival rate of 80% for LRD kidneys and 46% for cadaver donor kidneys in this age group. In children <6 years old, graft survival has also improved, to a 1-year survival rate of 90% with cadaver donor kidneys. Improvement in graft survival in the younger child has likely resulted from a number of factors, including improved medical and surgical management, the use of larger kidneys, and the use of anti–T cell preparations.

Donor age also contributes to outcome. Historically, for cadaveric donor renal transplantation, kidneys from young donors were given to young recipients. This practice has been shown to yield unacceptably high rates of graft failure due predominantly to graft thrombosis. One-year graft survival rates from donors 0 to 5, 6 to 10, and >10 years old were 63%, 73%, and 80%, respectively.

In the precyclosporine era, optimal HLA matching between donor and recipient was associated with improved graft survival in both the LRD and cadaver donor renal transplants. This has come into question with the advent of cyclosporin immunosuppression; however, precise HLA matching has the strongest influence on graft outcome, with a 17% advantage of identical matches at HLA-B and HLA-DR compared with mismatched grafts.

Recurrence of Primary Kidney Disease

In children, the causes of recurrence of kidney disease consist of metabolic and glomerular diseases and constitute up to 5% of graft losses. Inherited metabolic diseases that have the potential for graft involvement include cystinosis, oxalosis, and sickle cell anemia. Among the glomerular diseases, focal segmental glomerulosclerosis has the highest recurrence rate of almost 50%, with loss of graft in half of those. Membranoproliferative glomerulonephritis (MPGN) type 1 will recur in 30% to 70% of grafts, whereas MPGN type II will recur in 100% of transplanted kidneys. Other primary glomerular diseases with the potential for recurrence include IgA nephropathy, Henoch-Schönlein purpura nephropathy, hemolytic uremic syndrome, and, rarely, systemic lupus erythematosus.

In addition to the recurrence of glomerulonephritis, transplant recipients can develop a de novo glomerular lesion, most commonly in the form of a membranous nephropathy.

BIBLIOGRAPHY

Abitbol CL, Burke GW, Zilleruelo G, Montane B, Strauss J. Clinical management of the pediatric renal-allograft recipient. Child Nephrol Urol 11:169, 1991.

Ettenger RB. Children are different: the challenges of pediatric transplantation. Am J Kidney Dis 20:668, 1992.

10.4 Bone Marrow Transplantation

STANLEY CALDERWOOD, MD, FRCPC

A partial list of indications for bone marrow transplantation (BMT) in pediatric patients is given in Table 10–9. Preparation for BMT requires the administration of combinations of high-dose chemotherapy and/or radiation therapy (HDT). When treating malignant conditions, BMT overcomes the myeloablative effects of chemotherapy and allows significant dose escalation, with enhanced chance of cure. In nonmalignant conditions, the primary objective of BMT is replacement of diseased marrow with healthy donor marrow.

There are two distinct forms of BMT: *allogeneic*, in which the marrow is

Table 10–9. INDICATIONS FOR BMT IN PEDIATRICS

Malignant	Nonmalignant
Leukemia (acute and chronic)	Acquired marrow failure
Lymphoma (Hodgkin and non-Hodgkin)	Congenital marrow failure
Solid tumors	Red blood cell disorders
Brain tumors	Thalassemias
Sarcomas	Sickle cell anemia
Neuroblastomas	
Other	Neutrophil disorders
Myelodysplasias	Chronic granulomatous disease
Paroxysmal hemoglobinuria	Chédiak-Higashi
FEL	Migration/adhesion defects
	Monocyte/macrophage disorders
	Osteopetrosis
	Langerhan cell histiocytosis
	Platelet disorders
	Congenital immunodeficiencies
	Inborn errors of metabolism

obtained from a healthy volunteer donor, and *autologous*, in which the marrow is collected from the patient at an earlier time and stored, usually cryopreserved, until required for transplantation. Allogeneic BMT is used in treatment of both malignant and nonmalignant conditions, whereas the major indication for autologous BMT at present is treatment of malignancies. With the introduction of gene therapy, a discussion of which is beyond the scope of the chapter, autologous transplantation may find an extended role in the treatment of genetic diseases.

Donor Selection

ALLOGENEIC BONE MARROW TRANSPLANTATION

The ideal donor of bone marrow for allogeneic BMT is a sibling who is fully compatible at the human leukocyte antigen (HLA) locus. HLA antigens are broadly expressed on most tissues and are intricately involved in regulation of the immune response. Disparity for one or more genes in the HLA locus increases the risk of graft rejection and graft-versus-host disease (GVHD). Unfortunately, only about 30% of BMT candidates will have a suitable family donor. In an attempt to address this problem, large international registries of volunteer bone marrow donors have been established. These registries can be accessed through computerized data banks.

Placental blood is a rich source of lymphohematopoietic progenitors that can be used in allogeneic BMT. Attempts to establish banks of cryopreserved placental blood have begun in North America and Europe. These would represent an additional source of unrelated lymphohematopoietic stem cells for transplantation.

AUTOLOGOUS TRANSPLANTATION

The ideal candidate for autologous BMT would be a patient in whom the marrow is relatively free of contaminating tumor cells and whose disease is expected to be responsive to HDT. Unfortunately, in many childhood malignancies, there is a high risk of tumor contamination in the marrow. To address this problem, a number of different techniques have been established to "purge" the marrow of tumor cells; however, a discussion of these is beyond the scope of this chapter.

MARROW COLLECTION

With the donor under general anesthetic, the marrow is aspirated percutaneously from the marrow cavity of the iliac crest. The marrow is filtered to remove large particles and fat. If there is a red blood cell incompatibility between donor and recipient, red blood cells or plasma may need to be removed before administration of the marrow to the recipient. In the autologous setting, the marrow usually needs to be cryopreserved for storage before use.

Under normal circumstances, lymphohematopoietic stem cells, which are capable of restoring marrow function after HDT, circulate in the bloodstream in very low numbers. These numbers increase substantially in the recovery phase from myelosuppressive chemotherapy or after treatment with cytokines such as granulocyte colony-stimulating factor. They can be collected using a procedure known as leukapheresis. This represents an alternative method of "marrow" harvest.

Transplantation

Marrow is infused into the bloodstream via a large-bore central line. The lymphohematopoietic stem cells express intracellular adhesion molecules, which help them "home" to the marrow.

Concurrent with infusion of fresh marrow, which is anticoagulated with heparin, protamine neutralization is administered to prevent bleeding complications.

Dimethylsulfoxide (DMSO) is used to prevent damage to marrow during freezing and cryopreservation; however, it can cause histamine release and hemolysis of red blood cells. Premedication is necessary with an antihistamine and a glucocorticoid, in addition to twice-maintenance intravenous fluids to prevent renal damage from free hemoglobin. An anaphylaxis kit is kept at the patient's bedside because DMSO may cause anaphylaxis.

Post-Transplant Care

GENERAL SUPPORTIVE MEASURES

General supportive measures depend on the type of HDT used and the indication for transplant. *Antiemetics, narcotic analgesics,* and *anxiolytics* may be indicated. *Fluids* are usually administered at twice-maintenance levels, and allopurinol (4 mg/kg/dose, max 200 mg/dose, TID) is given to prevent tumor lysis syndrome and renal damage. *Bladder catheterization* or 2-mercaptoethane sulfonate sodium is used to prevent hemorrhagic cystitis, which may accompany high-dose cyclophosphamide. Phenytoin may be indicated to prevent seizures, which may be induced by high-dose busulfan.

ISOLATION

Patients are significantly immunosuppressed after HDT. To reduce the risk of infection, especially fungal infection, most centers isolate patients from day 0 (i.e., from the day of marrow infusion) until neutrophils have recovered to $>0.5 \times 10^9$. Commonly used protective isolation methods include laminar air flow (LAF) rooms or high-efficiency particulate air (HEPA) filters. Barrier isolation techniques vary considerably between centers, ranging from careful hand washing to full surgical scrub with boot and head covers, masks, sterile gowns, and gloves.

TRANSFUSIONAL SUPPORT

Transfusion with packed red blood cells to maintain a *hemoglobin level of ≥ 70 g/L* and with platelet concentrates to maintain platelet levels of $\geq 10 \times$

10^9/L are usually recommended. Higher platelet counts may be needed in bleeding patients or patients at risk of bleeding. All blood products should be irradiated to reduce the risk of transfusion-induced GVHD. Patients who are seronegative for cytomegalovirus should receive only cytomegalovirus-negative blood products. Intravenous pooled immunoglobulin is usually administered weekly or to maintain IgG levels of ≥ 6.0 g/L.

IMMUNOSUPPRESSION

Immunosuppression to prevent graft rejection is incorporated into the HDT given in preparation for BMT and is required only in the allogeneic setting. Cyclosporine, methotrexate, and steroids are given alone or in combination to prevent GVHD in the allogeneic setting.

INFECTION PROPHYLAXIS

Profound neutropenia and immunosuppression, which accompany HDT, result in susceptibility to viral, parasitic, fungal, and bacterial infection. Common infections and prophylactic measures are as follows:

Cytomegalovirus. Patients who are seropositive for CMV or whose marrow donor is CMV positive routinely receive antiviral prophylaxis. Choices include *acyclovir* (1500 mg/m^2/day IV divided BID day 0 through day 100; switch to oral dosing as soon as patient is tolerating oral intake), *ganciclovir* (10 mg/kg/day IV divided BID, starting with recovery of absolute neutrophil count [ANC] to >0.5 $\times$ 10^9/L and continuing through day 100; discontinue if ANC drops to <0.5 $\times$ 10^9/L), and *preemptive therapy.* (Monitor for signs of asymptomatic CMV reactivation, usually by bronchoalveolar lavage, and treat only patients who have viral shedding.)

Herpes Simplex Virus. Patients who are seropositive for herpes simplex virus receive prophylaxis with *acyclovir* (750 mg/m^2/day divided BID), beginning with administration of HDT and continuing until neutrophil recovery.

Pneumocystis carinii. Prophylaxis with *trimethoprim/sulfamethoxazole* (3 to 5 mg/kg/day OD or divided BID), beginning with HDT and continuing until 1 year after the transplantation. The drug should be discontinued if the ANC drops to <0.5 $\times$ 10^9/L. *Pentamidine* (4 mg/kg IV every 2 weeks) may also be used in patients intolerant to trimethoprim/sulfamethoxazole.

Fungus. Prophylaxis with *oral fluconazole* (5 mg/kg rounded to nearest 75 mg OD) starting on day 0 and continuing until ANC recovery to >0.5 $\times$ 10^9/L. Neutropenic patients with persistent fever of undetermined etiology are started on *amphotericin B IV* (see Febrile Neutropenia).

Bacteria. *Penicillin VK* (125 or 300 mg BID) through 1 year after transplantation. All patients with fever and neutropenia are treated prophylactically with *broad-spectrum antibiotics* (see Febrile Neutropenia).

NUTRITIONAL SUPPORT

Almost all patients who receive HDT develop gastrointestinal complications, including nausea, vomiting, anorexia, and mucitis. Oral caloric intake may therefore be severely limited. Patients in a negative nitrogen balance are at a greater risk of infection, organ toxicity as a result of the HDT, and delayed marrow recovery. Consequently, virtually all patients will require nutritional support with total parenteral nutrition.

Management of Common Complications

A number of complications occurring after BMT may require intensive care unit support. The more common of these are outlined in Table 10–10. Space constraints do not allow for an in-depth discussion of all complications, so only the more common clinical syndromes peculiar to BMT are discussed in the following section. Congestive cardiac failure and acute renal failure are discussed in Chapters 7.3 and 9.4.

FEBRILE NEUTROPENIA

Febrile neutropenia is defined as a persistent core temperature of $>38.3°C$ occurring in a patient with an absolute neutrophil count of $<0.5 \times 10^9/L$. A number of factors place BMT patients at risk of developing bacterial or fungal sepsis, including alteration of normal skin and gut flora; disruption of normal barriers, including skin and mucous membranes; and neutropenia and immunosuppression.

For these reasons, fever in a neutropenic patient should be assumed to be bacterial sepsis until proved to be otherwise. Fever may also result from fungal, viral, or parasitic infection or from mucitis, drugs, and radiation.

Table 10–10. NONMYELOID COMPLICATIONS OF HDT

Pulmonary	Diffuse and focal pulmonary infiltrates
	Pulmonary emboli
	Pleural effusions
Gastrointestinal	Nausea, vomiting, anorexia
	Mucitis
	Neutropenic enterocolitis
	Veno-occlusive disease of the liver
	Ascites
Cardiac	Myocarditis, cardiomyopathy
	Pericarditis, pericardial effusion
	Endocarditis
	Arrhythmias
Genitourinary	Acute renal failure, tumor lysis syndrome
	Renal tubulopathy
	Hepatorenal syndrome
	Hemorrhagic cystitis
Central nervous system	Encephalopathy
	Meningoencephalitis
	Stroke

All patients with febrile neutropenia should have a complete physical examination with careful evaluation of vital signs to rule out hypotension and impending shock. A focus for the fever should be sought, keeping in mind that due to the neutropenia localizing signs could be minimal. Investigations should include the following: (1) cultures of blood, urine, and stool in all patients and skin and oral lesions if present. Lumbar puncture with culture of spinal fluid is not routine and should be performed only in patients with signs and symptoms of meningitis or encephalitis. (2) Chest radiographs (two views) should be obtained in all patients because signs and symptoms of pneumonia may be very subtle in neutropenic patients. (3) Limited computed tomography scan of sinuses and abdominal ultrasound or computed tomography scan should be obtained in patients with persistent fever of undetermined origin. Gallium scan and ocular examination for retinitis may also be helpful in these patients.

The management of febrile neutropenia is outlined in Figure 10–5. Septic shock should be treated aggressively, with attention paid to the ABCs and vigorous fluid replacement. It is important that broad-spectrum antibiotics are started without delay because patients may develop septic shock very rapidly.

NEUTROPENIC ENTEROCOLITIS (TYPHLITIS, ILEOCECAL SYNDROME, NECROTIZING COLITIS)

Neutropenic enterocolitis commonly presents with fever, diarrhea, abdominal pain, and tenderness. It is characterized by necrosis of the colonic mucosa without an inflammatory infiltrate. It most commonly involves the cecum, although the entire colon and terminal ileum may be involved. Perforation of the intestine may occur in severe cases.

The differential diagnosis includes infectious gastroenteritis, especially caused by *Clostridium difficile,* acute GVHD, lactose intolerance, and malabsorption.

Patients should have a thorough evaluation for signs of peritonitis, which may be minimal due to neutropenia. A surgical consult should be obtained on all patients, even if signs are minimal.

Investigations should include cultures (stool and blood), abdominal radiographs (three views) looking for air fluid levels, intraluminal gas, and free air in the peritoneum. Endoscopy may be indicated to rule out GVHD or pseudomembranous enterocolitis. In patients with typical signs and symptoms or intraluminal gas, endoscopy should be avoided owing to risk of perforation.

All patients should be placed NPO. A nasogastric tube should be inserted and attached to low intermittent suction for persistent vomiting, abdominal distention, or intraluminal gas. Patients with perforation will require surgical intervention after stabilization. If no perforation is seen, conservative management with intravenous antibiotics may be appropriate. Patients need to be covered for enteric organisms, including gram negatives and anaerobes. Coverage is usually begun with piperacillin, gentamicin, and metronidazole. Clindamycin should be avoided unless *Clostridium difficile* has been ruled out. With early aggressive management, perforation can usually be avoided.

DIFFUSE PULMONARY INFILTRATES

Pulmonary disease may develop in 40% to 60% of BMT patients, with up to 40% of these ultimately requiring intensive care unit support. Typical signs and

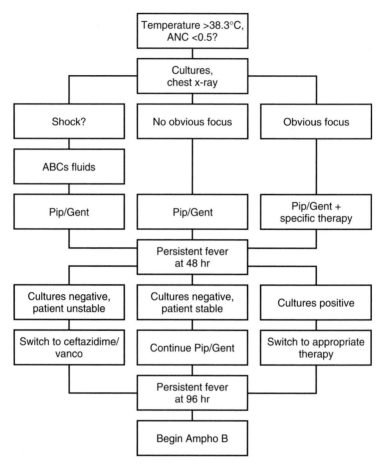

Figure 10–5. Approach to Febrile Neutropenia. Pip, piperacillin; Gent, gentamicin; vanco, vancomycin; Ampho. B, amphotericin B.

symptoms include fever, cough, tachypnea, and progressive respiratory distress. Diffuse pulmonary infiltrates (DPIs) are usually bilateral and may represent interstitial disease, air space disease, or a combination of the two. The differential diagnosis of DPIs is outlined in Table 10–11. DPIs interfere with gas exchange and pulmonary perfusion. Resultant respiratory failure with hypoxia, hypercarbia, and acidosis must be treated aggressively.

Clinical Evaluation of Patients with DPI Should Include ABCs

Investigations should include (1) arterial blood gases, serum electrolytes, and albumin; (2) blood cultures and viral studies (including nasopharyngeal swab, viral serologies, culture of buffy coat and urine for CMV); (3) chest radiographs (two

Table 10–11. CAUSES OF DIFFUSE PULMONARY INFILTRATES

Pulmonary edema
   Fluid overload
   Congestive cardiac failure
   Adult respiratory distress syndrome
   Leaky capillaries syndrome
Diffuse pulmonary hemorrhage
Infection
   Viral: cytomegalovirus, Epstein-Barr virus, respiratory
   syncytial virus, influenza, parainfluenza, adenovirus
   Fungal: *Aspergillus, Candida, Pneumocystis carinii*
   Other: *Mycoplasma,* Legionnaires' disease
Leukoagglutination reactions
Idiopathic pneumonia syndrome

views); (4) computed tomography scan of chest (may give better resolution in difficult cases); (5) bronchoalveolar lavage if infiltrates are unresponsive to diuretics; and (6) open lung biopsy (*this is controversial and should not be performed for the sole purpose of confirming a diagnosis of idiopathic interstitial pneumonia*).

Initial management of DPI is outlined in Figure 10–6. Specific measures to be taken depend on etiology but may include (1) intubation and ventilation to manage respiratory failure; (2) fluid and sodium restriction, diuretics, and/or digitalis to treat edema; (3) steroids and positive pressure ventilation (may be beneficial in adult respiratory distress syndrome); (4) treatment of infection (specific therapy as indicated by culture results, empiric therapy in deteriorating patient if etiology is unclear); (5) if diffuse pulmonary hemorrhage is suspected, treatment of coagulopathy and transfusion to keep platelets at $>50 \times 10^9/L$ (intubation with positive pressure ventilation may provide some "tamponade"); (6) for leukoagglutination reactions, use of only Pall-filtered or leukocyte-poor blood products; and (7) management of idiopathic interstitial pneumonia (supportive). Steroids do not appear to be beneficial and may increase the risk of infection.

VENO-OCCLUSIVE DISEASE OF THE LIVER

Veno-occlusive disease (VOD) is a common complication in the setting of HDT. Signs and symptoms of VOD include right upper quadrant pain and tenderness, weight gain, ascites, edema, and jaundice. VOD has specific pathologic correlates, and the diagnosis should only be made in the absence of other causes of liver disease or with histologic confirmation.

Mild cases of VOD may be confused with viral or drug-induced hepatitis, congestive cardiac failure, acute GVHD, and portal vein thrombosis. Multiple microabscesses in the liver, especially fungal, can also present with tender hepatomegaly, elevated GGT, and cholestatic jaundice.

Clinical evaluation of patients with suspected VOD should include complete physical examination looking for edema, ascites, tender hepatomegaly, jaundice, signs of coagulopathy (bruising and bleeding), and signs of encephalopathy.

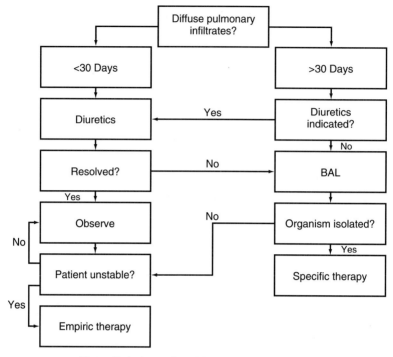

Figure 10–6. Approach to diffuse pulmonary infiltrates.

Investigations should include serum electrolytes, ALT, GGT, bilirubin (conjugated and unconjugated), prothrombin time, activated partial thromboplastin time, total protein, albumin, and NH_3. Also, an abdominal ultrasound should be done to document ascites and hepatomegaly and exclude liver abscesses. Doppler ultrasound may show reversal of flow in the portal vein; however, this is a late finding, and its absence does not rule out VOD. Computed tomography of the abdomen may give better resolution to rule out abscesses. Percutaneous liver biopsy may confirm the diagnosis in difficult cases; however, involvement may be patchy.

In all except mild cases, VOD should be managed in the intensive care unit. Several major concerns should be considered. First, for *intravascular volume depletion*, sodium-free albumin or pooled immune globulin may be helpful in maintaining intravascular volume. Renal-dose dopamine has been used in an attempt to maintain renal perfusion and reduce fluid retention; however, it may have deleterious effects on sodium retention. Second, for *fluid retention*, restrict fluid to two thirds of maintenance and strict sodium restriction to <1 to 2 mEq/ kg/day to aid in controlling weight gain, edema, and ascites. Sodium diuresis with an aldosterone inhibitor may be indicated. Ascites causing respiratory compromise but unresponsive to fluid and sodium restriction may be treated with paracentesis. Repeated paracentesis or surgical shunt may rarely be indicated. Attempts to

Table 10–12. STAGING SYSTEM FOR ORGAN INVOLVEMENT
IN ACUTE GRAFT-VERSUS-HOST DISEASE

Skin Rash (% of body surface area)	Diarrhea (mL/kg/day)	Bilirubin (μmol/l)	Stage
25	<5	12–20	1
25–50	5–10	20–50	2
>50	>10	>50	3
Bullae	Paralytic ileus	elevated AST/ALT	4

control fluid retention should be secondary to maintaining intravascular volume. Fluid resuscitation should be given to patients with hypotension unresponsive to albumin. Third, to maintain *renal function*, hemodialysis may be required to maintain intravascular volume while controlling extravascular and third-space fluids. Renal failure secondary to hepatorenal syndrome may also require dialysis. Fourth, to maintain *hepatic function*, vitamin K supplementation and fresh frozen plasma, cryoprecipitate, or coagulation factor concentrates may be indicated to control coagulopathy. General measures to control encephalopathy, including protein restriction and lactulose, may be indicated. Fifth, *reestablish hepatic perfusion.* Tissue plasminogen activator and prostaglandin E_1 infusions have been tried in some patients in an effort to dissolve thrombi and reestablish liver perfusion. Hemorrhage is the major risk with the use of tissue plasminogen activator.

With supportive management, patients with mild or moderate VOD have a good prognosis; however, patients with severe disease, as marked by renal failure requiring dialysis or liver failure with encephalopathy, have a case fatality rate of $\approx$90%.

ACUTE GRAFT-VERSUS-HOST DISEASE

Acute graft-versus-host disease (GVHD) is the antithesis to organ rejection after solid organ transplantation in that donor immune cells react against and attempt to reject host tissues. GVHD is characterized by *exfoliative skin rash, diarrhea,* and *cholestatic jaundice.* A grading system for organ involvement and overall severity of GVHD is outlined in Tables 10–12 and 10–13. Initially, each

Table 10–13. OVERALL GRADE OF GRAFT-VERSUS-HOST DISEASE
BASED ON INDIVIDUAL ORGAN STAGE

Skin	Gut	Liver	Grade
1–2	0	0	I
1–3	1	1	II
2–3	2–3	2–3	III
2–4	2–4	2–4	IV

organ is staged separately. An overall grade is then defined by the pattern and severity of individual organ involvement.

The pattern of organ involvement (skin, biliary tree, and gut) reflects the high level of HLA expression in these tissues. The skin rash typically begins on the palms and soles. The rash may be maculopapular or violaceous and may be painful. It may become confluent over the cheeks, ears, and neck and may spread to involve the entire body. In severe cases, bullae formation is noted. Biliary tree epithelium is the next most frequent target, and its involvement is associated with cholestatic jaundice. Gastrointestinal tract involvement is usually in the terminal ileum and colon and presents with watery diarrhea, hematochezia, and abdominal pain. In up to 13% of patients, GVHD of the gut may involve the upper gastrointestinal tract alone and present with persistent anorexia, nausea, and vomiting.

GVHD usually begins around day 20 after marrow infusion, and when typical signs and symptoms are present, the diagnosis is not difficult to establish. The differential diagnosis of skin GVHD includes viral exanthemas and toxic or allergic drug eruptions (especially cyclophosphamide). Early in its course, GVHD of the liver may be confused with VOD; however, GVHD is rarely associated with liver failure or hepatorenal syndrome. The differential diagnosis of gut GVHD includes HDT-induced gastrointestinal toxicity and infectious enteritis.

Investigations should include skin biopsy; ALT, GGT, and bilirubin (conjugated and unconjugated); percutaneous liver biopsy in difficult cases; and stool volume (24-hour stool collection for α_1-antitrypsin, barium swallow with small bowel follow-through, and rectal biopsy in difficult cases).

Management

Prevention. Select an HLA-identical donor whenever possible. Cyclosporine, methotrexate, and steroids have been administered alone or in combination as prophylaxis against GVHD. Despite prophylaxis, 30% to 40% of patients may develop some GVHD.

Treatment. Prednisone (2 to 4 mg/kg/day) should be started in all patients with GVHD of >Grade 1. Patients who progress after 5 days of prednisone or who have not improved after 7 days should receive second-line therapy. This may include pulsed steroids (methylprednisolone 30 mg/kg/day IV daily for 3 days), antithymocyte globulin (10 to 40 mg/kg/day for 3 or 4 days), or azathioprine 1 mg/kg/dose PO BID). Other second-line therapies, including monoclonal anti–T cell antibodies, are still experimental.

Prognosis

The prognosis for BMT patients varies considerably depending on the type of transplant and the indications for transplantation. The estimated procedure-related mortality ranges from 5% to 10% in the autologous setting and from 10% to 15% in the allogeneic setting. Overall disease-free survival rates range from 30% for certain solid tumors such as stage IV neuroblastoma to >80% for matched sibling transplants for aplastic anemia.

BIBLIOGRAPHY

Armitage JO, Antman KH (eds): High-Dose Cancer Therapy: Pharmacology, Hematopoietins, Stem Cells. Baltimore, Williams & Wilkins, 1992.

Forman S, Blume K, Thomas ED (eds): Bone Marrow Transplantation. Boston, Blackwell Scientific Publications, 1994.

Treleaven J, Barrett J (eds): Bone Marrow Transplantation in Practice. New York, Churchill Livingstone, 1992.

11

Pediatric Emergency Procedures

11.1 Intraosseous Infusions

MICHELLE McNEILL, MD

Indications

- After several attempts at peripheral access in a child (<6 to 8 years) in shock or impending arrest
- When other methods fail

Contraindications

- Active infection at insertion site
- Known or suspected fracture
- Known or suspected osteopetrosis or osteogenesis imperfecta

Procedure

Sites

- Proximal tibia (most common)
- Distal femur
- Distal tibia
- Humerus
- Sternum (adolescents and adults)
- Iliac crest
- Greater trochanter

Equipment

- Intraosseous needles, bone marrow biopsy needles, or spinal needles
- Syringe for flush
- Lidocaine (Xylocaine) 1%
- Tape

Technique

This technique is for the tibia, but the principles apply to any site used.

- With sterile precautions, the needle is inserted 2 cm below and medial to the tibial tuberosity (Fig. 11–1).
- The tip of the needle is directed away from the growth plate by aiming slightly caudal.
- The needle is advanced with a firm boring or screwing motion until a decrease in resistance is felt. Bone marrow is not always obtained on aspiration.
- Standard intravenous tubing is attached, and drugs and fluids may be given.
- Heparinized saline will cleanse the needle of clotted marrow and bone spicules.
- A hand can be placed behind the limb during infusion to ensure needle placement and that infusion does not go into the muscle.

Alternative Sites

- Distal femur: the insertion is made in the midline 2 to 3 cm above the external condyles, and the needle is directed cephalad to avoid the growth plate.
- Distal tibia: the needle is inserted 1 cm proximal to the medial malleolus

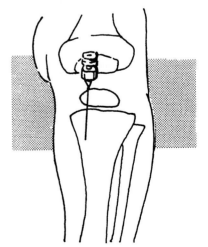

Figure 11–1. Insertion of intraosseous needle in the upper end of the tibia.

and posterior to the saphenous vein and directed cephalad (for infants and neonates).

Complications (Very Rare)

- Extravasation of fluid or medications (most common)
- Local cellulitis
- Subcutaneous abscess
- Compartment syndrome
- Osteomyelitis
- Sepsis
- Fracture at site
- Growth plate injury
- Fat or bone marrow embolization

11.2 Endotracheal Intubation

MICHELLE McNEILL, MD

Indications

See Chapter 2.

Contraindications

- Craniofacial trauma
- Upper airway trauma
- Complete airway obstruction
- Basal skull fracture (nasal intubation)

Procedure

Equipment

- Cardiorespiratory monitor
- Suction catheter
- Endotracheal tubes of the appropriate size:

$$\text{Estimated tube size} = (16 + \text{age [yr]})/4$$
or size of patient's little finger
or size of patient's nares

■ Tube length:

$$\text{Oral} = (12 + \text{age [yr]})/2$$

$$\text{Nasal} = (15 + \text{age [yr]})/2$$

■ Always have a tube one size smaller and one size larger than estimated.
■ Laryngoscope blade, straight or curved
■ Stylet
■ Magill forceps
■ Bag-and-mask apparatus
■ Drugs (see Chap. 2)

Technique

Oral Intubation

■ Position the patient properly in the sniffing position with the head extended on the neck and the neck slightly flexed in relation to the trunk (do not hyperextend).
■ Preoxygenate with 100% O_2.
■ Drugs: atropine, sedation, muscle relaxant (if necessary).
■ Laryngoscopy: open the mouth with the scissors technique, with the right thumb on the lower teeth and the index finger on the upper teeth
■ With the laryngoscope in the left hand, introduce the blade into the right side of the mouth and displace the tongue to the left by moving the laryngoscope toward the center of the mouth.
■ The straight laryngoscope blade is introduced all the way and gradually withdrawn until the vocal cords are seen.
■ The curved blade is introduced until the epiglottis is seen; the blade is inserted in the vallecula, and traction applied along the body of the scope will elevate the epiglottis and allow visualization of the cords (Fig. 11–2).
■ The orotracheal tube is inserted at the right corner of the mouth and gently advanced through the vocal cords.
■ Gentle cricoid pressure may bring anteriorly placed cords into view.
■ Failure to intubate the patient in a reasonable time should be followed by abortion of the attempt and a reattempt after preoxygenation.

Nasotracheal Intubation

■ Provides better immobilization of the tube
■ The tube is lubricated with mucus and passed through the nares into the posterior pharynx.
■ Laryngoscopy is performed as above, the vocal cords are visualized, and the tip of the tube is then picked up with the Magill forceps (placed through the mouth) and guided through the vocal cords.

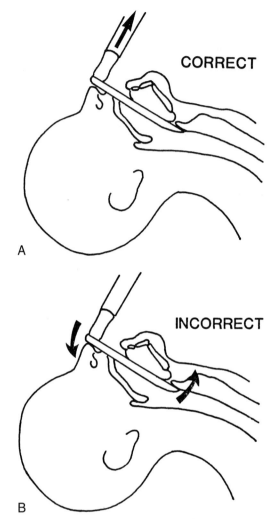

CORRECT

A

INCORRECT

B

Figure 11–2. Correct and incorrect applications of force during laryngoscopy.

Ascertain Tube Position

- Watch for chest wall movement with breaths.
- Listen for equal breath sounds on both sides.
- Listen in epigastrium to ensure that no breath sounds are heard.
- Condensation may be seen in tube with exhalation.
- There is improvement in heart rate, blood pressure, color, and O_2 saturation.
- Confirm position with chest radiography.
- Secure the tube when correct placement is ensured.

Complications

- Trauma to oropharynx, teeth, vocal cords
- Intubation of stomach, gastric distention, vomiting, and aspiration

11.3 Needle Cricothyroidotomy

B. LOUISE PARKER, MD, FRCPC

Indications

- Upper airway obstruction (i.e., facial trauma, foreign body, epiglottitis) with inability to secure airway by conventional methods

Procedure

Equipment

- 14- to 20-gauge needle (Angiocath)
- 10-mL syringe
- 3.0 or 3.5 endotracheal tube adapter
- Ventilating equipment and O_2

Technique

- Place the patient in a supine, head-neutral position (Fig. 11–3).
- Palpate the cricothyroid membrane in midline.
- Attach the needle to the syringe.
- Insert the needle in midline at a 45° angle caudally.
- Rapid aspiration for air indicates entry to the trachea.
- Withdraw the needle slowly while advancing the catheter.
- Attach the hub of the catheter to the endotracheal tube adapter.
- Oxygenation and ventilation can now be performed.

Complications

- Perforation of the posterior tracheal wall
- CO_2 retention
- Failure to oxygenate (may require additional catheter insertions)

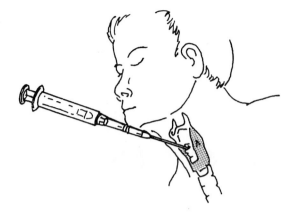

Figure 11–3. Insertion of needle through the cricothyroid membrane.

11.4 **Tracheostomy**

B. LOUISE PARKER, MD, FRCPC

Indications

- Upper airway obstruction: when endotracheal intubation is not possible (due to trauma) or impossible (due to epiglottitis), it is preferable to perform a needle cricothyroidotomy in the pediatric patient

Procedure

Equipment

- General surgical tray
- Scalpel
- Lidocaine (Xylocaine) 1%
- Suture
- Flexible tracheostomy tube (or endotracheal tube)

Technique

- Clean area with patient supine and head in a neutral position.
- Infiltrate with lidocaine if time permits.

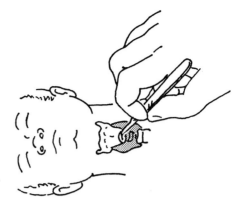

Figure 11–4. Insertion site for performing a tracheostomy.

- Make a horizontal skin incision and then a vertical tracheal incision from the third to the fifth tracheal rings (Fig. 11–4).
- Place tube into trachea once airway has been suctioned.
- Stabilize with suture or tie tapes.
- Obtain a radiograph to confirm position.

Complications

- Accidental decannulation
- Bleeding
- Pneumothorax/pneumomediastinum
- Tracheoesophageal fistula
- Subcutaneous emphysema
- Cardiorespiratory arrest
- Long term: atelectasis, occlusion, ulceration, granuloma, stenosis

11.5 Needle Thoracentesis and Chest Tube Insertion

B. LOUISE PARKER, MD, FRCPC

Needle Thoracentesis

INDICATION

- Life-threatening tension pneumothorax

PROCEDURE

Equipment

- 16- to 20-gauge needle with catheter
- Three-way stopcock
- 20-mL syringe

Technique

- Enter second intercostal space at midclavicular line and allow for drainage of air.
- Once air is evacuated, this should be followed by chest tube insertion.

Chest Tube Insertion

INDICATIONS

- Pneumothorax (tension, spontaneous, traumatic)
- Hemothorax
- Pleural effusion
- Emphysema
- Chylothorax

PROCEDURE

Equipment

- Lidocaine (Xylocaine) 1%
- 25-gauge needle
- 3-mL syringe
- No. 15 scalpel
- Kelly forceps

- Suture
- Pleurovac/Heimlich valve
- Chest tube: No. 12 newborn, No. 16 infant, No. 22 small child, No. 24 child (may be smaller if air versus fluid being evacuated)

Technique

- Choose site (fifth or sixth intercostal space mid or anterior axillary line).
- Clean area and infiltrate skin, subcutaneous tissue, and periosteum with lidocaine.
- Make skin incision (1 to 1.5 cm) at bottom edge of rib (Fig. 11–5).
- With Kelly forceps, bluntly dissect to create an oblique passage up and over the rib. Spread forceps to create a sufficiently large passage for the chest tube.
- With tips of forceps together, enter pleural space just above the rib. Considerable force may be required. Place the index finger 0.5 to 1 cm (see Fig. 11–5) from the tip of the forceps to avoid damage to the lungs with sudden entry into the pleura. Spread the membrane open with the forceps.
- Grasp the tip of the chest tube with the forceps and direct it through the path already made.
- Clamp the chest tube with Kelly forceps.
- Advance the chest tube *anterior for air and posterior for fluid collections.*
- Suture the chest tube and secure; apply dressing.
- Connect to drainage system.
- Obtain a chest radiograph to confirm placement.

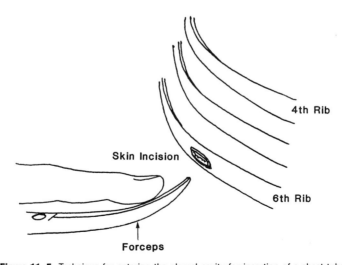

Figure 11–5. Technique for entering the pleural cavity for insertion of a chest tube.

Complications

- Secondary pneumothorax
- Infection
- Damage to underlying visceral tissues
- Failure to drain loculated fluid
- Subcutaneous emphysema

11.6 Pericardiocentesis

B. CATHERINE ROSS, MD

Indications

- Cardiac tamponade
- Diagnostic testing of pericardial effusion
- Elective removal of pericardial fluid in presence of chronic or recurrent effusion leading to impaired cardiac output
  - □ Note: Nonemergency cases should be done with echocardiographic guidance.

Procedure

Equipment

- ECG monitor
- 20-gauge Angiocath
- Lidocaine (Xylocaine) 1%
- 20- to 50-mL syringe
- Three-way stopcock

Technique

- Use ECG monitor.
- Sedate the patient if required (may need airway management).
- Clean the precordium with povidone-iodine and drape.
- Anesthetize just below the xiphoid process with local anesthetic.
- Insert the needle just below the xiphoid process at ≈30° (Fig. 11–6).
- Aim toward the left shoulder.
- Aspirate with the syringe while advancing the needle until fluid is obtained.

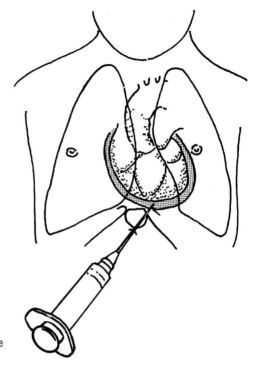

Figure 11-6. Technique for drainage of the pericardial space.

- Remove the trocar of the Angiocath and reattach the syringe to the catheter to remove effusion.
- Monitor ECG for changes in ECG complex, which indicates penetration beyond pericardium into myocardium. If this occurs, withdraw the needle until baseline ECG pattern returns.
- Remove the needle and cover site.
- Obtain chest radiograph or/and echocardiogram to look for an accumulation or complications.
  - ☐ Note: If ongoing drainage is required, pigtail catheter may be inserted with the Seldinger technique.

Complications

- Myocardial penetration or puncture
- Cardiac arrhythmias
- Development of hemopericardium, pneumothorax, pneumopericardium, infection, cutaneous fistula, or pericardial peritoneal fistula

11.7 **Lumbar Puncture**

B. CATHERINE ROSS, MD

Indications

- Conditions requiring cytologic or biochemical assessment of cerebrospinal fluid
- Instillation of intrathecal chemotherapy

Contraindications

- Bleeding diathesis
- Platelet count of <20,000
- Intracranial pressure (papilledema)
- Infection of skin along needle insertion site
- Critically ill child with cardiorespiratory compromise

Procedure

Equipment

- Lumbar puncture tray
- Lumbar puncture needle with stylet
- 21- to 23-gauge short needle for infants, 20- to 21-gauge long needle for older children
- Three-way stopcock with manometer

Preferred Sites

- Intervertebral space L3-4 or L4-5 (see method below)

Technique

- With sterile techniques (Fig. 11–7), place the patient with the back fully flexed.
  - □ On side with hips, knees, and head flexed
  - □ Sitting with hips, knees, and head flexed
- Monitor the patient's cardiorespiratory status closely.
- Draw an imaginary line between two iliac crests and the intervertebral space at or below this line, i.e., L3-4 or L4-5 (see Fig. 11–7).
- Anesthetize skin and underlying tissue with local anesthetic.

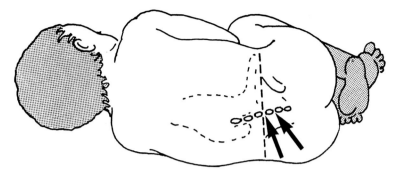

Figure 11–7. Patient position and landmarks for performing a lumbar puncture.

- With a spinal needle with stylet, aim the needle toward the umbilicus in the midsagittal plane (ensure that there is no prior rotation of torso).
- Advance the needle and stylet slowly.
- Withdraw stylet, check for CSF, reinsert stylet and advance so needle enters dura—a "pop" may be felt (may use manometer and three-way stopcock to measure opening pressure).
  - ☐ Note: **Do not aspirate fluid.**
- Replace the stylet and withdraw the needle while applying pressure.
- Bandage and place the patient on his or her back for several hours after the procedure.

Complications

- Transtentorial or tonsillar herniation
- Bleeding
- Infection
- Headache
- Subarachnoid epidermal cyst
- Local back pain
- Cardiorespiratory arrest (if patient was too unstable to have procedure performed)

11.8 Central Venous Access

BRYAN D. MAGWOOD, BSc, MD, FRCPC

Indications

- Infusion of fluids and drugs
- Measurement of central venous pressure
- Sampling of blood

Procedure

Equipment

- Catheter kit (syringe, needle, guidewire, dilator, catheter, hubs, and so on)
- Sterile tray (forceps, needle-driver, scissors, No. 11/15 scalpel blade, sutures, gauze, drapes)
- Lidocaine (Xylocaine) 1%

Technique

The most frequently used approach to insertion is the percutaneous Seldinger technique:

- Identify site and landmark.
- Inspect the catheter kit for defects and completeness.
- Infiltrate insertion site with lidocaine 1%.
- Puncture vessel at 30° to 40° with the needle on saline-loaded syringe.
- When blood aspirates easily, remove the syringe and reconfirm flow.
- Thread guidewire into vessel and expose adequate wire to thread catheter.
- Remove needle while applying pressure over insertion site.
- Make small skin incision at puncture site to accommodate dilator/catheter.
- If required, pass and withdraw dilator over wire; ensure access to one end of the wire.
- Pass catheter over wire through distal port; ensure access to one end of the wire.
- Pull wire out through placed catheter; ensure blood flow through all ports.
- Suture catheter in place.
- Obtain radiograph of catheter position.

Specific Site Considerations

1. Umbilical (not done by the Seldinger technique): rapidly obtained and useful in infants up to 1 week of age
   - Catheter length: umbilicus to clavicle measurement +4 (in cm)

- Radiograph location: above diaphragm to avoid intrahepatic infusion
2. Femoral (Fig. 11–8A): simplest route of central access; less effective during cardiopulmonary resuscitation (CPR).
   - Insertion site: below inguinal ligament 0.5 to 1 cm; medial to femoral artery
3. Internal jugular (Fig. 11–8B): optimal site, requiring experienced operator owing to risk of airway compression, hemothorax, or pneumothorax
   - Position: Trendelenburg 20° to 30°
   - Insertion site: right side provides straight path to superior vena cava; turn head left
   - Three approaches:
     - □ Anterior: lateral to right carotid artery and medial to right sternocleidomastoid muscle; gently retract carotid artery with left hand; aim for right nipple
     - □ Posterior: beneath point where external jugular vein crosses sternocleidomastoid muscle; aim for suprasternal notch
     - □ Central: apex of sternal and clavicular heads of sternocleidomastoid muscle; aim for right nipple
       Obtain radiograph of location: junction of superior vena cava and right atrium

4. Subclavian (Fig. 11–8C): optimal site, requiring experienced operator owing to risk of airway compression, hemothorax, or pneumothorax
   - Position: Trendelenburg 20° to 30°
   - Insertion site: at crossing of clavicle and first rib; enter at distal margin of medial third of clavicle and, while guiding the needle under, aim towards suprasternal notch
   - Obtain radiograph of location: junction of superior vena cava and right atrium

Complications

- Hemorrhage
- Infection
- Embolization
- Dysrhythmias

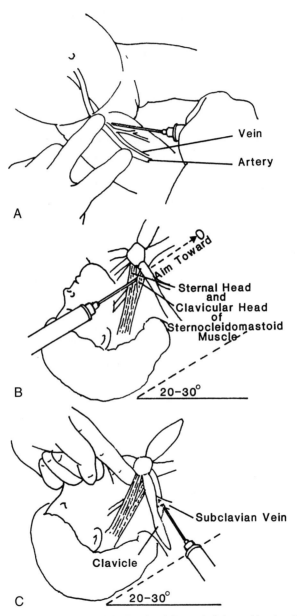

Figure 11–8. Central venous sites and landmarks. *A*, Femoral. *B*, Internal jugular. *C*, Subclavian.

11.9 **Pulmonary Artery Lines**

BRYAN D. MAGWOOD, BSc, MD, FRCPC

Indications

Measurement of:

- Pulmonary artery (PA) and PA wedge (PAW) pressures
- Cardiac output (CO)
- Mixed venous O_2 saturation (Svo_2)
- Shock unresponsive to volume and inotrope resuscitation
- Septic shock with low CO and systemic vascular resistance (SVR)
- Left ventricular function requiring close monitoring (PAW pressure reflects left ventricular end-diastolic pressure)
- To monitor O_2 delivery (a function of CO $\times$ O_2 content)
- Elevated PA pressures

Consider the Following Precautions

- Severe dysrhythmias, which may be exacerbated by catheter placement
- Coagulopathy
- Large intracardiac shunts with risk of left-side catheterization
- Very low CO (hampers placement of catheter in PA)

Technique

The approach and equipment for PA line insertion are similar to those for central venous catheterization (see "Central Venous Access" for general details).

- Select catheter (<15 kg, 5F catheter and 6F introducer; ≥15 kg, 7F catheter and 8.5F introducer).
- Select site (internal jugular, subclavian, or femoral).
- Use modified Seldinger technique.
  - ☐ Introducer sheath is placed before the catheter.
  - ☐ The catheter is inserted into the introducer through a sterile sheath.
- Place the catheter.
  - ☐ Advance the catheter while transducing pressure at distal port.
  - ☐ Look for characteristic central venous and right ventricular pressure waves (see Chapter 7.1, Cardiovascular Monitoring).
  - ☐ When right ventricular waves appear, inflate the balloon per instructions.
  - ☐ Advance the catheter until PA pressure waves appear (see Chapter 7.1, Cardiovascular Monitoring).

- ☐ Monitor the ECG closely for ventricular dysrhythmias; discontinue if they are persistent.
- ☐ When PA waves appear, deflate the balloon and reinflate briefly to obtain PAW pressure.
- ☐ *Never leave the balloon inflated.*
- ☐ Note the insertion length marked on catheter for placement in PA.
- ☐ Obtain a chest radiograph as for any central line.

Complications

See "Central Venous Access" for details.

- Obstruction of right ventricular outflow
- Knotting of catheter during manipulations
- Pulmonary infarction
- Structural heart damage if catheter is pulled back with the balloon inflated

11.10 Arterial Line Insertion

B. CATHERINE ROSS, MD

Indications

- Continuous arterial pressure monitoring
- Frequent blood sampling (e.g., blood gas)

Contraindications

- Poor collateral blood flow
  - ☐ Note: No medications or hyperosmolar solutions are to be administered via the arterial line.

Procedure

Equipment

- Arterial catheter (size is dependent on size of vessel)
- 18- to 24-gauge needle

- Lidocaine (Xylocaine) 1%
- Suture
- Arterial pressure monitor
- Syringe
- Isotonic heparinized flush
- Arm/leg board

Preferred Sites

- Radial
- Posterior tibial
- Dorsalis pedis
- Femoral (see "Central Venous Access" for Seldinger technique)

Technique (Radial Artery)

- Perform modified Allen test to assess collateral flow from ulnar artery.
- In infants, transilluminate wrist to visualize vessels (Fig. 11–9).

Figure 11–9. Technique for insertion of radial arterial line. See text for description of A, B, and C.

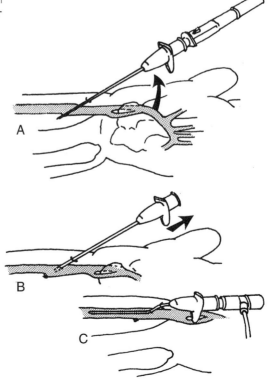

- To secure, supinate and extend wrist to 45° over small rod of gauze tape.
- With sterile precautions, puncture *skin* with 18-gauge needle.
- Introduce catheter and stylet at a 15° to 30° angle through skin puncture (less-acute angle is used for young patients) (Fig. 11–9A).
- Advance the catheter and stylet until the vessel is punctured; then either
  - □ Remove the stylet if there is good pulsatile flow; advance the catheter into the artery.
  - □ Advance the catheter and stylet until the artery is transfixed (Fig. 11–9B). Remove the stylet and slowly withdraw the catheter until there is pulsatile flow; then advance the catheter into the artery (Fig. 11–9C).
- Attach transducer for continuous mean arterial pressure monitoring.
- Suture, tape to arm board.
- Closely monitor the site.

Complications

- Ischemic damage to extremities
- Thrombosis, emboli
- Pseudoaneurysm formation
- Sepsis, infection
- Hemorrhage
- Skin necrosis

11.11 Temporary Cardiac Pacing

MARC D. LeGRAS, BSc, MD, CM, FRCPC, FACC

Indications

- Varying degrees of atrioventricular block with inadequate hemodynamic response
- Inadequate heart rate (bradycardia unrelated to atrioventricular node dysfunction)
- Inadequate cardiac output ("relative" bradycardia after surgery)
- Overdrive pacing (termination of atrial flutter, atrioventricular node reentry, and both preexcited or concealed accessory pathways; suppression of junctional ectopic tachycardia)
- Prevention (ventricular arrhythmias, long QT syndrome, digoxin toxicity)

Methods

- Transvenous
- Transthoracic temporary epicardial leads
- Transcutaneous (Zoll) and transesophageal: both cause discomfort and are not as reliable

Temporary Transvenous Pacing: Femoral Approach

Disclaimer

- Ideally an individual experienced in cardiac catheterization should perform this procedure.

Equipment

- Bipolar pacing catheter (4F for infants, 5F for children)
- Temporary pacemaker
- Portable fluoroscopy equipment and lead gown (may not be needed if experienced with balloon-tipped catheter)
- Femoral sheath and kit, catheter contamination shield
- Sterile drapes and skin prep, local anesthetic

Technique

- Position fluoroscopy equipment.
- After appropriate prepping, draping, and infiltration of local anesthesia, place femoral vein sheath and suture in place. If unsure whether in the vein or artery, use fluoroscopy to check the wire position in relation to the spine before inserting the sheath.
- Pass the pacing catheter through the catheter contamination shield before inserting in femoral vein. Do not extend the shield until the catheter is finally positioned in the heart.
- Advance catheter to right atrium, taking care not to push against resistance; should this occur, free up the catheter tip by pulling back and then advance while imaging.
- Enter the right ventricle by turning the catheter tip medial and advance so the tip moves downward in the direction of the right ventricular apex. Place the tip in the right ventricular apex and leave a well-rounded curve on the catheter as it courses through the heart to permit adequate slack; a temporary pacing catheter is very easily displaced. If a balloon-tipped pacing catheter is being used, the balloon may be used to float the catheter into the right ventricle. Once in the right ventricle, deflate the balloon to advance the catheter to the right ventricular apex.
- Connect to the pacemaker. Turn output to minimum and rate slower than

that of the patient. Turn on the pacemaker and determine at what millivolt level the QRS is sensed—set the sensitivity to half this value. Then, set the pacemaker rate at faster than that of the patient and gradually increase the output until ventricular capture occurs, noting the output value. Set the pacemaker output to three times higher than the observed capture value (minimum, 5 mA). Set the pacing rate to a physiologic age-related value or as desired.

■ Carefully extend the catheter contamination shield and then form a loop with the catheter and shield and tape to the adjacent thigh area with waterproof tape. Tighten the ends of the shield. Use additional means of securing the pacemaker catheter so that patient movement will not dislodge it.

■ Check the pacing catheter position in the heart with fluoroscopy before completing the procedure. *Again, ensure that pacing is evident.*

Pacemaker Settings

The National American Society for Pacing and Electrophysiological Pacemaker (NASPE) code governs three parameters. The first indicates the chamber or chambers being paced (atrium [A], ventricle [V], or both [D]). The second indicates the chamber or chambers being sensed (A, V, or D). The third indicates the response to the chamber being sensed (I = inhibits, T = triggered, D = triggered and inhibits, and O = asynchronous).

A summary of the NASPE code is as follows:

DDD: Dual-chamber pacer, dual-chamber sensor, and can be inhibited or triggered.

DVI: Dual-chamber pacer, only the ventricle is sensed, and the pacemaker can inhibit.

VVI: The ventricle is paced and sensed and the pacemaker can inhibit.

AAI: The atrium is paced and sensed and the pacemaker can inhibit.

AOO: The atrium is paced asynchronously and there is no sensing.

1. Mode
   ■ Normal AV node function
     □ AAI: the most physiologic. Cardiac output is better with AAI than with DDD.
   ■ Abnormal AV node function
     □ DDD or VVI: DDD is preferable to VVI.
2. Rate
   ■ Low rate: minimum heart rate for acceptable cardiac output.
   ■ Use ECG age norms as a starting point.
   ■ Upper rate: maximum acceptable heart rate; will be well above normal ECG age range after severe physiologic stress.
   ■ In the presence of poor contractility, heart rate may be main determinant of cardiac output. Ensure the low rate and upper rate are far apart in DDD mode; otherwise, Wenckebach phenomenon will occur.

3. AV interval
   - Set it longer than PR interval when ventricular sensing of conducted beats is desired.
   - Usual range is 100 to 180 milliseconds.
   - Observe arterial line blood pressure for hemodynamic effect of AV interval and pacing rate and readjust.
4. Refractory periods
   - Default values are ≈300 milliseconds.
   - Shorten refractory period (±AV interval) to permit high rate P-wave tracking in DDD.
5. Output
   - Output is determined by combination of pulse width (duration of pacing spike delivered) and volts or current (amplitude of pacing spike).
   - Typical default values are pulse width of 0.5 milliseconds and current of 5.0 mA.
   - Determine the minimum energy at which capture occurs and triple the current. This provides three times the safety margin.
   - Check safety margin every 24 hours or sooner with worsening myocardial or lead function.
6. Sensing
   - Decreasing the numbers makes the pacemaker more sensitive.
   - Determine the highest value at which sensing still occurs and set to 50% of this value (default A = 0.5 mV, V = 4.0 mV).
   - Loss of sensing: leads to inappropriate pacemaker function such as intermittent noncapture and possibly pacemaker-induced arrhythmias.

Pacemaker Care

- Changes in settings must be ordered in writing to minimize errors and communication problems.
- Check capture threshold and sensing daily. Adjust settings to adapt to changing physiology.
- All leads and pacemakers must be firmly secured to prevent dislodgment.
- Display last date of battery change on the pacemaker. All individuals must be briefed and know how to change battery.
- The cardiac monitor may not alarm if pacing spikes are sensed but noncapture is occurring; use of a pulse oximeter will permit detection of noncapture and asystole.

Troubleshooting

- Irregular pacing, violating low rate
  - ☐ Rule out loss of sensing.
  - ☐ Rule out loss of capture.
  - ☐ Ensure that low and upper rates are not too close—otherwise, Wenckebach phenomenon or low rate violation occurs.
- High capture thresholds

   ☐ High-output pacemaker or new leads may be required.
   ☐ Consider alternate pacing mode or method.
- Asystole in the presence of appropriate pacemaker function
   ☐ Is output adequate?
   ☐ Are all lead connections tight?
   ☐ Have the leads dislodged?
   ☐ Is the battery worn out? Has the battery been properly replaced?

BIBLIOGRAPHY

Ellenbogen KA: Cardiac Pacing. Boston, Blackwell Scientific Publications, 1992.
Fish F, Benson DW Jr: Disorders of cardiac rhythm and conduction. *In* Emmanouilides GC, Riemenschneider TA, Allen HD, Gutgesell HP (eds): Moss and Adams Heart Disease in Infants, Children, and Adolescents Including the Fetus and Young Adult, 5th ed. Baltimore, Williams & Wilkins, 1995.

11.12 Jugular Bulb Catheterization

NARENDRA C. SINGH, BSc, MB, BS, FRCPC, FAAP

Indications

- Monitor cerebral venous oxygen saturation measurement
- Cross-brain oxygen extraction (with measurement of cerebral blood flow)
- Cross-brain glucose and lactate utilization

Contraindications

- Local infection
- Local neck trauma
- Impairment of cerebral venous drainage

Procedure

Sites

- Right jugular bulb is recommended for right-sided, diffuse, or multifocal bihemispheric disease since it is larger with higher flow.
- Left jugular bulb is suggested for left-sided focal lesions, open neck trauma, and right-sided ventriculoperitoneal (VP) shunt.

Equipment

- Antiseptic solution
- Sterile drapes
- 21-gauge needle
- 3-mL syringe
- Local anesthetic (2%)
- Guidewire (0.45 mm)
- Polyethylene catheter (2.5–8 cm)
- Heparinized saline (1 U/mL)
- Suture
- Sterile dressing

Technique

Technique A: Horizontal Supine Head Turn

- After appropriate sterile precautions are taken, the carotid artery is palpated and displaced medially at the midpoint of a line connecting the suprasternal notch and the tip of the mastoid (local anesthetic may be used if clinically indicated).
- A 21-gauge needle is then used to pierce the skin at a 30 to 40 degree angle from the horizontal plane and directed cephalad towards the foramen magnum.
- When the internal jugular is entered, the syringe is disconnected and the 0.45, mm guidewire is inserted in a retrograde fashion.
- The needle is then removed and the catheter is inserted until it meets resistance at the superior bulb of the vein.
- The guidewire is then removed, and the catheter is sutured in place and maintained with 1 mL/hr of heparinized saline (1 U/mL).
- A lateral skull x-ray is then done to confirm the position.

Technique B: Head-Up Position

- This technique is preferable in patients with suspected or confirmed cervical spine injury.
- The patient is positioned with the head slightly extended but otherwise central.
- After sterile precautions are taken, the puncture site is identified slightly lateral to the carotid impulse at the level of the inferior border of the thyroid cartilage.
- The subsequent steps are similar to those of technique A.

Complications

- Carotid puncture and hematoma
- Catheter malposition
- Catheter sepsis
- Venous thrombosis
- Phrenic and recurrent laryngeal nerve paralysis and Horner's syndrome

12

Pediatric Formulary

HEATHER J. VOSPER, BSc(Hon), BSc(Pharm), PharmD

The medication dosages are based on information available at the time of preparation of this text. To confirm drug dosages or to determine dosages of drugs not included, please refer to the manufacturer's package insert or to other pediatric drug dosing references that are frequently updated. It is safe practice to always check more than one reference when trying to select the dosage of a medication for an individual patient.

Note: When treating patients with liver and/or kidney impairment, consult additional references for possible dosage adjustments.

Legend: N, neonates; I, infants; C, children; A, adults; div, divided; conc, concentration; PCA, postconceptual age; PGA, postgestational age; PNA, postnatal age; AC, before a meal; QHS, every bedtime; OD, once a day; BID, twice a day; QID, four times a day; TID, three times a day; qh, every hour; HS, bedtime; ET, endotracheal; IM, intramuscular; IV, intravenous; PO, by mouth; PR, per rectum; PRN, as necessary; SL, sublingual.

Drug	Comments	Age/Dose/Route/Frequency
Acetaminophen		10–15 mg/kg/dose PO/PR q4–6h **Maximum, 65 mg/kg/day**
Acetylsalicylic acid (aspirin)	For juvenile rheumatoid arthritis, pericarditis, rheumatic fever	60–100 mg/kg/day div QID
	For Kawasaki disease	
	Acute stage	80–100 mg/kg/day in 4 div doses until 14th illness day
	Convalescent stage (after 14th day in afebrile patient)	3–5 mg/kg/day in single dose, discontinue 6–8 weeks after onset of illness (after verifying no coronary abnormalities)
	Chronic therapy (for patient with coronary abnormalities)	3–5 mg/kg/day in single dose; some add dipyridamole in selected patients deemed to be at high risk

Drug	Comments	Age/Dose/Route/Frequency
Acyclovir	Herpes simplex virus (HSV) in immunocompromised host (localized, progressive, or disseminated)	C <1 yr except N: 15–30 mg/kg/day IV in 3 div doses for 7–14 days C ≥1 yr: 750 mg/m²/day IV in 3 div doses for 7–14 days; 1000 mg/day PO in 3–5 div doses for 7–14 days
	Prophylaxis of HSV in immunocompromised HSV-seropositive patient	600–1000 mg/day PO in 3–5 div doses; 750 mg/m²/day IV in 3 div doses during risk period
	HSV encephalitis	C <1 yr: 30 mg/kg/day IV in 3 div doses for a minimum of 14 days C ≥1 yr: 1500 mg/m²/day in 3 div doses for 14–21 days
	Neonatal HSV	30 mg/kg/day IV in 3 div doses for 14–21 days For premature I, 20 mg/kg/day IV in 2 div doses is recommended for 14–21 days
	Varicella or zoster in immunocompromised host	C <1 yr: 30 mg/kg/day IV in 3 div doses C ≥1 yr: 1500 mg/m²/day IV in 3 div doses for 7–10 days
	Zoster in immunocompetent host	IV same as zoster in immunocompromised host; 4000 mg/day PO in 5 div doses for 5–7 days for patients ≥12 yr
	Varicella in immunocompetent host	80 mg/kg/day PO in 4 div doses for 5 days; maximum dose 3200 mg/day
	Prophylaxis of cytomegalovirus infection in immunocompromised host	50–80 mg/kg/day PO in 4 div doses during risk period **or** 1500 mg/m²/day IV in 3 div doses during risk period
Adenosine	In an emergency drug of choice for paroxysmal supraventricular tachycardia in C <1 yr	0.1 mg/kg IV followed by 0.2 mg/kg IV in 1–2 min if needed **Maximum single dose, 12 mg**
	Antiarrhythmic for conversion of supraventricular tachycardia to sinus rhythm	*Initial dose:* 0.10 mg/kg IV by rapid bolus injection with large flush; increase by increments of 0.05 mg/kg **Maximum, 0.25 mg/kg (timing of doses q1–2 min)** Note: Give as centrally as

Drug	Comments	Age/Dose/Route/Frequency
Adenosine (Continued)		possible; **antagonized by theophylline**
Aldactazide		1–4 mg/kg/day PO div q8–24h **(usually q12h)**
Aminophylline	Apnea of prematurity	*Loading dose:* 5–6 mg/kg IV/PO
		Maintenance dose: 1.5–2 mg/kg/dose IV/PO q6–8h
	Status asthmaticus	C: *Loading dose:* 6 mg/kg IV *Maintenance dose:* 0.8–1.5 mg/kg/hr IV (or equivalent dose intermittently)
Amiodarone	Intravenous preparation	*Loading dose:* 5 mg/kg IV over 1 hr
		Maintenance dose: 5–15 µg/kg/min IV; **Note:** May decrease blood pressure, may require digoxin dose reduction
	Oral preparation	*Loading dose:* 10 mg/kg/day PO div BID for 7–10 days
		Maintenance dose: 5.0 mg/kg/day PO (may decrease to 2.5 mg/kg/day **or** increase to 10 mg/kg/day for long term)
Amoxicillin		C: 20–50 mg/kg/day PO div q8h; **subacute bacterial endocarditis prophylaxis 50 mg/kg 1 hr before procedure; 25 mg/kg 6 hr later**
Amoxicillin-clavulanate		C <40 kg: 20–40 mg (amoxicillin)/kg/day div q8h
Amphotericin B	Dilute to conc of 0.1 mg/mL with D₅W (do not use saline or bacteriostatic solutions); maximum conc 0.25 mg/mL (for fluid-restricted patient)	*Initial dose:* 0.25 mg/kg/dose IV over 4–6 hr daily
		Range: increase by 0.25 mg/kg/dose increments up to 0.5–1.0 mg/kg/dose q1–2 days
		Maximum dose, 1.5 mg/kg/24 hr
		Total cumulative dose: I: 15–30 mg/kg over 1 month C: 1.5–2 gm over 6–10 weeks
	Bladder irrigation	5–10 mg/L in sterile water *Pediatric:* 1 L via continuous

Drug	Comments	Age/Dose/Route/Frequency
Amphotericin B (Continued)		irrigation over 24 hr or instill appropriate volumes (for size of child) for dwell time of 60–90 min q4–6h daily (**maximum, 1 L/day**) for 2–3 days A: instill 200–300 mL of solution, cross-clamp the catheter for 60–90 min and then allow bladder to drain, repeat the procedure daily for 2–3 days
Ampicillin		N <1 week <2000 gm: 50 mg/kg/day IV div q12h; **meningitis,** 100 mg/kg/day IV div **q12h** N <1 week >2000 gm: 75 mg/kg/day IV div q8h; **meningitis,** 150 mg/kg/day IV div **q8h** N >1 week <2000 gm: 75 mg/kg/day IV div q8h; **meningitis,** 150 mg/kg/day IV div **q8h** N >1 week >2000 gm: 100 mg/kg/day IV div q6h; **meningitis,** 200 mg/kg/day IV div **q6h** I and C: 100–200 mg/kg/day IV div q4–6 h; **meningitis,** 200 mg/kg/day IV div **q4–6h** **Maximum dose, 12 gm/day**
Amrinone		*Loading dose:* 0.75–3 mg/kg IV over 3–10 min *Infusion:* N: 3–5 μg/kg/min IV I and C: 5–20 μg/kg/min IV
Atracurium		0.3–0.5 mg/kg/dose IV, followed by 0.1–0.5 mg/kg/dose q1h PRN
Atropine (resuscitation)	Undiluted	0.02 mg/kg (minimum, 0.1 mg) ET/IV **Maximum single dose, 0.5 mg** (C) and **1 mg** (adolescent); repeat q5min to **maximum total dose of 1 mg** (C) and **2 mg** (adolescent)

Drug	Comments	Age/Dose/Route/Frequency
Budesonide suspension for nebulization		*Initial dose:* 500–1000 μg BID *Maintenance dose:* 250–500 μg BID
Caffeine	Apnea of prematurity	Dose of **caffeine base**: *Loading dose:* 10 mg/kg IV/PO × 1 *Maintenance dose:* 2.5 mg/kg/day IV/PO q24h
Calcium chloride (resuscitation) (10 mL = 6.8 mmol Ca²⁺)	Undiluted or further dilute to 2–10% solution	0.2 mL (20 mg)/kg IV of 10% calcium chloride (5.4 mg/kg elemental calcium)
Captopril		*Initial dose:* 0.5 mg/kg/day PO div TID *Maintenance dose:* 0.5–6 mg/kg/day PO div TID (q12h in renal impairment)
Carbamazepine		N: 10–40 mg/kg/day PO div q12–24h C 6–12 yr: 20–30 mg/kg/day PO div q6–8h C >12 yr: 600–1200 mg/day PO div q6–8h
Cardiac cocktail (1 mL contains 25 mg meperidine, 6.25 mg promethazine, 6.25 mg chlorpromazine)	Sedation	0.1 mL/kg deep IM 1 hr before procedure **Maximum, 2 mL as a single dose**
Cefazolin		N ≤1 week: 40 mg/kg/day IV div q12h N >1 week <2000 gm: 40 mg/kg/day IV div q12h N >1 week ≥2000 gm: 60 mg/kg/day IV div q8h I and C: 50–100 mg/kg/day IV div q8h **Maximum, 6 gm/day**
Cefotaxime		N ≤1 week: 100 mg/kg/day IV div q12h N >1 week <2000 gm: 100 mg/kg/day IV div q12h N >1 week >2000 gm: 150 mg/kg/day IV div q8h I and C <50 kg: 100–200 mg/kg/day IV div q6–8h **Maximum, 8 gm/24 hr**

Drug	Comments	Age/Dose/Route/Frequency
Cefotaxime (Continued)		**Meningitis** I and C <50 kg: 200 mg/kg/day IV div q6h C >50 kg: moderate to severe infection: 1–2 gm/dose IV q6–8 h; life threatening: 2 gm/dose IV q4h **Maximum, 12 gm/day** C >12 yr and A: 1–2 gm/dose IV q6–8h **Maximum, 12 gm/day**
Ceftazidime		N ≤1 week: 100 mg/kg/day IV div q12h N >1 week <2000 gm: 100 mg/kg/day IV div q12h N >1 week >2000 gm: 150 mg/kg/day IV div q8h I and C (1 month–12 yr): 150 mg/kg/day IV div q8h **Maximum, 6 gm/day** A: 1–2 gm IV q8–12h
Ceftriaxone		N ≤1 week: 50 mg/kg/day IM/IV q24h N >1 week <2000 gm: 50 mg/kg/day IM/IV q24h N >1 week >2000 gm: 75 mg/kg/day IM/IV q24h I and C: 50–75 mg/kg/day IM/IV div q12h–24h I >3 mo and C: **meningitis,** IV route preferred 100 mg/kg/day div q12h × 3 doses, then q24h **Maximum, 2 gm/24 hr**
Cefuroxime		N <1 week: 60 mg/kg/day IV div q12h N >1 week <2000 gm: 60 mg/kg/day IV div q12h N >1 week >2000 gm: 90 mg/kg/day IV div q8h I and C: 75–150 mg/kg/day IV div q8h **Maximum, 6 gm/day**
Cefuroxime axetil (oral)		<2 yr: 125 mg PO BID 2–12 yr: 250 mg PO BID A: 250–500 mg PO BID
Chloral hydrate	Hypnotic	50–100 mg/kg/dose PO/PR given 30 min before procedure **Maximum single dose, 2 gm**
	Sedation	15–25 mg/kg/dose q6–8h PRN PO/PR

Drug	Comments	Age/Dose/Route/Frequency
Chloral hydrate *(Continued)*		**Maximum single dose, 500 mg**
Chloramphenicol	Monitoring of serum levels recommended in neonate	N <1 week: 25 mg/kg/day IV div q24h N >1 week <2000 gm: 25 mg/kg/day IV div q24h N >1 week >2000 gm: 50 mg/kg/day IV div q12h I and C: 75 mg/kg/day IV div q6h
Chlorpromazine (questionable utility in pulmonary hypertension of the newborn)		*Loading dose:* 0.13–0.88 mg/kg IV over 1 hr *Maintenance dose:* 0.03–0.21 mg/kg/hr continuous infusion
Cimetidine		20–40 mg/kg/day PO/IV div q6–8h
Cisapride		0.2–0.3 mg/kg/dose PO TID/QID **Maximum, 5–10 mg PO QID; give 15 min AC**
Clindamycin		N ≤1 week <2000 gm: 10 mg/kg/day IV div q12h N ≤1 week >2000 gm: 15 mg/kg/day div q8h N >1 week <2000 gm: 15 mg/kg/day div q8h N >1 week >2000 gm: 20 mg/kg/day div q8h I >1 mo and C: 20–40 mg/kg/24 hr div q6–8h
Clobazam		C: *Initial dose:* 0.5 mg/kg/24 hr PO QHS *Maintenance dose:* 0.5–2.9 mg/kg/24 hr PO QHS or BID (usually 1–1.3 mg/kg/24 hr) A: *Initial dose:* 10 mg PO QHS *Maintenance dose:* 10–40 mg/24 hr PO div OD/TID **Maximum,** 80 mg/24 hr (give higher proportion of divided dose at HS); increase slowly every 5 days by 5–10 mg/24 hr
Cloxacillin		N <1 week <2000 gm: 50 mg/kg/day div q12h

Drug	Comments	Age/Dose/Route/Frequency
Cloxacillin *(Continued)*		N <1 week >2000 gm: 75 mg/kg/day div q8h N ≥1 week 1200–2000 gm: 90 mg/kg/day div q8h N ≥1 week >2000 gm: 150 mg/kg/day div q6h I and C: 100–200 mg/kg/day div q6h
Coumadin (warfarin)		I and C: 0.1 mg/kg/day with a range of 0.05–0.34 mg/kg/day (adjust to achieve desired prothrombin time) A (adolescents): 5–15 mg/day for 2–5 days; then adjust dose according to prothrombin time
Desmopressin (DDAVP)	Diabetes insipidus	C: 5–10 µg/dose *nasal* q12–24h A: 10–20 µg/dose *nasal* q12–24h C: 0.25–1 µg/dose IM/IV q12–24h A: 1–2 µg/dose IM/IV q12–24h **Maximum, 4 µg/dose**
	Coagulopathy: to increase factor VIII levels	0.3 µg/kg/dose IV **Maximum, 25 µg**
Dexamethasone	Anti-inflammatory or immunosuppressive	0.03–0.2 mg/kg/day IV div q6–12h
	Airway edema	0.25–0.5 mg/kg/dose IV q6h
	Meningitis: Administration of the first dose of steroids before or with the initial antibiotic dose has been shown to be beneficial	I and C: 0.15 mg/kg/dose IV q6h × 4 days
	In patients who are difficult to wean from ventilator	0.5 mg/kg/day IV × 72 hr; then 0.3 mg/kg/day IV × 72 hr; decrease by 10% of current dose every 3 days until 0.1 mg/kg/day is reached; then given on alternate days × 1 week and then discontinue Continue for 20 days of therapy; if no improvement in *6 days*, discontinue trial
Diazepam	Status epilepticus	I and C: 0.2–0.5 mg/kg/dose IV/PR (may repeat q15–30 min to **maximum dose of 5–10 mg**)
	Sedation or muscle relaxation	C: 0.04–0.25 mg/kg/dose IV/PR q2–4h

Drug	Comments	Age/Dose/Route/Frequency
Diazepam (Continued)		**Maximum, 0.6 mg/kg within 8-hr period** C: 0.12–0.8 mg/kg/day PO div q6–8 hr
Diazoxide	Hypertensive crisis	1–5 mg/kg/dose IV, may repeat in 15 min, then q4–24h PRN
	Hyperinsulinemic hypoglycemia	N and I: 8–15 mg/kg/day PO div q8–12h C: 3–8 mg/kg/day PO q8–12h
Digoxin	Digitalizing dose (three doses: first **STAT**, second in 6 hr, third in another 6 hr)	*Digitalizing dose* (repeat three times): <37 weeks PCA: 0.007 mg/kg/dose PO, 0.005 mg/kg/dose IV ≥37 weeks PCA–2 yr: 0.017 mg/kg/dose PO, 0.012 mg/kg/dose IV >2 yr: 0.013 mg/kg/dose PO, 0.01 mg/kg/dose IV **Dose limit:** total digitalizing dose = 1 mg *Maintenance dose:* <37 weeks PCA: 0.004 mg/kg/day PO div q12h, 0.003 mg/kg/day IV div q12h ≥37 weeks PCA–2 yr: 0.01 mg/kg/day PO div BID or in a single dose >2 yr: 0.008 mg/kg/day PO div BID or in a single dose **Dose limit:** maintenance dose = 0.25 mg/day

Do not administer IM; reduce dose by 50% during concurrent indomethacin therapy. When digitalizing to terminate tachycardia, total digitalization dose is divided into one half, one fourth, and one fourth. Digoxin dose should be adjusted in renal impairment. Reduce dose by 50% during concurrent administration of amiodarone, propafenone, or quinidine. Conversion of PO to IV: decrease dose by 25%.

Drug	Comments	Age/Dose/Route/Frequency
Dimenhydrinate		C: 5 mg/kg/day PO/PR/IM/IV div q6h **Maximum, 300 mg/day** A: 50–100 mg q4–6h PO/PR/IM/IV **Maximum, 400 mg/day**
Diphenhydramine		5 mg/kg/24 hr PO/IM/IV div BID/QID PRN **Maximum, not to exceed 300 mg/day**

Drug	Comments	Age/Dose/Route/Frequency
Dobutamine		*Initial dose:* 1–2 μg/kg/min IV *Usual range:* 3–10 μg/kg/min IV **Maximum, 15–40 μg/kg/min**
Docusate		I and C: <3 yr, 10–40 mg/day PO 1–4 div doses; 3–6 yr, 20–60 mg/day PO 1–4 div doses; 6–12 yr, 40–150 mg/day PO 1–4 div doses Adolescents/A: 50–400 mg/day PO 1–4 div doses
Dopamine	Dopaminergic β₁ Stimulation α-Adrenergic stimulation	2–5 μg/kg/min IV 5–15 μg/kg/min IV >20 μg/kg/min IV **Maximum, 20–50 μg/kg/min**
Enalapril **(experience is limited in pediatrics)**		*Initial dose:* 0.1 mg/kg/day PO increased over 2 weeks to 0.12–0.43 mg/kg/day has been used to treat severe congestive heart failure, 5–10 μg/kg/dose IV has been administered q8–24h for neonatal hypertension
Epinephrine (resuscitation); for 0.01 mg/kg, use 0.1 mL/kg of 1:10,000; for 0.1 mg/kg, use 0.1 mL/kg of 1:1000	Bradycardia Asystole or pulseless arrest	0.01 mg/kg (1:10,000) IV, 0.1 mg/kg (1:1000) ET *First dose:* 0.01 mg/kg (1:10,000) IV/IO, 0.1 mg/kg (1:1000) ET *Second and subsequent doses:* 0.1 mg/kg (1:1000) IV/IO/ET every 3–5 min: doses up to 0.2 mg/kg (1:1000) may be effective N: 0.01–0.03 mg/kg
Epinephrine (inotrope)	Support cardiac output	*Initial dose:* 0.05 μg/kg/min IV; *range dose:* 0.1–1.0 μg/kg/min IV **Maximum, 2 μg/kg/min**
Erythromycin	Estolate salt Gluceptate salt	15–40 mg/kg/day PO div q6–12h N <1 week: 20 mg/kg/day IV div q12h N 1–4 weeks: 30–40 mg/kg/day IV div q8h C: 20–50 mg/kg/day IV div q6h
Esmolol		*Loading dose:* 500 μg/kg IV over 3 min; then 100 μg/kg/min (may be adjusted)

Drug	Comments	Age/Dose/Route/Frequency
Fentanyl		*Bolus:* 1–2 μg/kg IV *Infusion:* 0.5–1.0 μg/kg/hr IV (variable, may require 5–10 μg/kg/hr)
Fluconazole	Doses as high as 12 mg/kg/day have been used in immunocompromised children	I (case reports only): 5 mg/kg/day IV/PO q24h C >3 yr: 3–6 mg/kg/day IV/PO q24h
Flucytosine		N: 12.5–37.5 mg/kg/dose PO q6h I and C: 12.5–37.5 mg/kg/dose PO q6h
Flumazenil		I and C: 0.005–0.1 mg/kg/dose IV, repeat q5min as necessary **Maximum dose 1 mg, usual dose 0.01 mg/kg***
	Resedation	Repeat doses at 20-min intervals A: 0.2 mg IV, repeat at 1-min intervals up to cumulative dose of 1 mg
	Resedation	Repeat doses at 20-min intervals as needed; no more than 3 mg/hr
Furosemide: *continuous infusion*, monitor electrolytes, especially potassium q4h for at least the first 24 hr of Lasix infusion		*Bolus dosing: initial dose:* N: 1–2 mg/kg/dose IV q12–24h (oral bioavailability poor) I and C: 1 mg/kg/dose IV **or** 2 mg/kg/dose PO q6–12h *Maintenance dose:* may increase by 1 mg/kg/dose increments to a **maximum of 6 mg/kg/dose** *Continuous infusion: loading dose:* 0.1 mg/kg IV; *maintenance dose:* 0.1 mg/kg/hr IV to be doubled q2h if urine output is <1 mL/kg/hr to a **maximum of 0.4 mg/kg/hr** (higher doses have been used in oliguric states)

*Continuous infusions have been used at 0.005–0.01 mg/kg/hr.

Drug	Comments	Age/Dose/Route/Frequency
Ganciclovir	Cytomegalovirus retinitis	I >3 mon, C, and A: *induction:* 5 mg/kg/dose IV q12h (14–21 days); *maintenance dose:* 5 mg/kg/day IV q24h (7 days/week) or 6 mg/kg/day IV q24h (5 days/week)
	Other cytomegalovirus infections	5 mg/kg/dose IV q12h (14–21 days) or 2.5 mg/kg/dose IV q8h; *maintenance dose:* 5 mg/kg/day IV (7 days/week) or 6 mg/kg/day IV (5 days/week)
Gentamicin		PCA ≤29 weeks, PNA 0–28 days: 2.5 mg/kg/dose IV q24h, or significant hypoxia >28 days: 3.0 mg/kg/dose IV q24h
		PCA 30–36 weeks, PNA 0–14 days: 3.0 mg/kg/dose IV q24h
		PCA 30–36 weeks, PNA >14 days: 2.5 mg/kg/dose IV q12h
		PCA ≥37 weeks, PNA 0–7 days: 2.5 mg/kg/dose IV q12h
		PCA ≥37 weeks, PNA >7 days: 2.5 mg/kg/dose IV q8h
		Older I and C <5 yr: 2.5 mg/kg/dose IV q8h
		6–10 yr: 2 mg/kg/dose IV q8h
		≥10 yr: 1.5 mg/kg/dose IV q8h
Glucagon (1 unit = 1 mg)	Hypoglycemia or insulin shock therapy	N: 0.3 mg/kg/dose IM/IV/SC **Maximum, 1 mg/dose**
		C: 0.025–0.1 mg/kg/dose, not to exceed 1 mg/dose; repeated in 20 min as needed
Glucose (resuscitation)	$D_{25}W$ (N:$D_{10}W$)	0.5–1 gm/kg IV (2–4 mL of 25% solution/kg/dose)
Glycopyrrolate	Control of oral secretions	40–100 µg/kg/dose PO TID/QID, 4–10 µg/kg/dose IM/IV every 3–4 hr
Hepatitis B immunoglobulin	Perinatal	0.5 mL/dose IM within 12 hr of birth
Hepatitis B vaccine		0.5 mL IM
Hydralazine	Hypertensive crisis	0.1–0.5 mg/kg/dose IV PRN q4–6h **Maximum of 2 mg/kg/dose**

Drug	Comments	Age/Dose/Route/Frequency
Hydralazine (Continued)	Chronic hypertension	0.75–7.0 mg/kg/day PO div q6–12h
Hydrocortisone	Adrenal insufficiency	*Acute:* 5 mg/kg/dose IV bolus, then I and young C: 50–200 mg/day IV/PO div q6h; older C: 200–400 mg/day IV/PO div q6h *Maintenance dose:* 20 mg/m^2/day PO div q8h **or** cortisone acetate 25 mg/m^2/day PO div q8h
	Anti-inflammatory **or** immunosuppressive	0.8–4.0 mg/kg/day PO div q6h
	Status asthmaticus	*Loading dose:* 5–10 mg/kg IV × 1 *Maintenance dose:* 5–10 mg/kg/dose IV q6h × 5 days, then taper
Hydroxyzine		2–4 mg/kg/24 hr IM div q6h PRN, 2 mg/kg/24 hr PO div q6–12h PRN
Imipenem-cilastatin		N <1 week: 50 mg/kg/day IV div q12h I and C <3 yr: 100 mg/kg/day IV div q6h C >3 yr: 60 mg/kg/day IV div q6h **Maximum, 2 gm/24 hr** A: 2 gm/24 hr IV div q6h
Immune globulin	Hypogammaglobulinemia	600 mg/kg/dose IV once monthly
	Idiopathic thrombocytopenic purpura	1 gm/kg/dose IV as single daily dose × 1–2 days
	Kawasaki disease	400 mg/kg/day IV as single daily dose × 4 days
Indomethacin	Anti-inflammatory	C >4 yr: 1.5 mg/kg/24 hr PO/PR div TID/QID
	Patent ductus arteriosus closure	0.1–0.3 mg/kg/dose IV q12–24h up to a total of three doses
Ipratropium bromide *via nebulizer*		0.5–1.0 mL (125–250 μg) solution diluted to 2 mL with normal saline q4–8h
Isoproterenol		*Initial dose:* 0.05–0.1 μg/kg/min IV *Range:* 0.2–0.5 μg/kg/min IV **Maximum, 2 μg/kg/min**
Ketamine	To facilitate intubation of patients in status	1–2 mg/kg IV

Drug	Comments	Age/Dose/Route/Frequency
Ketamine (Continued)	asthmaticus or with cardiovascular compromise	
	Sedation	0.5–1.0 mg/kg IV over 2–3 min followed by continuous infusion of 10 μg/kg/min **(caution: premedicate with benzodiazepine)**
Ketorolac		I and C: 0.5–1.2 mg/kg/dose IV/IM q6–8h or IV bolus 1.0 mg/kg followed by continuous infusion of 0.2 mg/kg/hr
Ketotifen		>3 yr: 1 mg PO BID; <3 yr: 0.5–1 mg PO BID
Labetalol (for hypertension)		*Initial dose:* 0.2–1.0 mg/kg slow IV over minimum 5 min followed by:
		Bolus: 0.4 mg/kg IV q10min **up to maximum dose 3–4 mg/kg** or
		Continuous infusion: 0.25–1.5 mg/kg/hr IV **up to maximum of 3 mg/kg/hr (neurosurgery patients may require larger doses)**
		Maintenance dose: 20 mg/kg/ day PO div q6–8h
Lactulose		I: 2.5–10 mL/day PO div TID/ QID
		C: 40–90 mL/day PO div TID/QID
Lidocaine (resuscitation)	Ventricular tachycardia with pulse (2% solution = 20 mg/mL)	1 mg/kg IV/ET followed by infusion of 20–50 μg/kg/ min
Lidocaine (antiarrhythmic)		*Bolus:* 1 mg/kg/dose IV q5min **up to maximum 5 mg/kg**
		Infusion: 10–50 μg/kg/min IV
Prevent increased intracranial pressure in head-injured patients *before suctioning*	Neonates and premature infants should receive doses of no more than 1.0 mg/kg	1 mg/kg/dose IV
Lorazepam	Status epilepticus	N: 0.05 mg/kg/dose IV
		I and C: 0.05–0.1 mg/kg/dose IV
		0.1 mg/kg/dose PR (dilute 1:1 with normal saline)
	Sedation	0.05–0.1 mg/kg/dose IV/PR
Magnesium (oral)		20–40 mg elemental magnesium (0.4–0.8 mmol)/ kg/day PO div TID

Drug	Comments	Age/Dose/Route/Frequency
Magnesium sulfate (IV) 50% solution 2 mmol Mg/mL	Hypomagnesemia	N: 25–50 mg IV (0.1–0.2 mmol/kg/dose) every 8–12 hr for 2–3 doses C: 25–50 mg/kg/dose IM/IV (0.1–0.2 mmol) q4–6h × 3–4 doses; may repeat Doses of 100 mg/kg/dose (0.4 mmol Mg/kg/dose) have been used **Maximum single dose, 2000 mg (8 mmol)** *Maintenance dose:* 60–120 mg/kg/day IV (0.24–0.48 mmol/kg/day) *Infusion:* dilute 20 mmol Mg in 50 mL at 1 mL/hr = 0.4 mmol Mg/hr; titrate accordingly, start at 0.4 mmol/kg/day
Mannitol	Cerebral edema	0.25 gm/kg IV, may be repeated q1–2h PRN, may increase dose stepwise to 1 gm/kg/dose
Meperidine		I: 0.5 mg/kg IV/IM repeat PRN (usually q4h) **Maximum dose, 2 mg/kg IV** C: 1–2 mg/kg IV/IM repeat PRN (usually q4h) **Maximum dose, 2 mg/kg IV**
Methylprednisolone	Anti-inflammatory or immunosuppressive Status asthmaticus	0.4–1.6 mg/kg/day IV div q6–12h *Loading dose:* 1–2 mg/kg IV × 1 *Maintenance dose:* 0.5–1 mg/kg dose IV q6h × 5 days, then taper
Metoclopramide	Gastroesophageal reflux Antiemetic (chemotherapy induced)	0.4–0.8 mg/kg/day oral/IV in 4 div doses (efficacy beyond 12 weeks questionable) 1–2 mg/kg/dose IV q2–4h
Metolazone		0.2–0.4 mg/kg/day PO div q12–24h
Metronidazole		PNA 0–7 days (all wt): 10 mg/kg/day IV/PO q24h PNA >1 week <2000 gm: 15 mg/kg/day IV/PO q12h PNA >1 week >2000 gm: 30 mg/kg/day IV/PO q12h

Drug	Comments	Age/Dose/Route/Frequency
Metronidazole *(Continued)*		I and C: 30 mg/kg/day IV/PO q6h *Clostridium difficile* infection: 20 mg/kg/day PO q6h
Midazolam		*Loading dose:* 0.1–0.2 mg/kg IV (over 20–30 sec) *Infusion:* 0.5–5 µg/kg/min IV
Morphine		*Bolus:* I: 0.1 mg/kg IV, repeat PRN (usually q4h) C: 0.1–0.2 mg/kg IV *Infusion:* 10–30 µg/kg/hr IV
Naloxone		N (narcotic induced asphyxia): 0.01–0.1 mg/kg IV/IM/ET C <20 kg: 0.1 mg/kg/dose IV/IM/ET, repeat q2–3min PRN C ≥20 kg: 2 mg/dose IV/IM/ET, repeat q2–3min PRN A: 0.4–2 mg/dose IV/IM/ET, repeat q2–3min PRN *Infusion:* Repeat above as load. Then infuse two thirds of load per hour. For recurring respiratory depression, increase infusion rate by 50% increments. Precede all increments with a bolus (50% of initial loading dose). Discontinue after 6–12 hr and reassess for respiratory depression.
Neomycin	Hepatic coma	2.5–7 gm/m²/day PO div q4–6h for 5–6 days; not to exceed 12 gm/day
Neostigmine (Give atropine first)	For reversal of nondepolarizing neuromuscular blockers	I: 0.05 mg/kg/dose IV C: 0.07–0.08 mg/kg dose IV **Maximum, 2.5 mg/dose**
Nifedipine	Hypertensive emergencies Hypertension	0.25–0.5 mg/kg SL 0.5–1.5 mg/kg/day PO div q8h
Nitroglycerin		0.5–20.0 µg/kg/min IV
Nitroprusside		*Initial dose:* 0.1–1.0 µg/kg/min IV (usually 0.5–1.0 µg/kg/min) *Range:* 0.5–10 µg/kg/min **Recommended not to exceed 8–10 µg/kg/min for >10 min or 2 µg/kg/min for prolonged treatment** **Total maximum dose 3 mg/kg**

Drug	Comments	Age/Dose/Route/Frequency
Norepinephrine		*Initial dose: (dose of drug base):* 0.1 µg/kg/min IV *Usual range (dose of drug base):* 0.05–1.0 µg/kg/min IV
Omeprazole		C ≥3 yr: 10–20 mg PO/IV OD
Pancuronium		N: 0.03–0.09 mg/kg/dose IV q0.5–4h PRN I and C: 0.05–0.15 mg/kg/dose IV q0.5–4h PRN
Paraldehyde (available as 100%, 1 gm/mL)	Rectal administration	N, I, and C: 200–300 mg/kg/dose PR (0.2–0.3 mL/kg/dose), give as a 30–50% solution in olive or mineral oil or normal saline **Maximum, 5 mL/dose q4–8h PRN**
	IV administration*	N: 300 mg/kg IV infused over 2 hr (3 mL/kg/hr of a 5% solution q24h) I and C: 150 mg (0.15 mL)/kg/dose IV given once or q4–6h **or** *loading dose* 100–150 mg/kg/dose IV (2–3 mL of 5% solution/kg/dose over 15–20 min; then 20 mg/kg/hr (0.4 mL of a 5% solution/kg/hr) as a continuous infusion Refractory cases may require doses up to 50–200 mg/kg/hr (1–4 mL of a 5% solution/kg/hr)
Penicillin G		PNA 0–7 days <2000 gm: 50,000 units IV/IM div q12h PNA 0–7 days >2000 gm: 75,000 units IV/IM div q8h PNA >1 week <2000 gm: 75,000 units kg/day IV/IM div q8h PNA >1 week >2000 gm: 100,000 units IV/IM div q6h **Above doses should be doubled for central nervous system infections**

---

*Must dilute before IV use to a 5% solution (5 mL of 100% paraldehyde diluted to a total of 100 mL with D$_5$W or normal saline gives a 5% solution).

Drug	Comments	Age/Dose/Route/Frequency
Penicillin G (*Continued*)		I and older C: 200,000–300,000 units/kg/24 hr div q4–6h × 10–14 days
Pentobarbital	Preop for patient >6 mo Sedation	1–3 mg/kg IV, 2–6 mg/kg IM/PO/PR **Maximum dose, 120 mg**
	Cardiac catheterization	*Symptomatic:* 2 mg/kg PO/IM *Nonsymptomatic:* 4 mg/kg PO/IM **Maximum dose, 200 mg**
	Anticonvulsant Sedative	3–5 mg/kg/dose IV/IM 2–6 mg/kg/day in 3 div doses PO/PR **Maximum dose, 100 mg/day**
	Induction of coma (for treatment of increased intracranial pressure	10–20 mg/kg IV administered over 2 hr followed by *infusion* of 1 mg/kg/hr (blood level 20–35 mg/L or 88.4–132 µM/L)
Phenobarbital		*Loading dose:* 15–30 mg/kg/dose × 1 IV or div to total of 30 mg/kg *Maintenance dose:* I: 5–8 mg/kg/day IV/PO div q12–24h C: 3–5 mg/kg/day IV/PO div q12–24h
Phenoxybenzamine		1 mg/kg IV load over 1 hr, then 0.5–2.0 mg/kg/day div q6–12h 0.2 mg/kg PO OD (increase by 0.2 mg/kg) **Maximum, 10 mg** *Usual maintenance dose:* 0.4–1.2 mg/kg/day div q6–8h
Phentolamine	Pheochromocytoma (diagnosis) Hypertension	0.05–0.1 mg/kg/dose IM/IV **Maximum single dose, 5 mg** 0.05–0.1 mg/kg/dose IM/IV given 1–2 hr before the procedure, repeat if needed until hypertension is controlled **Maximum single dose, 5 mg**
Phenytoin (do not exceed maximum rate of 1 mg/kg/min)		N: *Loading dose:* 15–20 mg/kg/dose IV × 1 or div to total of 20 mg/kg *Maintenance dose:* 5–8 mg/kg/day IV div q12h (**not absorbed well orally**) I and C: *Loading dose: 10–20*

Drug	Comments	Age/Dose/Route/Frequency
Phenytoin (Continued)		mg/kg/dose IV × 1 or div to total 20 mg/kg *Maintenance dose:* 4–7 mg/kg/day IV/PO div q12h
Phosphate	Treatment of hypophosphatemia	*Low dose:* 0.08 mmol/kg IV over 6 hr *Intermediate dose:* 0.16–0.24 mmol/kg over 4–6 hr *High dose:* ≤0.36 mmol/kg over 6 hr Dilute 15 mmol (Na or K phosphate) in 50 mL, run at 1 mL/hr = 0.3 mmol phosphate/hr, titrate accordingly (0.04–0.08 mmol phosphate/kg/hr)
Piperacillin		N ≤30 days: 100–200 mg/kg/day div q8–12h I and C >30 days (moderate infection): 100–200 mg/kg/day div q6h I and C >30 days (severe infection): 200–300 mg/kg/day div q4–6h **Maximum, 18 gm/24 hr**
Procainamide		<1 yr: *Loading dose:* 6 mg/kg >1 yr: *Loading dose:* 10–15 mg/kg All ages: *maintenance dose: infusion* 20–80 μg/kg/min **No faster than 0.5 mg/kg/min**
Propafenone	**Note:** Can enhance atrioventricular conduction in presence of primary atrial tachyarrhythmias	*Loading dose:* 2 mg/kg IV over 90 min *Maintenance dose:* 4–7 μg/kg/min IV
Propranolol		0.01–0.1 mg/kg IV over 3 min (slow IV push) **Maximum of 1 mg/dose** I: 0.5–4 mg/kg/day PO div q6h C: 0.5–4 mg/kg/day PO div q8h
Prostaglandin E_1		0.05–0.1 μg/kg/min IV, may reduce dosage to 0.025 μg/kg/min by titrating the patency of patent ductus arteriosus
Prostaglandin E_2		50–200 μg/kg PO every 2–3 hr (with titration as above)

Drug	Comments	Age/Dose/Route/Frequency
Racemic epinephrine (via nebulizer)		N: 0.05 mL/kg diluted to 2 mL with normal saline q30min–2h I <1 yr: 0.25 mL diluted to 2 mL with normal saline q30min–2h I >1 yr and C: 0.5 mL diluted to 2 mL with normal saline q30min–2h
Ranitidine		N: 2–4 mg/kg/day IV div q8h I and C: 2–6 mg/kg/day IV div q6h or *Loading dose:* 1 mg/kg × 1 followed by infusion *Infusion:* 0.1–0.2 mg/kg/hr *Maintenance (oral) dose:* 2.5–5 mg/kg/day PO div q12h
Ribavirin (6-gm vials)	Reconstituted to a concentration of 20 mg/mL given as an aerosol daily for 3–7 days	6 gm/day over 24 hr (continuous inhalation)
Rifampin	Prophylaxis *Neisseria meningitidis*	N: 10 mg/kg/day PO div q12h × 2 days I and C: 20 mg/kg/day PO div q12h × 2 days **Maximum, 600 mg/dose** A: 600 mg PO BID × 2 days
	Prophylaxis *Hemophilus influenzae*	N: 10 mg/kg/day PO q24h × 4 days I and C: 20 mg/kg/day PO q24h × 4 days **Maximum, 600 mg/dose** A: 600 mg PO OD × 4 days
Salbutamol		*Loading dose:* 10 µg/kg IV over 10 min *Maintenance dose:* 0.2–4.0 µg/kg/min IV **Maximum, 10 µg/kg/min IV**
	By nebulizer	0.03 mL/kg/dose inhalation solution diluted to 2 mL with normal saline **Maximum q2h (maximum 1 mL/dose)** May also be given by continuous inhalation
Sodium bicarbonate	Undiluted 1 mmol/mL (C ≥2 yr) or diluted to 0.5 mmol/mL with D₅W (N and I <2 yr)	1 mmol/kg IV

Drug	Comments	Age/Dose/Route/Frequency
Sodium cromoglycate inhalation	Solution for inhalation: 10 mg/mL	20 mg inhaled QID
Sodium polystyrene sulfonate		1 gm/kg/dose PO q6h or PR q2–6h (mix with water, D$_5$W, normal saline)
Spironolactone		1–4 mg/kg/day PO div q8–24h (usually q12h)
Succinylcholine (always give atropine before giving succinylcholine)		*Initial dose:* N and I: 2 mg/kg/dose IV C: 1 mg/kg/dose IV *Maintenance dose:* 0.3–0.6 mg/kg/dose IV q5–10min PRN
Sucralfate		1–10 kg: 250 mg PO q6h 10–20 kg: 500 mg PO q6h >20 kg: 1 gm PO q6h
Thiopental	Seizures	C: 2–4 mg/kg/dose IV Adolescents and A: 75–250 mg/dose IV (repeat as needed)
	Increased intracranial pressure in children	1.5–5 mg/kg/dose IV (repeat as needed to control pressure); **or** 5 mg/kg × 2 doses, then 5 mg/kg/hr by continuous infusion **Maximum 20 mg/kg/hr**
	Intubation	C: 2–4 mg/kg IV
Tobramycin		N ≤7 days 800–1500 gm: 3 mg/kg/dose IV q24h N ≤7 days 1500–2000 gm: 2.5 mg/kg/dose IV q18h N ≤7 days >2000 gm: 2.5 mg/kg/dose IV q12h N >1 week PGA 30–34 weeks: 2.5 mg/kg/dose IV q18h N >1 week PGA 34–38 weeks: 2.5 mg/kg/dose IV q12h N >1 week PGA >38 weeks: 2.5 mg/kg/dose IV q8h I and C: 2.5 mg/kg/dose IV q8h A: 3.5 mg/kg/day IV div q8h
Trimethoprim (TMP)/ sulfamethoxazole (SMX)	C >2 mon: Mild to moderate infection Serious infection (*Pneumocystis carinii pneumonia* [PCP])	6–12 mg TMP/kg/day IV/PO div q12h 15–20 mg TMP/kg/day IV/PO div q6h

Drug	Comments	Age/Dose/Route/Frequency
Trimethoprim (TMP)/ sulfamethoxazole (SMX) (*Continued*)	Urinary tract infection prophylaxis PCP prophylaxis	2 mg TMP/kg/dose IV/PO OD 5–10 mg TMP/kg/day **or** 150 mg TMP/m²/day IV/PO div q12h 3 days/week **Dose should not exceed 320 mg TMP/1600 mg SMX 3 days/week**
	A: Urinary tract infection/ chronic bronchitis	1 double-strength tablet PO q12h for 10–14 days
Tromethamine (alkalinizes without increased PCO_2 and sodium)	Usual dose depends on buffer base deficit *When known*	Number of mL of 0.3 M solution = body wt (kg) × base deficit (mEq/L) × 1.1 given IV
	When not known	3–6 mL/kg/dose IV (1–2 mEq/kg/dose) **Note:** 1 mM = 120 mg = 3.3 mL = 1 mEq of tromethamine
	Metabolic acidosis with cardiac arrest	3.5–6 mL/kg (1–2 mEq/kg/dose) IV into a large peripheral vein; IV: continuous drip: infuse slowly by syringe pump over 3–6 hr **Maximum rate 1 mL/min**
Ursodiol		15 mg/kg/day PO div TID
Valproic acid	Status epilepticus	C: 10–20 mg/kg PR × 1 (dilute syrup 1:1 with water) *Maintenance dose:* N: 15–40 mg/kg/day PO div q12–24h I and C: 30–60 mg/kg/day PO div q8–24h
Vancomycin		≤7 *days PNA* (based on body weight): 800–1500 gm: 20 mg/kg/dose IV q24h 1500–2000 gm: 20 mg/kg/dose IV q18h >2000 gm: 15 mg/kg/dose IV q12h >7 *days PNA* (based on PCA in weeks): 27–30 weeks: 20 mg/kg/dose IV q24h 30–34 weeks: 20 mg/kg/dose IV q18h

Drug	Comments	Age/Dose/Route/Frequency
Vancomycin (*Continued*)		34–38 weeks: 15 mg/kg/dose IV q12h >38 weeks: 15 mg/kg/dose IV q8h I and C: 40 mg/kg/24 hr div q6h **Maximum, 2 gm/24 hr**
	Meningitis	I >1 mon and C: 60 mg/kg/24 hr div q6h
	Colitis	I >1 mon and C: 40–50 mg/kg/24 hr PO div q6h **Maximum, 2 gm/24 hr**
Varicella-zoster immunoglobulin	Within 48 hr but not later than 96 hr after exposure	0–10 kg: 125 units = 1 vial IM 10.1–20 kg: 250 units = 2 vials IM 20.1–30 kg: 375 units = 3 vials IM 30.1–40 kg: 500 units = 4 vials IM >40 kg: 625 units = 5 vials IM
Vasopressin (aqueous) 20 pressor units/mL	Diabetes insipidus; IM/SC dosage is highly variable; titrate based on serum and urine sodium and osmolality, as well as fluid balance and urine output.	C: 2.5–5 units (2–4 × per day) IM/SC A: 5–10 units (2–4 × per day) IM/SC *IV continuous infusion*: *Initial dose:* 0.5 milliunits/kg/hr (0.0005 units/kg/hr), titrate to 2 milliunits/kg/hr) **Maximum, 10 milliunits/kg/hr**
	Gastrointestinal hemorrhage	C: 0.1–0.3 units/min (100–300 milliunits) IV continuous infusion, then titrate dose as needed Adolescents and A: 0.2–0.4 units/min, titrate dose as needed
	Abdominal distention	A: *Loading dose:* 5 units IM, then 10 units q3–4h
Vecuronium		0.1 mg/kg/dose IV q1h PRN *Continuous infusion:* 0.1 mg/kg × 1, then 0.05–0.1 mg/kg/hr
Verapamil (**contraindicated in newborns; do not use in children ≤1 yr**)		C ≥2 yr: 0.1–0.15 mg/kg IV over 2 min (**do not exceed 5 mg**), may repeat × 1 after 30 min (**do not exceed 10 mg**)
	Oral maintenance	1–5 yr: 4–10 mg/kg/day div q8h or 40–80 mg TID

Drug	Comments	Age/Dose/Route/Frequency
Verapamil *(Continued)*		>5 yr: 4–10 mg/kg/day div q6–8h or 80 mg TID/QID
Vitamin K	Vitamin K deficiency due to drugs, malabsorption, or decreased synthesis of vitamin K	N: 1.0 mg given once at birth and IM/IV/SC PRN I and C: 1–2 mg/dose as a single dose IM/IV **or** 2.5–5 mg/24 hr PO

13

Reference Tables

Table 13–1. PEDIATRIC TRAUMA SCORE (PTS)

Component	Category +2	+1	-1
Size	≥20 kg	10–20 kg	<10 kg
Airway	Normal	Maintainable	Unmaintainable
Systolic blood pressure	≥90 mm Hg	90–50 mm Hg	<50 mm Hg
Central nervous system	Awake	Obtunded/loss of consciousness	Coma/decerebrate
Open wound	None	Minor	Major/penetrating
Skeletal	None	Closed fracture	Open/multiple fractures
		Sum _____ (PTS)	

If proper-sized blood pressure cuff is not available, blood pressure can be assessed by assigning the following values: +2, pulse palpable at wrist; +1, pulse palpable at groin; -1, no pulse palpable.
Modified from Tepas JJ III, Alexander RH, Campbell JD, et al: An improved scoring system for assessment of the injured child. J Trauma 25:720, 1985.

Table 13–2. MODIFIED GLASGOW COMA SCALE

Eye-opening Response	
Spontaneous	4
To speech	3
To pain	2
None	1
Verbal Response	
Oriented	5
Confused conversation	4
Inappropriate words	3
Incomprehensible sounds	2
None	1
Best Upper Limb Motor Response	
Obeys	6
Localizes	5
Withdraws	4
Abnormal flexion	3
None	1
Verbal Response for Young *** Childen and Adults***	
Appropriate words or social smiles, fixes and follows	5
Cries, not consolable	4
Persistently irritable	3
Restless, agitated	2
None	1

A score of ≤8 indicates severe head injury; 9 to 12, moderate head injury; and 13 to 15, mild head injury.
This is not uniformly accepted as the definitive grading system for children.
Modified from Luerssen TG: Acute traumatic cerebral injuries. *In* Cheek WR (eds): Pediatric Neurosurgery, 3rd ed. Philadelphia, WB Saunders, 1994, p. 274.

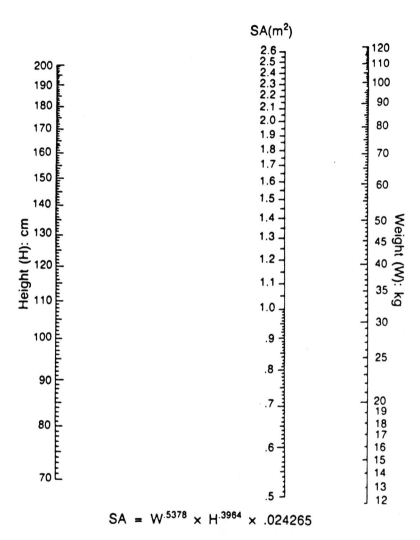

$$SA = W^{.5378} \times H^{.3964} \times .024265$$

To use the nomogram, a ruler is aligned with the height and weight on the two lateral axes. The point at which the center line is intersected gives the corresponding value for surface area.

Figure 13–1. Body surface area nomogram for children and adults. (From Haycock GB, Schwartz GJ, Wisotsky DH: Geometric method for measuring body surface area: A height-weight formula validated in infants, children, and adults. J Pediatr 93:62, 1978.)

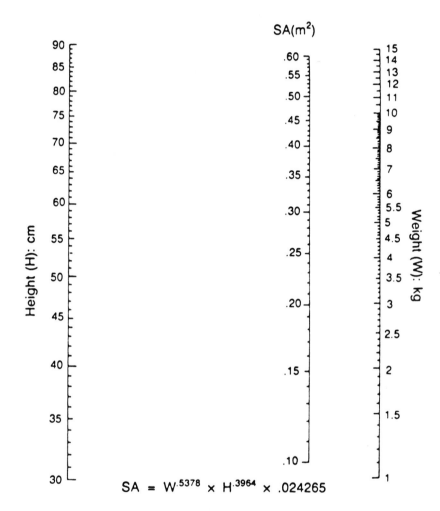

To use the nomogram, a ruler is aligned with the height and weight on the two lateral axes. The point at which the center line is intersected gives the corresponding value for surface area.

Figure 13–2. Body surface area nomogram for infants. (From Haycock GB, Schwartz GJ, Wisotsky DH: Geometric method for measuring body surface area: A height-weight formula validated in infants, children, and adults. J Pediatr 93:62, 1978.)

Table 13–3. PEDIATRIC ECG INTERPRETATION

In the development of the heart of an infant or a child, the ECG changes until an "adult" pattern emerges. Consult Table 13–4 for age-related normal ranges. Approach interpretation systematically:

Rate

A small box duration is 0.04 sec (40 msec); a big box duration is 0.20 sec (200 msec).
Mnemonic: 300–150–100–75–60–50 bpm counting big boxes between QRS complexes
Precise measure of heart rate: 60,000 msec in 1 min divided by the msec of the RR interval; i.e., 60,000/(RR [in msec]) = HR (in bpm).

Rhythm

In sinus rhythm, the P-wave axis is 0° to 90°, P positive in leads I, II, and aVF. Each QRS is preceded by a P wave with a constant PR. The computer rhythm interpretation is often wrong. Some possibilities are normal sinus rhythm, sinus arrhythmia, low right atrial rhythm, left atrial rhythm, wandering atrial pacemaker, and junctional rhythm.

Axis

Use the **approximation method;** establish the quadrant using lead I and aVF. Then, look for an isoelectric lead (axis is 90° to this) or one in which the QRS is the most positive or negative. Axis deviation is an axis outside the normal range for age.

Hypertrophy

Voltage criteria change with age.
Hypertrophy with "strain"; T-wave inversion or ST changes in the ipsilateral leads.
Bundle-branch block or WPW preclude reliable assessment of hypertrophy.
Some criteria are less equal than others; the listings below are in order of specificity for each criterion.

RVH	*LVH*
+ve T wave age 3 days to 7 yr	R V_6 > 98th
qR V_1 or V_3R, V_4R	S V_1 > 98th
R V_1 > 98th	Deep Q waves II, III, aVF, and V_6
Pure R wave	
S V_6 > 98th	

BVH	*RAE*
Obvious hypertrophy criteria in both ventricles	<1 mon: P > 2.5 mm any lead
R > mean in the presence of hypertrophy of the contralateral ventricle	>1 mon: P > 3 mm any lead
Katz Wachtel phenomenon V_4; RV_4 + SV_4 > 98th	*LAE*
	Deep negative terminal portion V_1 1 box by 1 box
	Notched and wide P II > 120 msec

Bundle-Branch Block

Cannot assess axis, hypertrophy, or ischemia in presence of BBB
    Right BBB
        QRS > 100 msec, RSR V_1, slurred R V_1, slurred S V_6
    Left BBB
        QRS > 100 msec, slurred R V_6, slurred S V_1
    Intraventricular conduction delay
        Also known as "incomplete BBB"; does not satisfy QRS > 100 msec or definite R or L pattern

Table continued on following page

Table 13–3. PEDIATRIC ECG INTERPRETATION *(Continued)*

Repolarization Abnormalities

Also caused by **depolarization abnormalities;** so ischemia, strain, and assessment of QT_c are not valid in presence of BBB, IVCD, WPW, or pacing

$$QT_c = \frac{QT\ (\text{in sec})}{\sqrt{(RR\ [\text{in sec}])}}$$

Male, ≤ 0.425; Female, ≤ 0.440

ST depression	Early repolarization
ST elevation	Strain
Patterns of ST changes	Cardiomyopathy
Pericarditis	Electrolytes

Infarct

Q wave pattern and ST changes, at least 1 box wide and 1 box deep
Kawasaki, anomalous origin of left coronary from pulmonary artery, surgical or cardiac catheterization, dyslipidemia

Classic ECGs

Cyanotic Heart Disease

Transposition: RVH
Tricuspid atresia: LAD, $\downarrow$ RV forces, LVH
Tetralogy: RAD, RVH
Pulmonary atresia VSD: RAD, RVH
Pulmonary atresia intact septum: LAD or normal, or LVH, ST Δs, $\downarrow$ RV forces
Double-outlet right ventricle: RAD, severe RVH: qR V_1
TAPVD: severe RVH, qR V_1, $\pm$ RAE
Pulmonary stenosis: RAD, RVH
Ebstein's: 1° AVB, RAE, BBB, $\downarrow$ RV forces, possible WPW
Truncus arteriosus: BVH, LVH, ST Δs

Left Heart Disease

HLHS: RAD, RVH, $\pm$ $\downarrow$ LV forces
Aortic stenosis: LVH, $\pm$ ST Δs
Mitral stenosis: LAE, $\pm$ RVH
Coarctation: neonate RVH, older LVH

Other

Preexcitation aka WPW: short PR, delta
Long QT syndrome: long QT_c, abnormal T waves, T alternans, pause-dependent T Δs, dextrocardia: $\uparrow$ R V_3R–V_1, $\downarrow$ R V_3–V_6, P axis $>90°$
Pericarditis: early; $\uparrow$ STs, later T flat or inverted
ALCPA: Q I, aVL, V_3–V_6, later presentation: smaller Qs + LVH

By Marc D. LeGras, BSc, MD, CM, FRCPC, FACC.
ALCPA, anomalous left coronary artery from pulmonary artery; AVB, atrioventricular block; BBB, bundle-branch block; BVH, biventricular hypertrophy; HLHS, hypoplastic left heart syndrome; IVCD, intraventricular conduction defect; LAD, left axis deviation; LAE, left atrial enlargement; LV, left ventricular; LVH, left ventricular hypertrophy; QT_c, corrected QT; RAD, right axis deviation; RAE, right atrial enlargement; RV, right ventricular; RVH, right ventricular hypertrophy; TAPVD, total anomalous pulmonary venous drainage; VSD, ventricular septal defect; WPW, Wolff-Parkinson-White.

Table 13–4. ECG VALUES IN CHILDREN

Age	HR (bpm)	Frontal QRS (°)	QRS 98th V$_5$ (msec)	PR 98th (msec)	R V$_1$ 98th (mm)	S V$_1$ 98th (mm)	R V$_6$ 98th (mm)	S V$_6$ 98th (mm)	R + S V$_4$ 98th (mm)
< 1 Day	93–154 (123)	+59 to 190	75	160	26 (14)	23 (8)	11 (4)	10 (3)	52
1–2 Days	91–159 (123)	+64 to 199	66	138	27 (14)	21 (9)	12 (5)	10 (3)	53
3–6 Days	91–166 (129)	+77 to 197	68	136	24 (13)	17 (7)	12 (5)	10 (4)	49
1–3 Weeks	107–182 (148)	+65 to 161	78	137	21 (11)	11 (4)	16 (8)	10 (3)	48
1–2 Mon	121–179 (149)	+31 to 113	76	130	18 (10)	12 (5)	21 (12)	7 (3)	54
3–5 Mon	106–186 (141)	+7 to 104	78	145	20 (10)	17 (6)	22 (13)	10 (3)	58
6–11 Mon	109–169 (134)	+6 to 97	76	157	20 (10)	18 (6)	23 (13)	7 (2)	50
1–2 Yr	89–151 (119)	+7 to 101	76	148	18 (9)	21 (8)	23 (13)	7 (2)	48
3–4 Yr	73–137 (108)	+6 to 104	72	162	18 (8)	21 (10)	24 (15)	5 (2)	53
5–7 Yr	63–133 (100)	+11 to 143	78	164	14 (7)	24 (12)	27 (16)	4 (1)	54
8–11 Yr	62–130 (91)	+9 to 114	85	172	12 (6)	25 (12)	25 (16)	4 (1)	50
12–15 Yr	60–119 (85)	+11 to 130	87	175	10 (4)	21 (11)	23 (14)	4 (1)	50

The ranges represent the 2nd and 98th percentiles. Upper limits represent the 98th percentile; mean values are in parentheses.

Values are from percentile data from Davignon A, et al: Normal ECG standards for infants and children. Pediatr Cardiol 1:123, 1979/80, and modifications to Garson A, Jr: The electrocardiogram in infants and children: A Systematic Approach. Philadelphia, Lea & Febiger, 1983, Table A-17, p. 404.

Suggested readings: Park MK: How to Read Pediatric ECGs. Chicago, Year-Book Medical Publishers, 1987; and Garson A Jr: The Electrocardiogram in Infants and Children: A Systematic Approach. Philadelphia, Lea & Febiger, 1983.

Table 13–5. QUICK GUIDE TO DRUG INFUSIONS IN PEDIATRICS

Desired Infusion Rate (μg/kg/min)		
Required Infusion Rate (1 mL/hr equals)	*Drug (mg) Added to 50 mL IVF*	*Drug and Usual Dosage (μg/kg/min)*
		Norepinephrine 0.05–1.0
0.1 μg/kg/min	0.3 × body wt	Epinephrine 0.05–1.0
0.5 μg/kg/min	1.5 × body wt	Isoproterenol 0.10–1.0
1.0 μg/kg/min	3.0 × body wt	Nitroglycerin 0.5–10
2.0 μg/kg/min	6.0 × body wt	Nitroprusside 0.5–10
5.0 μg/kg/min	15.0 × body wt	Dopamine 1.0–20
10.0 μg/kg/min	30.0 × body wt	Dobutamine 1.0–20
		Midazolam 0.5–0.4
		Salbutamol 0.2–5.0

Example: 8-kg patient required dopamine at a rate of 10 μg/kg/min
6.0 × 8 (body wt) = 48 mg dopamine added to 50 mL IVF at 5 mL/hr
(1 mL/hr = 2 μg/kg/min)

Desired Infusion Rate (μg/kg/hr)

Morphine: Body wt ÷ 2 = drug (mg) added to 50 mL IVF (1 mL/hr = 10 μg/kg/hr)

Fentanyl: Body wt × 50 = drug (μg) added to 50 mL IVF (1 mL/hr = 1 μg/kg/hr)

Prostaglandin E$_1$ supplied in 225 μg/vial

$$\frac{225}{0.05 \times \text{body wt} \times 60} = \text{mL of IVF to dilute one vial (1 mL/hr} = 0.05\ \mu\text{g/kg/min)}$$

IVF, intravenous fluid.

Table 13–6. NEONATAL AVERAGE DAILY FLUID REQUIREMENTS (mL/kg/day)

Birth Weight	Day 1	Day 2	Day 3	Day 4	Day 5	> Day 5
600–800 g	80–100	100–125	130	130	150	150–200
800–1000 g	60–100	90–115	120	130	150	150–200
1–1.5 kg	60	70	100	120	150	150–200
1.5–2.0 kg	60	70	100	120	140	150–180
>2.0 kg	60	75	90	120	140	160–180

These are only guidelines; adjust for urine output, weight changes, electrolytes, and so on.
Other adjustments: (1) add 30% to 50% for radiant heaters; (2) add 10% to 50% for phototherapy; (3) subtract ≈10% for Saran Wrap/heat shields; (4) subtract ≈20% to 30% for endotracheal intubation plus assisted ventilation; and (5) <600 g start at rates as per 600–800 g and adjust as appropriate.

Table 13–7. MAINTENANCE FLUID REQUIREMENTS IN CHILDREN

Weight	Formula
Body Weight Daily Maintenance Formula	
0–10 kg	100 mL/kg
11–20 kg	1000 mL for first 10 kg + 50 mL/kg for 11–20 kg
21–30 kg	1500 mL for first 20 kg + 25 mL/kg for 21–30 kg
Body Weight Hourly Maintenance Formula	
0–10 kg	4 mL/kg/hr
11–20 kg	40 mL/hr for first 10 kg + 2 mL/kg/hr for 11–20 kg
21–30 kg	60 mL/hr for first 20 kg + 1 mL/kg/hr for 21–30 kg
Body Surface Formula	
1500 mL/m² body surface area/day	
Insensible Water Losses	
300 mL/m² body surface area plus urine output/day	

Table 13–8. NUTRITIONAL REQUIREMENTS

Age	Protein (gm/kg/day)	Energy (kcal/kg/day)
0–6 mon	2.5	100–120
6–12 mon	2.5	90–100
1–2 yr	2.0	80–90
2–13 yr	1.5	1000 + 100 (age in yr)
>13 yr	1.0	1000 + 100 (age in yr)

Protein

Neonates	Begin with 0.5 gm/kg/day
Infants	Begin with 1 gm/kg/day; ↑ by 0.5–1.0 gm/kg/day

Lipid

Begin with 1.0 gm/kg/day; ↑ by 0.5–1.0 gm/kg/day to a maximum of 4 gm/kg/day (monitor lipid levels)

Carbohydrate

6–8 mg/kg/min; maximum of 12 mg/kg/min

INDEX

Note: Page numbers in *italics* indicate figures; those followed by t indicate tables.

A

A-aDO$_2$ (alveolar-to-arterial oxygenation difference), 98–99
Abdominal distention, mechanical ventilation with, 66
  vasopressin for, 397
Abdominal trauma, 34, 35–36
ABR (auditory brain stem responses), 188, 189t
ACE (angiotensin-converting enzyme) inhibitors, for cardiovascular disease, 178
Acetaminophen, dosage of, 375
  for bacterial pneumonia, 86
  for hepatic failure, 245
  for pain, 286, 286t
  intoxication with, 257–258, *258*
N-Acetylcysteine, for acetaminophen intoxication, 257–258
Acetylsalicylic acid, dosage of, 375
Acid-base balance, after liver transplantation, 323
  in diabetic ketoacidosis, 263, 265t
  in renal failure, 251
Acidosis, lactic, 274, *276*
  metabolic, 274, *275*
    with cardiac arrest, tromethamine for, 396
Activated clotting time (ACT), with extracorporeal membrane oxygenation, 101
Acute renal failure (ARF), 247–252
Acyclovir, after bone marrow transplantation, 339
  dosage of, 376
  for encephalitis, 204
Adenosine, dosage of, 376–377
  for arrhythmia, 133t
Adrenal insufficiency, hydrocortisone for, 387
Adrenergic receptors, in cardiogenic shock, 147
Adult respiratory distress syndrome (ARDS), 92–97, *93*, 95t

Adult respiratory distress syndrome (ARDS)
  (Continued)
  clinical manifestations and diagnosis of, 92–93
  defined, 92
  management of, 93–96, 95t
  mechanical ventilation for, 94–95
  monitoring for, 94
  novel therapy for, 95–96, 95t
  outcome of, 96–97
  pathophysiology of, 92, *93*
  with septic shock, 230–231
Advanced trauma life support (ATLS), 31
AET (atrial ectopic tachycardia), management of, 137–138
  pathophysiology of, *129*
Afterload, 22
  after surgical repair of congenital heart disease, 154
  indirect measures of, 120t
Agonists, for status asthmaticus, 90
Airway, oropharyngeal, 17
  soft nasopharyngeal, 17
Airway edema, dexamethasone for, 382
Airway management, 12–21
  drugs to facilitate intubation for, 12–16, 15t, 16t
  equipment for, 12, 14t
  in trauma, 31, 32t
  intubation in, 18–21, 18t, 20t
  oropharyngeal airway in, 17
  oxygen in, 17
  pathophysiology of child and, 12, *13*, 13t
  positioning in, 16, *17*
  soft nasopharyngeal airway in, 17
  suctioning in, 16
Airway obstruction, *17*
  acute upper, 69–79
  defined, 69–70